ISBN 978-0-260-23736-1
PIBN 11013185

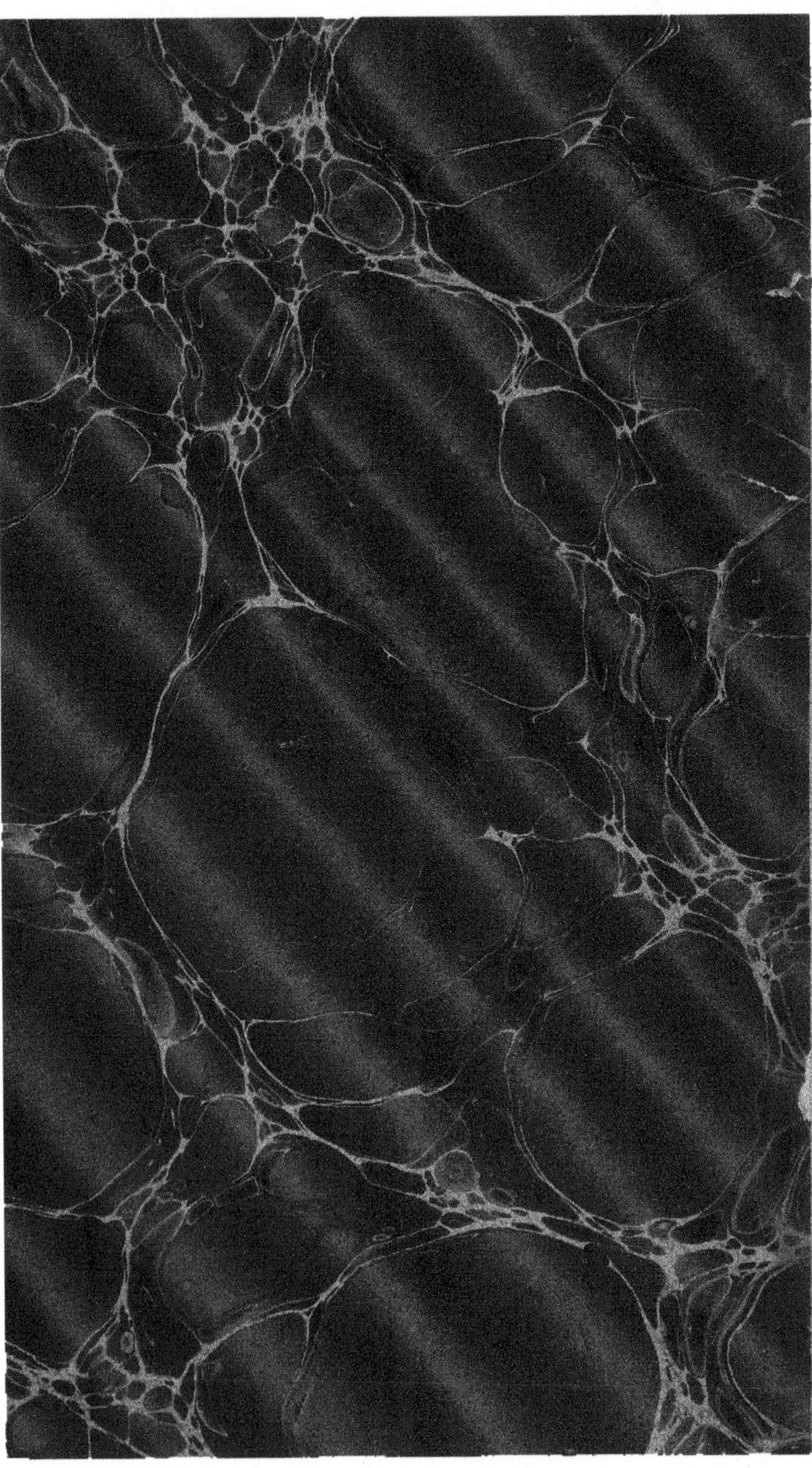

SYSTEM

OF

DENTAL SURGERY.

IN THREE PARTS.

I. DENTAL SURGERY AS A SCIENCE.

II. OPERATIVE DENTAL SURGERY.

III. PHARMACY CONNECTED WITH DENTAL SURGERY.

BY

SAMUEL SHELDON FITCH, M. D.

SURGEON-DENTIST.

Dentium curam habeto ut bene digeras et diu vivas. laxatis dentibus laxantur et chyloseos officinæ: hinc mille malorum occasiones.—*Baglivi* XIII.

NEW YORK:

G. & C. & H. CARVILL—108 BROADWAY.

1829.

R. & G. S. WOOD, PRINTERS.

William Stevenson
Phil^a

AS

A SMALL TESTIMONY OF RESPECT,

FOR THAT URBANITY

WHICH CHARACTERISES THE ACCOMPLISHED GENTLEMAN

IN PRIVATE LIFE;

AND FOR THOSE SPLENDID TALENTS

AND EXTENSIVE ACQUIREMENTS WHICH HAVE EXALTED HIS PUBLIC CHARACTER

TO AN ENVIABLE HEIGHT OF REPUTATION;

THIS WORK IS RESPECTFULLY DEDICATED TO

NATHANIEL CHAPMAN, M. D.

PROFESSOR OF THE THEORY AND PRACTICE OF MEDICINE

IN THE UNIVERSITY OF PENNSYLVANIA:

BY

HIS FRIEND AND HUMBLE SERVANT,

THE AUTHOR.

PREFACE.

In presenting the following "System of Dental Surgery," to the American Medical Public, the Author feels himself called upon to apologize for so bold an undertaking, before his temples were frosted by experienced years, or his dicta had become "law" in his profession. Conscious of the great want of a good work upon this subject, and anxious to fill in some degree a hiatus in English Medical Literature; the production was undertaken, not so much that itself would affect all these objects, but that by uniting a part of what is now known upon it, the defects might attract the notice of some more intelligent eye, and arouse a spirit that would approximate the science to some degree of perfection. Pursuing this object, the author has, in nearly all cases, adopted the language and opinions of those writers upon the different parts of this science and art, which are in accordance with his own: he has done this, that the authorities might be known, and his own responsibility diminished: for why should he tempt the bow of Ulysses alone? If, at any time, he has differed from the opinions of others, he has done it without giving definite reasons, which are still left to the judgment of the reader.

Perhaps it may not be amiss in this place to mention a few of the names whose opinions have been noticed, and from whose writings, to a considerable extent, materials for this work have been drawn.

Of the French. Martin, Fauchard, Bourdet, Jourdain, Duval, La Forgue, Dellabarre, Le Maire, Baumes, Audibran, Rousseau, &c. &c. &c.

Latin. Baglivi, Bartholinus, and others.

Of the English. Hunter, Blake, Fox, Murphy, Parmly, Koecker, Darwin' Rush, Chapman, Horner, Coates, &c. &c. &c.

The French translations the reader will indulge; as the limited time the author could devote to the subject, prevented any other than a plain and literal version without attempting ornament of diction.

He takes this opportunity to present his most cordial and sincere thanks to the many gentlemen who have most generously co-operated in promoting this publication; of whom he will only mention Drs. Chapman and Jackson, distinguished Medical Professors, in the University of Pennsylvania; who, by their patronage, have imposed upon him a lasting obligation. Mr. Eleazar

Parmly, Dentist, of New York, himself an easy and intelligent writer, with that urbanity and ingenuousness so peculiar to him, has added to my admiration and respect, the most heartfelt gratitude for his cheerfully-rendered assistance to the publication of this volume.

In consequence of the work's being published in New York, and the author resident here, a few errors have obtained, which are noticed in an Errata.

To conclude: the work, with no small degree of solicitude, is humbly presented to the medical public, hoping that it may be treated with kindness, and prove a small addition to the medical literature of our country.

S. S. FITCH.

Philadelphia, January 22d, 1829. *No.* 171, *Walnut-street.*

CONTENTS.

PART I.

CHAPTER VI.

PART II.

CHAPTER I.

CHAPTER II.

PART III.

CHAPTER I.

CHAPTER II.

DENTAL SURGERY.

PRELIMINARY DISCOURSE.

If the value of any science is to be estimated by its comparative utility, Dental Surgery will hold a distinguished place in the esteem of mankind. When we consider the extensive influence which the state of the teeth exerts upon the functions of the stomach and the organs of digestion, this subject rises in importance, and assumes a character and consequence, not usually ascribed to it.

This science dates its origin from remote antiquity, and is coeval with the first families of the earth. From the moment that the principles of mortality were impressed upon the organs of man, those destined for the comminution of his food, became implicated in the common frailty, and, sympathizing with all the other members of his body, were found subject to disease, decay, and dissolution.

It is easy for us to conceive, that among the most rude nations, and in the earliest state of society, many important facts connected with this subject, were well understood. The Natural History of the Teeth, as far as regarded their development; and their Anatomy, so far as concerned their form, external appearance, and insertion in the jaws, must necessarily have been known to the earliest races of men. If, prompted by affection, feeling, or the dictates of religion, they had burned their dead, or had inhumated them from their sight, still, comparative anatomy would, perhaps, have given them more just notions of the Teeth, than of any other organs of the animal system. Long before a prying curiosity, or an anxious thirst for knowledge, had induced their sages to dissect the bodies of animals to learn their structure, their bleached bones would have taught them the formation of their osseous frame: and the teeth of most mamiferous animals are inserted, nearly in the same manner as those of man, and must have attracted immediate notice. Again, a peculiarity connected with them, not found in any other organs of the body, must have taught the first parents of the human race, that the teeth of their children might be lost and be replaced again, by a larger, firmer, and better set. This taught them their development, and a constant observance of the crowns and nearly all the bodies of the teeth, made them familiar with their external appearance. So that it amounts to almost a certainty, that mankind acquired a general knowledge of the teeth as soon if not sooner than of any other organs. They must, at a very early period, have appreciated their great utility in masticating their food, and their immense influence in modifying the expression of the human countenance; either by their regularity and perfection, producing a pleasing appearance; or, by their irregularity or deformity, giving it an aspect at once displeasing and repulsive to the most casual observer. It would have been seen that they gave the countenance a youthful appearance, whilst their loss indicated the approach of age. Consequently as soon as the human family began to increase to large societies, and a mutual dependance to be felt, the teeth became an object of attention; as materially adding to the beauty of the countenance, and, thereby, greatly promoting the power of pleasing. Hence in almost every epoch of civilization and refinement, and strikingly in proportion to the degree of their advancement, have the teeth been an object of attention, their regular arrangement and beautiful formation viewed with pleasure, and the means of their preservation considered a desideratum. But as the records of the past, previously to the invention of the art of printing, were made with much difficulty, and at a great expense of time and labour; they are necessarily scanty in number, and very general in their delineations; whilst the frequent overthrow of the luxurious, refined, and polished nations, by barbarians, who paid no respect to learning, the learned, or their works, contributed to a great, and, in many cases, almost overwhelming extent, to dissipate and nearly extinguish, the few lights of learning, that had shone during the long period antecedent to the discovery of the art of printing. And when it is considered that, probably, an account of very few of the great revolutions, which at different and remote periods, have convulsed the natural and moral world, has ever reached us, we need not be surprised at finding no elaborate works upon the teeth amongst the writings of antiquity; but are left to glean a few observations upon this subject, from the writings of their poets; and to draw conclusions upon it, from the customs of succeeding generations. The Bramins of India, at this day, make the cleaning of their teeth a matter of religious observance. "As this custom," says Mr. Murphy,* "is coeval with the date of their religion and government, it exhibits a curious proof of the regard which this scientific people had for the purity and beauty of the mouth; when this practice is inculcated as a law, and rendered indispensable as a religious duty." I scarcely need remark, that the Bramins are considered as the remnant of one of the oldest polished nations upon the earth; and

* See Murphy, page 151.

whose origin and history are lost in the lapse of ages. During the brighter periods of Egyptian greatness, we are assured that they regarded the teeth with peculiar attention; and that our art was carried to a considerable extent in Memphis, their ancient capital; and was thence diffused to the surrounding nations. The written records of the customs, habits, history, and learning of the Egyptians, were nearly all lost when their grand library was burned at Alexandria, A. D. 860, by which about 700,000 volumes of ancient writings were lost to the learned world; and, with them, nearly all traces of the learning and ancient history of the Egyptians: save what is to be found in detached fragments of authors, inferred from their public works, or gathered in the explanation of obscure hieroglyphics. Among the Hebrews many phenomena connected with the teeth were well understood; and their regularity and healthy state considered as peculiarly necessary in the perfection of beauty. Solomon in complimenting an illustrious woman, and in admiration of those charms, conferred by a beautiful set of teeth, says: "Your teeth are like a flock of sheep, that are even shorn, which come up from the washing; whereof every one bear "twins, and none are barren among them."* At once conveying to us an idea of a full and perfect set of regular, even, and clean teeth, by a figure as delicate, chaste, and lovely, as any that the customs or peculiarities of that pastoral people, could afford. He likewise seemed well aware that the loss of the teeth often occurred in old age; for, in remarking the characteristics of the decline of life, among others he says; "The grinders cease because they are few." The Hebrew writers appear to have clearly understood, that, in some animals, their teeth gave to them a hideous and

* See Canticles of Solomon, Chap. iv. verse 2.

frightful appearance; and were terrible instruments either for defence or attack; for says Daniel,* "after this I saw in the night visions, and behold, a fourth beast, dreadful and terrible, and strong exceedingly; and it had great iron "teeth; it devoured and brake in pieces, &c." Their loss was punished by the law of retaliation, an eye for an eye, and a tooth for a tooth.

The Poets of India occasionally delight to refer to the beauty and cleanliness of the teeth, in most pleasing images, as;†

"The Cunda blossom yields to the whiteness of the Teeth: speak but one mild word, and the rays of thy sparkling teeth will dispel the gloom of my fears!"

The Ancient Greeks and Romans acknowledged the importance of the teeth; and, so far had the principles and practice of Dental Surgery advanced amongst them, that their natural history was considerably understood, and almost every part of this science and art was known and practised by their physicians, and persons with whom it was a particular profession. Galen speaks of this last class of practitioners, and calls them Α'τρθσ 'ο δσντιχοσ, (Médicins Dentaires) Physicians, or Surgeon Dentists. Hippocrates, who has justly been styled the "Father of Medicine," has transmitted to us an account of many operations upon the teeth, or, as the French with great propriety term them, "Operations Odontotecniques." But we have never received from the Greeks or Romans, any works especially devoted to this branch of Surgery or Medicine. The Greek and Latin poets have refered to the teeth at almost every period of their growth and age. They have spoken of artificial teeth

* Chap. 7. verse 7. † Gitazovinda. Murphy, page 152.

as a common occurrence, and likewise have noticed the effects of the teeth upon the countenance, and upon the address and appearance of the individual. (*a*) Thus Ovid recommends as a remedy " against love, to make her smile who has bad teeth. We find Palladius (*b*) joking a superannuated coquette, in saying to her, that, " for the price of her hair, with that of her paint; her wax, her honey, and her teeth, she might have bought an entire mask.'

Martial, the Greek Poet, addressing himself to Lelius, says, (*c*) " you are not ashamed to purchase teeth and hair but what will you do for an eye ; as there are none to sell." The toothless mouth of Egle was repaired by bone and ivory; (*d*) and Galla more refined, removed her artificial teeth, during the night. (*e*) Horace cites the case of the sorceresses Canidia and Sagana, running through the city and losing, the one her teeth, and the other her false hair. (*f*)

Macedonius said to an old lady ; " What medical art can ever be able to fasten your teeth ?" Martial answered, " Cascellius is in the habit of fastening as well as extracting the teeth." I need not extend the subject any farther; enough has been said, and much more might be, if necessary, to prove clearly and conclusively that the odontotechny of the Greeks and Romans was advanced to a considerable degree of perfection: and that the toilet of the politer part of these people, was not considered as in any degree perfected, when their teeth were dirty, or their mouths in an unpleasant state. Catulus delights to say, that, " when Julia presented herself to Manlius, she shone by a flowery mouth. (*g*) She doubtless possessed those teeth of snow, so sung by the favorite of the muses; (*h*) or that row of pearls so extolled by Lu-

---

(*a*) See Dentiste Jeunesse, page 63, (*b*) 22, (*c*) 23, (*d*) 24, (*e*) 25, (*f*) 34, (*g*) , 60(*h*) 62,

cian; (i) the lustre of which was esteemed by Theocritus as above that of the finest marble of Paros.

As we have noticed that traces of our science and art are to be found in every epoch of civilization and refinement, so on the contrary, when the institutes of polished society began to fail, virtuous and enlightened communities to sink into ignorance and debauchery, or were overwhelmed by barbarians, it declined with them; not to revive again, until raised by the hands of more enlightened men, to fulfil the wants and complete the attractions of polite society.

Although nursed in the lap of Grecian and Roman refinement, this happy condition was not always to remain; Grecian strength was broken by Roman power; and her states became Roman provinces. The Roman Empire, enervated by luxury and weakened by intestine broils, gradually sunk under its own weight, until the northern barbarians, flushed with success, and lured by the spoils of conquest, carried their arms to the heart of Rome itself; and at length wasted by repeated ravages, nothing remained of this once proud mistress of the world, save the grandeur of her splendid ruins.

A night of ignorance and barbarism succeeded, and continued, during the lapse of some centuries, which have been appropriately termed, "sæcula atrocea, The Dark Ages." It was as the sun eclipsed, between a bright morning and a subsequently beautiful day. Our science and art, during the greater part of these ages, found a resting place only in those records, which detailed the customs, and portrayed the refinement of ancient days. "Hic currus fuit hic ilius arma."

(i) See Dentiste Jeunesse. page 63.

With the revival of learning and letters in the xivth, xvth, and xvith centuries, this subject became an object of attention with the learned, and obtained the notice of Falopius, Eustachius, and Ambrose Pare. The latter described the manner of replacing the teeth, and the use of obturateurs.

Eustachius published the first edition of his Opusculum de Dentibus in the year 1563;* which appears to be the first work of consequence upon this subject, of which any account has ever reached us.†

Urbain Hemard,‡ published a work entitled, Researches upon the true Anatomy of the Teeth, their nature, and properties, with an account of those diseases to which they are subject, at Lyons, by Benoit Rigaud, in 1582. "These Researches," says Fauchard, "which are very good and useful, plainly evince that this surgeon had read the Greek and Latin Authors, whose writings he has judiciously incorporated into his own work." Mr. Blake calls Urbain Hemard an ingenuous surgeon and a great man.‖ Mr. Audebran observes that, "he was the first to unite in "a body those precepts upon the teeth, which before had not been well considered." He was surgeon to the Cardinal Georges of Armignac. The next work upon this subject was published by Benjamin Martin; printed in Paris by Thiery, in the year 1679, entitled, "A dissertation upon the teeth," forming a small volume, in 12mo. of 136 pages. In which he treats of the nature of the teeth, their sensibility, their development, diseases, &c. &c.; but does not describe those methods by which they are preserved and rendered healthy. He was apothecary to one of the French princes.

---

* Ruff a German. Wurtzburgh, 1548.
† Blake, page 4.
‡ Fauchard, Preface, page 10.
‖ Page 6—32.

Fauchard,* in speaking of the state of dental surgery, in his time, remarks, that in France, " the most celebrated surgeons, having abandoned this branch of surgery, or having but little cultivated it, their negligence gave rise to a class of persons who without theoretic knowledge or experience, and without being qualified, practised it at hazard, having neither principles nor system. It was only since the year 1700, that the intelligent in Paris opened their eyes to these abuses: When it was provided, that those who intended practising dental surgery, should submit to an examination by men, learned in all the branches of medical science; who should decide upon their merits." Mr. Blake concurs in these remarks, and observes,† that about the year 1700, the necessity of some artificial mode of preserving the teeth attracted particular attention in Paris, and a few surgeons there began to confine their attention to diseases of the mouth and teeth alone; from which period may be dated the commencement of useful knowledge in that branch, founded on experience."

It appears that at this time dental surgery was at a very low ebb in England, being little understood either in theory or practice; and as bad, or even worse, amongst the other European nations. Our science and art obtained a gradual amelioration in Paris, and, in the year 1728, Fauchard published his justly celebrated work: a work which has only to be read to be admired; and has justly obtained for him the title of " the Father of Modern Dentists." He lived in the reign of Louis XVth, and was one of the most distinguished dentists of his time. His work proves him to have been learned in the medical sciences. Mr. Andibran, says, " it

---

* Preface, page XI—XII. † Page 5.

is in effect impossible to expose with more clearness, and to demonstrate with more evidence, the precepts of an art which partakes at the same time of medicine and surgery."*

It is entitled, "Le Chirugien Dentiste ou Traite des Dents, ou L'on Enseigne les moyens de les entretenir propre et saines, de les embellir, d'en reparer la perte et de remedier à leur maladies, à celles des gencives et aux accidens qui peuvent survenir aux autres parties voisines des dents.

Avec des observations et des Reflexions sur plusiers cas singuliers."

It is enriched with 42 engraved plates.

This work is far from being faultless, but allowances being made for the infancy of the science, and few works upon this subject will be found to surpass it. From this time, the knowledge and precepts of dental surgery, assumed the form of a regular body of science, destined to be enriched by the researches and contributions of future practitioners, and to be of immense benefit to mankind. A second edition of this work was published in 1746. I will continue this subject a little farther, and mention a few of the many writers, that have appeared among the French and English, without, however, presuming to trespass so much upon the time of the reader, as to fatigue him with the names of all those who have contributed, directly and indirectly, to the advancement of our science. The French, who have ever been celebrated for their attention to the graces and elegance of their persons, have contributed more to the advancement of this science, especially in the "la pratique," than any other nation.

---

* Audibran, page 8—9.

Bunon, published a work, entitled, "Essai sur les maladies des Dents. Paris, 1743."

Mouton, wrote a small work upon this subject, entitled, "Essai d' odontotechnie, ou Dissertation sur les dents artificielles, 1746." Written in an elegant but not in a methodical manner.

Bourdet, published his work upon this subject, in Paris, 1757, entitled, "Recherches et Observations sur toutes les Parties de L' Art du Dentiste."

It is enriched with some valuable plates and contains many correct observations.

Jourdain published two works upon this subject: the first was printed in Paris, 1761, and is entitled, "Traite des depots dans les sinus Maxillaires des fractures et des caries suivi des reflexions sur toutes les operations de L' Art du Dentiste."

The second is entitled, "Traite des maladies et des operations réellement chirurgicales de la bouche et des autres parties qui y correspondent." Paris, 1778. In 8vo. 2 Volumes.

These works have enjoyed a considerable reputation.

Gariot, published a work entitled, "Traite des Maladies de la bouche d'apres l'etat actuel des connaissances en medécine et en chirurgie qui comprend la structure et les fonctions de la Bouche, l'histoire des maladies des dents les moyens d'en conserver la sante et la beautie et les operations particulieres a l' Art du dentiste." In 8vo. Paris, 1805.

Baumes. Traite de la premiere Dentition et des Maladies souvent tres-graves qui en dependent." In 8vo. Paris, 1805.

I could proceed to mention pages of names, and title pages of works, with which our present subject has been enriched from the pens of eminent French dentists, physicians, and surgeons; but I will merely suffer myself to mention the names of Tenon, Hebert, Fourdain, Laforgue, Duval, Mahon, Delabarre, Andibran, Lemaire, &c. &c.; besides the French Dictionary of the Medical Sciences, and a host of French Surgeons and Anatomists, who have directly and indirectly, poured a flood of light upon this subject. Many of whose observations and precepts will be found incorporated into the subsequent work. Among the English, it must be acknowledged, that there has been, and continues to be, rather a paucity of works upon this subject; and especially the practical part. Thomas Berdmore published a practical work upon the teeth in the reign of George the Third, to whom he was Dentist. This work contains nearly as much practical matter, as any subsequent English writer.

Mr. John Hunter, published his work upon Odontotechny, in London, 1771, entitled, "The Natural History of the Human Teeth, explaining their Use, Formation, Growth, and Diseases; illustrated with copper plate engravings."

A second part of the work was entitled: "A Practical Treatise on the Diseases of the Teeth, and the consequences of them, &c. &c."

This work is highly esteemed in some respects, and has passed through several editions. It is enriched with some valuable plates. Mr. Hunter advocated the practice of transplanting the teeth; but which in consequence of the numerous accidents arising from it and its frequent failures, is at present nearly abandoned. Mr. Blake remarks,* "that Mr. Hunter did not confine his attention to the teeth alone, but procured much of his knowledge from Dentists of his acquaintance; consequently, his opinions were not always the result of his own experience and were not always to be trusted."

---

* Blake, page 6.

Mr. Robert Blake wrote an Essay upon the Structure of the Teeth in man and various animals, illustrated with engravings, published in Dublin, 1801, having before been the subject of an inaugural dissertation, published in Edinburgh, 1799. This work is justly esteemed. Mr. Fox observes,* that we are indebted to Mr. Blake, for the first correct account of the manner in which the permanent teeth are formed." By others this discovery has been ascribed to Hebert, a Frenchman.

Mr. Joseph Fox published the first part of his work entitled, Natural History, and Diseases of the Human Teeth, in 8vo. London, 1803."

The second part, "History and Treatment of the Diseases of the Teeth and Gums." London, 1806.

This work of Mr. Fox, is at present a standard in the language; is enriched with many valuable engravings, and reflects much credit upon the talents of its amiable and learned author. In it Mr. Fox was guilty of a great error or oversight, in asserting,† that Mr. Hunter's book was the first scientific work ever published upon the teeth, when those of Fauchard, Bourdet and Jourdain had preceded it. A second edition appeared in 1814. Rushini produced a small Essay upon this subject, London, 1797. Mr. Charles Bew, a popular Treatise upon the Teeth, with an account of the cause of Caries, London. A work of little merit.

Fuller, "A Popular Essay on the Structure, Formation and Management of the Teeth, Illustrated by Engravings, London, 1810."

Mr. Joseph Murphy published, "A Natural History of the Human Teeth, with a Treatise on their Diseases from Infancy to Old Age, &c. &c. 8vo. London, 1811."

---

* Fox, page 21. † Preface page 9th.

This work is well written and displays much candour and intelligence, and is worthy of perusal. Considered as a literary work, it is perhaps not excelled by any on this subject in the English language. Several other small works have appeared in England, of which I will only mention that of Mr. Hertz. "A Familiar Dissertation on the Causes and Treatment of the Diseases of the Teeth," &c. &c.

In this country no extensive work has ever been published on Odontotechny.

To Mr. Eleazar Parmly of New York, we are indebted for a popular essay upon this subject, containing some valuable information. Mr. Flagg of Boston, and Mr. L. S. Parmly, have favoured us with their views upon it. Besides which we have been presented through the medium of the Medical Journals, some valuable papers upon different parts of our science, of which I will mention one by Dr. Trenor of New York, upon Tic Doloreaux; and another by the same gentleman upon the Structure, Organization, and nourishment of the teeth. Also a valuable paper upon transplanting of the teeth, by Mr. James Gardette of this city, one of our oldest and most respectable Dentists.

Finally, I will mention the work of Mr. Leonard Koecker, formerly of this city, but now residing in London. It comprises about 420 pages, 8vo. published in London, 1826, containing some valuable information, but upon the whole, has been rather coldly received in this country.

It would now be proper for me to say a few words upon the present state of Dental Surgery, in this country. In most parts of the United States, with the exception of some of the largest cities, it is very little understood. In some of our large towns, we have probably as ingenious and intelligent Surgeon Dentists as are to be found in the oldest cities of Europe. Men who are respectable for their literary, scientific, and professional acquirements. It is to be regretted that our subject has been neglected by a great proportion of the Medical Faculty. They, too generally, consider it as having little or no bearing upon their profession.

As an instance of the utter want of attention to this subject, by some medical men, I will take the liberty of mentioning the following case, which came to my knowledge.

A Lady having her mouth in a very unpleasant state, her gums inflamed and ulcerated, in consequence of an excessive accumulation of tartar upon the molar teeth of one side, applied to a physician who was a Professor in one of the Medical Universities of this country, for advice and relief from this disagreeable and somewhat alarming state of her mouth. The Surgeon was entirely at a loss to determine what was the real nature of the disease, or what the extraordinary tumour or concretion upon her teeth. The affection was finally decided to be cancerous, and in a state of great alarm, the lady was dismissed. She, however, did not entirely despair, but applied to some others of the Faculty, and was at last seen by one that had some little knowledge of the maladies of the mouth, who immediately quieted her fears, and, by the use of suitable remedies, relieved her from every symptom of disease.* At present, a spirit of inquiry is abroad, and I cannot but anticipate a period, when, upon this subject, prejudices shall be removed, mal practices cor-

* This ignorance is not peculiar to the physicians of this country. Duval says, page 80 Dentiste Jeunesse, "Far different was the conduct of a "provincial surgeon, who imagining that he had to remove a tumour which "greatly swelled the cheek, enlarged the opening of the mouth by incision. "This tumour, however, was nothing more than a mass of tartar, which "enveloped the teeth. He then attacked it with a hammer and chisel, "and the piece was sent to the Royal Academy of Surgery in 1789, where "may be seen the tooth of the patient, and the error of the surgeon."

rected, the darkness of ignorance be dispelled, and, commensurate with the talents and worth of many of its professors, its extensive bearing upon health, and its happy influence upon society, assume a correspondent rank among the Medical Sciences.

pages 25-28 missing

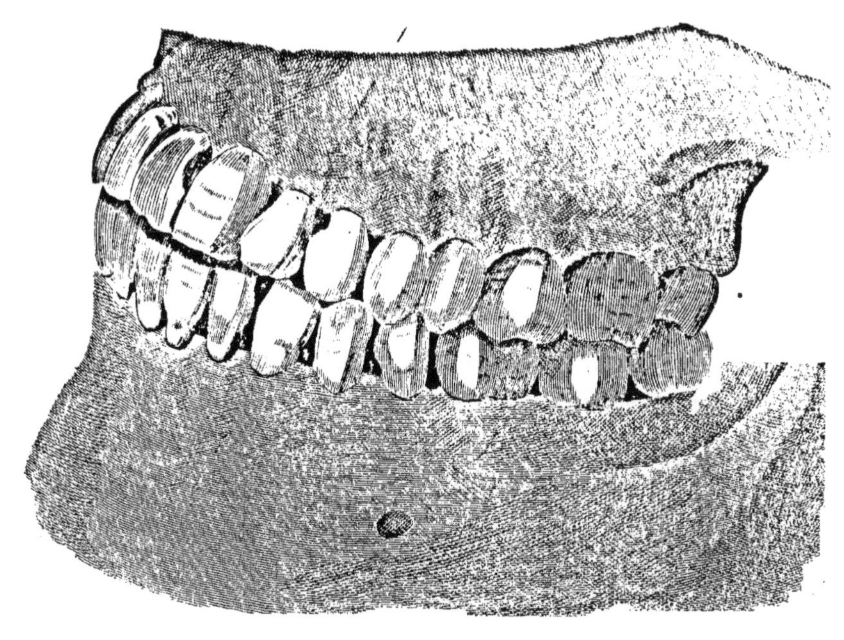

a b c e e
1

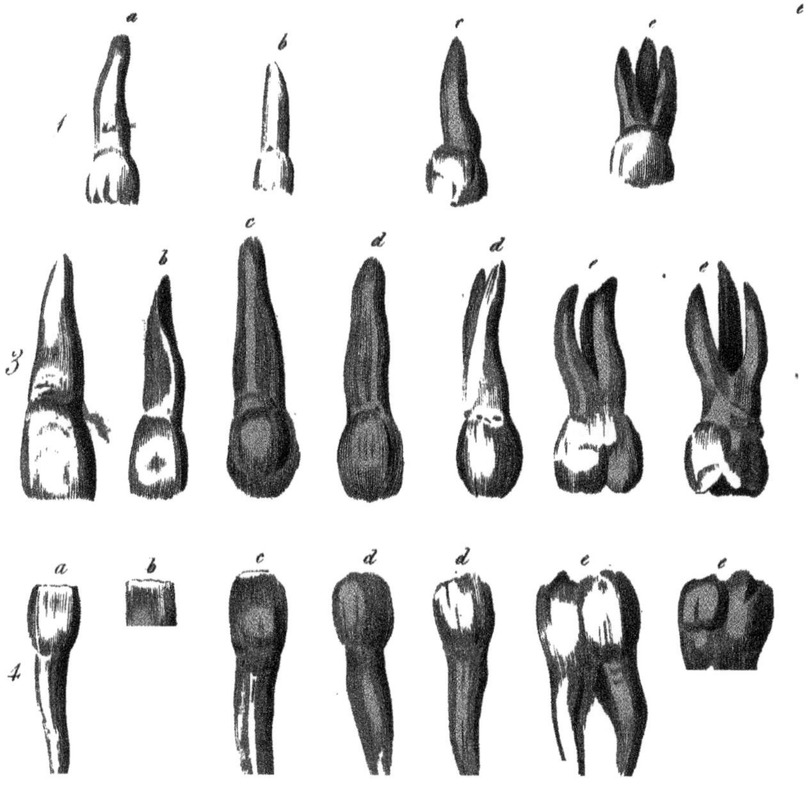

b c d d e e
3

a b c d d e e
4

SYSTEM OF DENTAL SURGERY.

CHAPTER I.

Assimilation is a term, which, when applied to the animal system, implies series of phenomena, by which the food is rendered subservient to the purposes of nutrition. The first of these, the comminution of the food is performed by a set of organs, that in man, not only enable him to masticate his food, but assist in the articulation of language, determine to some extent the expression of his features, and add dignity and beauty to his countenance. I need not for one moment detain the reader by enlarging upon the utility of these organs, or their influence upon the health of the animal, but merely remark that nearly all animals that subsist upon solid food, are provided with an apparatus for reducing and dividing it into small pieces, whereby it is rendered capable of being readily acted on by the digestive powers of the stomach. The maxillary bones with those muscles which give them motion, the teeth and their appendages, the alveoli, and gums, constitute the masticatory apparatus. The object of the present work, is to convey in a manner as clear and concise as possible, the Anatomy, Natural History, and Diseases of these organs. The effect of their diseases upon the general system, the means of preventing and curing those diseases, and a description of the mode by which some part of these organs may be substituted when lost, and to give a detailed account of the various articles of the materia medica used by the surgeon dentist.

4

PART I.

CHAPTER I.

SECTION I.

ANATOMY OF THE MAXILLARY BONES.

The Jaw Bones, technically termed the Maxillary, consist of four bones, two of which form the upper and two the under jaw, usually termed Maxillaria Inferiora and Superiora.

Upper Jaw.

Maxillaria superiora, or upper jaw, consists of two bones situated on the inferior and anterior surface of an irregular pile of bones which with the maxillaria superiora, constitute the bones of the face. The superior face of these bones is formed by a thin triangular plate which is the floor of the orbit. In the posterior part of this plate is a groove leading to a canal terminating in the front of the bone at the foramen infra orbitarium. This foramen is situated just below the middle of the lower margin of the orbit, and gives passage to the superior maxillary nerve and an artery. Externally the triangular plate is terminated by a rough surface, the malar process which articulates with the malar bone.

The nasal process arises by a thick strong root, from this front upper part of the bone at its upper side. Its front edge is thin, the posterior margin is thicker, and the upper edge is

The substance of this bone is externally hard and compact; internally there is a cellular structure, through the centre of which runs the canal, for the nerves and blood vessels. From this canal smaller ones are detached containing the vascular filaments which run to the roots of the teeth. The maxilla inferior articulates with the temporal bones by means of their glenoid cavities. Very marked differences in many individuals exist in the size and formation of these cavities, in consequence of which some persons are liable to a spontaneous dislocation of the jaw, in yawning, &c. when the condyle of the lower jaw, is slipped over the anterior rim of the glenoid cavity.*

SECTION II.

MUSCLES OF THE LOWER JAW.

Besides a very strong ligamentous connection of the lower jaw to the temporal and sphenoidal bones, it receives attachments from several of the strongest muscles of the system, by which its motions are affected and it becomes a powerful lever; the food being the resistance and the muscles the moving powers.

These muscles may be divided into two classes:

Firstly, Those which elevate the jaw and keep it in apposition to the other.

Secondly, Those which depress the jaw.

---

* See the Anatomy of Doctor Horner, Adjunct Professor of Anatomy in the University of Pennsylvania.

Rotation or a grinding motion and the extension and retraction of the jaw, are performed by some of the muscles acting singly, and by a compound motion of others.

First. Those which elevate the jaw and keep it in oppositiou to the other.

Masseter.

The masseter is placed between the chin and the ramus of the lower jaw; it is of an oblong shape and evidently consists of two portions, an external and an internal, which may be readily recognized by the course of their fibres as they decussate.

As a whole it arises tendinous and fleshy from the malar process of the upper maxilla; from the inferior edge of the malar bone between the maxillary and the zygomatic sutures, and from the zygomatic process of the temporal bone.

Of its two portions the internal is the smaller, and is inserted tendinous into the outer part of the root of the coronoid process of the lower jaw; while the external extends from the malar bone to the angle of the lower jaw, where it is inserted, tendinous, and fleshy. A part of the internal portion may be seen at the zygomatic suture, behind the external, without the latter being raised up. When both portions act together they close the jaws; the external alone draws the jaw forwards and the internal alone, will draw it backwards.

Temporalis.

The temporal muscle is placed on the side of the head and occupies its middle inferior region. It is covered externally by the fascia temporalis, a thick, dense, tendinous membrane; which arises by the semicircular ridge on the side of the cranium, and is inserted into the upper margin of the zygoma.

The temporal muscle arises from the inner face of this fascia; from the whole length of the semicircular ridge on the side of the os-frontis and parietale; and from the surface of the cranium between this ridge and the zygoma, including a part of the frontal bone of the parietal, and of the squamous portion of the temporal. This muscle also receives accession of fleshy fibres from the internal face of the zygoma.

From this extensive origin the fibres converge towards the zygoma, and passing beneath it, are inserted tendinous into the coronoid process of the lower jaw, so as to surround it on every side; some of the tendinous fibres go down in front almost to the last dens molaris. It pulls the lower jaw directly upwards.

Pterygoideus Externus.

The external pterygoid muscle, so called from its position, arises fleshy from the outer side of the external pterygoid process of the sphenoid bone; from the tuber of the upper maxilla; and from the under surface of the temporal process of the sphenoid bone.

It passes outwards and backwards horizontally, and is inserted into the inner side of the neck of the inferior maxilla, and into the capsular ligament of the articulation.

When the muscles of the opposite sides act together, they draw the lower jaw forwards, but if alternately, they give it a grinding motion.

Pterygoideus Internus.

The internal pterygoid muscle arises by tendinous and fleshy fibres from the internal plate of the pterygoid process of the sphenoid bone, along the outer margin of the eustachian tube.

It fills up the greater part of the pterygoid fossa; and passing downwards and backwards, is inserted tendinous and fleshy into the internal face of the angle of the lower jaw.

When the muscles of the opposite sides act, they close the jaw.

*Digastricus.**

It is situated immediately under, and a little upon the inside of the lower jaw, and outside of the fauces, extending from the mastoid process to the chin, nearly along the angle made by the neck and chin, or face. The name of this muscle expresses its general shape, as it has two fleshy bellies, and of course a middle tendon. Yet some of its anterior belly does not arise from the tendon of the posterior, but from the fascia, which binds it to the os-hyoides.

These two fleshy bellies do not run in the same line, but form an angle, just where the tendon runs into the anterior belly; so that this tendon seems rather to belong to the posterior, which is the thickest and longest.

This muscle arises from the sulcus made by the inside of the mastoid process, and a ridge upon the temporal bone, where it is united with the os occipitis. The extent of this origin is about an inch. It is fleshy upon its outer part, viz. that from the mastoid process; and tendinous on the inside from the ridge. From its origin it passes forwards downwards and a little inwards much in the direction of the posterior edge of the mammillary process, and forms a round tendon first in its centre and upper surface.

This tendon passes on in the same direction; and when got near the os-hyoides, it commonly perforates the anterior

* Hunter, page 24—32.

end of the stylo-hyoidæus muscle; and from the lower edge of this tendon, some fibres seem to go off, which degenerate into a kind of fascia, that binds it to the os-hyoides; and some of it goes across the lower part of the mylo-hyoideus binding the os-hyoides by a kind of belt. At this part the tendon becomes a little broader, makes a turn upwards, inwards, and forwards, and gives origin to the anterior belly, which passes on in the same direction, to the lower part of the chin, where it is inserted tendinous and fleshy, in a slight depression on the under, and a little on the posterior part of the lower jaw, almost contiguous to its fellow. Besides the attachment of the middle tendon to the os-hyoides, there is a ligamentous binding, which serves, in some measure, as a pulley. This is more marked in some subjects than in others; and this depends on the strength of the tendinous expansion which binds the tendon of the digastricus to the os-hyoides.

When we say that these parts are attached to the os-hyoides, we do not mean that they can be traced quite into it like some other tendons in the body; but the os-hyoides seem to be the most fixed point of attachment. Very often we find two anterior bellies to each muscle; the uncommon one, which is the smallest; does not pass to the chin, but joins with a similar portion of the other side, in a middle tendon, which is often fixed to the os-hyoides. At other times, we find such a portion on one side only; in which case it is commonly fixed to the middle tendon of the mylo-hyoideus.

The use of these muscles with regard to the lower jaw, is principally to depress it; but according as one acts a little more forcibly than the other, it thereby gives the jaw a small rotation; and becomes, in that respect a kind of antagonist to the pterygoideus externus. Besides depressing the lower jaw, when we examine the dead body they would appear to raise the larynx. But, although they have this effect, a proper attention to what happens in the living body will probably show, that their principal action is to depress the lower jaw; and that they are the muscles which are commonly employed for that purpose. Let a finger be placed on the upper part of the mastoideus muscle, just behind the posterior edge of the mastoid process, about its middle, touching that edge a little with the finger; then depress the lower jaw, and the posterior head of the digastric will be felt to swell very considerably, and so as to point out the direction of the muscle. In this there can be no deception; for there is no other muscle in this part that has the same direction; and those who are of opinion that the digastric does not depress the lower jaw, will more readily allow this, when they are told, that we find the same head of the muscle act in deglutition, but not with a force equal to that which it exerts in depressing the lower jaw. Further, if the sterno-hyoidæi, sterno-thyroidæa, and costo-hyoidæi, acting at the same time with the mylo-hyoidei, and genio-hyoidæi assisted in depressing the jaw, the os-hyoides and thyroide cartilage, would probably be depressed, as the bellies of the sterno-hyoidæi, and of the other lower muscles, are by much the longest; but, on the contrary, we find that the os-hyoides with the thyroide cartilage, is a little raised in the depression of the jaw, which we may suppose to be done by the anterior belly of the digastric: and secondly, if these muscles were to bring about this motion of the jaw, these parts would be brought forwards nearer to the straight line between the chin and sternum, which is not the case in this action whereas we find it to be the case in deglutition, in which these evidently act. By applying our fingers upon the genio-hyoidæus, and mylo-hyoidæus, near the os-hyoides, between the two anterior of the digastric, (not near the chin where the action of these two bellies may occasion a mistake,) we find these muscles quite flaccid; which is not the case in deglutition, nor in speaking, in which they certainly do act; nor do we find the muscles under the os-hyoides at all affected, as they are in the motion of the larynx.

It has been observed, that when we open the mouth, while we keep the lower jaw fixed, the fore part of the head or face is necessarily raised. Authors have been at a good deal of pains to explain this. Some of them considered the condyles of the jaw, as the centre of motion; but if this were the case, that part of the head, where it articulates with the spine, and, of consequence, the whole body must be depressed in proportion as the upper jaw is raised; which is not true in fact. Others have considered the condyles of the occiput as the centre of motion; and they have conceived the extensor muscles of the head to be the moving powers. The muscles which move the head in this case, are pointed out by two circumstances, which attend all muscular motion: in the first place, all actions of our body have muscles immediately adapted to them; and secondly when the mind wills no particular action, its power is applied by instinct to those muscles only which are naturally adapted to the motion, and further, the mind being accustomed to see the part move which is naturally the most moveable, attends to its motion in the volition, although it be in that instant fixed, and the other parts of the body move towards it; and although the other parts of the body might be brought towards it by other muscles, and would be so if the mind intended they should come towards it, yet these muscles are not brought into action. Thus the flexors of the arm commonly move the hand to the body, but if the hand be fixed, the body is moved by the same muscles to the hand. In this case, however, the mind wills the motion of the hand towards the body, and brings the flexors into action; whereas if it be wished to bring the body towards the hand, the muscles of the fore part of the body would be put into action, and this would produce the same effect.

To apply this to the lower jaw; when we attempt to open the mouth, while the lower jaw is immoveable, we fix our attention upon the very same muscles (whatever they are) which we call into action when we depress the lower jaw; and we find that we act with the very same muscles: for our mind attends to the depressing of the jaw, and not the raising of the face; and under such circumstances the mouth is actually opened. We find then by these means the head is raised, and the idea that we have of this motion is the same that we have in the common depression of the jaw; and we should not know except from circumstances, that the jaw was not readily depressed; and we find at this time too, that the extensors of the head are not in action: on the contrary, when the jaw is fixed in the same situation, if we have a mind to raise the head, or upper jaw, which of course must open the mouth; we fix our attention to the muscles that move the head backwards, without having the idea of opening our mouth; and at this time the extensors of the head act. This plainly shows that the same muscles which depress the jaw, when moveable, must raise the head when the jaw is kept fixed. This is a proof, too, that there are no other muscles employed in depressing the lower jaw, than will raise the head under the circumstances mentioned. This will further appear from the structure of the parts, wherein four things are to be considered, viz. the articulation of the jaw; the articulation of the head with the neck; the origin, and the insertion of the digastric muscle.

Suppose the upper jaw to be fixed, and the lower jaw to be movable on the condyle: if the digastric contracts, its origin and insertion will approach towards one another; in which case it is evident, that the lower jaw will move downwards and backwards. But if the lower jaw be fixed, as in the case supposed, and the vertebræ be also fixed, the condyle will move upwards and forwards upon the eminence in the joint, the fore part of the head will be pushed upwards and backwards by the condyle, and the hind part of the head will be drawn down, so that the whole shall make a kind of circular motion upon the upper vertebræ; and the digastric muscle, pulling the hind part of the head towards the lower jaw, and at the same time pushing up the condyles, against the fore part of the head, acquires by this mechanism, a very considerable additional power.

The action of the buccinator, and styloglossus, are of considerable use in mastication. The former arises from the back part of the upper and under jaw bones, and comes forward within the cheek ; a considerable portion of which is formed by it. It is of a triangular figure, is broadest behind, forwards it becomes narrower, and is inserted at the angle of the mouth inside. By its action in mastication, it contracts, and presses in the cheek, by which the food is kept between the teeth, from the exterior.

The stylo-glossus derives its name from its origin, which is on a process of the temporal bone called the styloid process, from which, extending forwards and downwards, in an oblique direction, it is inserted into the root of the tongue, and running along its sides forms a portion of it. The action of the stylo-glossus in mastication is opposed to that of the buccinator: it draws the tongue backwards, and gives it a lateral motion, by which the food is kept between the teeth internally.

SECTION III.

OF THE ARTICULATION OF THE LOWER JAW.*

Just under the beginning of the zygomatic process of each temporal bone, before the external meatus auditorius, an oblong cavity may be observed; in direction, length and breadth, in some measure corresponding with the condyle of the lower jaw. Before, and adjoining to this cavity, there is an oblong eminence, placed in the same direction, convex upon the top, in the direction of its shorter axis, which runs from behind forwards; and a little concave in the direction of its longer axis, which runs from within outwards. It is a little broader at its outer extremity, as the outer corresponding end of the condyle describes a larger circle in its motion than the inner. The surface of the cavity, and eminence, is covered with one continued smooth, cartilaginous crust, which is somewhat ligamentous; for, by putrefaction, it peels off like a membrane with the common periosteum. Both the cavity and eminence serve for the motion of the condyle of the lower jaw. The surface of the cavity is directed downward; that of the eminence downward and backward, in such a manner that a tranverse section of both would represent the italic letter *S*. Though the eminence may on a first view of it, appear to project considerably below the cavity, yet a line drawn from the bottom of the cavity to the most depending part of the eminence, is almost horizontal, and therefore nearly parallel with the line made by the grinding surfaces of the teeth in the upper jaw: and when we consider the articulation farther,

---

* Hunter, page 9—11.

we shall find that these two lines are so nearly parallel, that the condyle moves almost directly forwards, in passing from the cavity to the eminence; and the parallelism of the motion is also preserved by the shape of an intermediate cartilage.

In this joint there is a moveable cartilage which though common to both condyle and cavity, ought to be considered rather as an appendage of the former than of the latter, being more closely connected with it; so as to accompany it in its motion along the common surface of both the cavity and the eminence. This cartilage is nearly of the same dimensions with the condyle, which it covers; is hollowed in its inferior surface to receive the condyle; on its upper surface it is more unequal, being moulded to the cavity and eminence of the articulating surface of the temporal bone, though it is considerably less and is therefore capable of being moved with the condyle from one part of that surface to another. Its texture is ligamenta-cartilaginious. This moveable cartilage is connected with both the condyle of the jaw, and the articulating surface of the temporal bone, by distinct ligaments, arising from its edges all round. That by which it is attached to the temporal bone is the most free and loose; though both ligaments will allow an easy motion, or sliding of the cartilage on the respective surfaces of the condyle and the temporal bone.

These attachments of the cartilage are strengthened, and the whole articulation secured, by an external ligament, which is common to both, and which is fixed to the temporal bone, and to the neck of the condyle. On the inner surface of the ligament, which attaches the cartilage of the temporal bone, and backwards in the cavity, is placed what is commonly called the gland of the joint; at least, the ligament is there much more vascular than at any other part.

SECTION IV.

OF THE MOTION IN THE JOINT OF THE LOWER JAW.*

The lower jaw from the manner of its articulation, is susceptible of a great many motions. The whole jaw may be brought horizontally forwards by the condyles sliding from the cavity towards the eminences on each side. This motion is performed chiefly when the teeth of the lower jaw are brought directly under those of the upper, in order to bite, or hold any thing very fast between them. Or, the condyles only may be brought forwards, while the rest of the jaw is tilted backwards, as in the case when the mouth is open; for on that occasion the angle of the jaw is tilted backwards, and the chin moves downwards and a little backwards also. In this last motion, the condyle turns its face a little forwards; and the centre of motion lies a little below the condyle, iu the line between it and the lower angle of the jaw. By such an advancement of the condyles forwards, together with the rotation mentioned, the aperture of the mouth may be considerably enlarged; a circumstance necessary on many obvious occasions.

The condyles may also slide alternately backwards and forwards, from the cavity to the eminence, and vice versa; so that while one condyle advances the other moves backwards, turning the body of the jaw from side to side, and thus grinding, between the teeth, the morsel separated from the larger mass by the motion first described. In this case the centre of motion lies exactly in the middle, between the two condyles. And it is to be observed, that in these slidings of

---

* Hunter, 12—14.

the condyles forwards and backwards, the moveable cartilages do not accompany the condyles in the whole extent of their motion ; but only so far as to adapt their surfaces to the different inequalities of the temporal bone : for as these cartilages, are hollow on their lower surfaces where they receive the condyle, and on their opposite upper surfaces are convex where they lie in the cavity, but forwards, at the root of the eminence, that upper surface is a little hollowed, if they accompanied the condyles through the whole extent of their motion, the eminences would be applied to the eminences, the cavities would not be filled up, and the whole articulation would be rendered very insecure.

This account of the motion of the lower jaw, and its cartilages, clearly demonstrates the utility of these cartilages; namely, the security of the articulation; the surfaces of the cartilages accomodating themselves to the different inequalities, in the various and free motions of this joint. This cartilage is also very serviceable for preventing the parts from being hurt by the friction; a circumstance necessary to be guarded against, where there is so much motion. Accordingly, I find this cartilage in the different tribes of carniverous animals, where there is no eminence and cavity, nor other apparatus for grinding, and where the motion is of the true ginglimus kind only.

In the lower jaw, as in all the points of the body, when the motion is carried to its greatest extent, in any direction, the muscles and ligaments are strained and the person made uneasy. The state, therefore, into which every joint most naturally falls, especially when we are asleep, is nearly in the middle between the extremes of motion; by which means all the muscles and ligaments are equally relaxed. Thence it is, that commonly, and naturally the teeth of the two jaws are not in contact; nor are the condyles of the lower jaw, so far back in the temporal cavities as they can go.

SECTION V.*

OF THE INCREASE OF THE JAWS.

In a fœtus three or four months old, the rudiments of the teeth are placed nearly regular, but as they increase more rapidly than the arch of the jaws, we find some of them at birth as it were, pressed out of the circle for want of room, particularly the cuspidati; so that the sockets of the lateral incisores, and those of the anterior grinders nearly come in contact. However, the jaws gradually accomodate themselves to the teeth, and increase at this part nearly in proportion to the size of the cuspidati, becoming again regular, for indeed we seldom or ever meet with temporary teeth irregular. This Mr. Hunter allows, but says,† "The jaw still increases in all points till twelve months after birth, when the bodies of the six teeth are pretty well formed, but it never after increases in length between the symphysis and the sixth tooth; and from this time too, the alveolar process which makes the anterior part of the arches of both jaws, never becomes a section of a larger circle; and after this time the jaws lengthen only at their posterior ends." Mr. Hunter supposed, as the temporary grinders are larger than the bicuspides which succeed them, that the difference in size of these would be sufficient to allow the permanent in-

* Blake, Essay on the Teeth, in Man, &c. pages 47 to 55.

† Natural History, page 102.

cisores and cuspidati, which are much larger than their predecessors, to become regular, without any increase of the arch or circle. He was led into this opinion by comparing four lower jaws of different subjects, and at different periods of life; from the age when the five temporary teeth are completed, to that of the entire permanent set. He acknowledges, however, that it is impossible there should be a mathematical exactness in four different jaws; nor indeed is there a mathematical exactness in the lines drawn to support his theory, for they are by no means parallel.*

Indeed so varied are the dimensions of jaws, that the arch of one a year old may correspond, or even exceed the arch of an adult; and vice versa, the arch of an adult may be nearly as large again as that of a child; so it is not by comparing different jaws together that we shall be enabled to draw proper conclusions; but by comparing the permanent and temporary teeth of the same jaws.

It appears from my preparations, and experience convinces me, that the space occupied by the temporary teeth would not be sufficient to accommodate the same number of permanent teeth which succeed them, and which on the whole are so much larger, particularly in the upper jaw. This fact Mr. Hunter was aware of, and mentions that irregularities are more frequently met with in the upper, than in the lower jaw; so far I agree with him.

We have seen the rudiments of the permanent teeth at first placed nearly regular, but as ossification advances on them, they become crowded together for want of room. This irregularity particularly happens to the permanent teeth, because they are at first situated at the internal part of the

* Nat. Hist. Plate 16, Figure 2.

jaw, and of course in a much smaller circle than the temporary. As I have given an accurate representation of the jaws of a child about four years old, and the situation and connexion of both sets of teeth, in plate II.—figs. 1 and 2, very little is required to be said on this subject. In the under jaw, the lateral permanent incisores, hide nearly half the middle ones, and the lateral incisores and anterior bicuspides are so close together, that the cuspidati would not have near room enough to pass between them. In the upper jaw there is a much more confused appearance, and a more striking contrast with respect to the difference in size of both sets of teeth; the lateral incisores rest in part on the middle ones, and the sockets of the lateral incisores and anterior bicuspides nearly come in contact; so that the cuspidati are entirely thrown out of the circle.

We have seen also that the pulps and membranes of the permanent teeth were at first very small, and that the sockets were in proportion; but as the pulps enlarged and ossification advanced on them, the sockets increased likewise. It is but just therefore to suppose, that as the teeth rise and appear through the gum, the alveolar processes should accommodate themselves to them; which indeed will presently appear to be the case. If Mr. Hunter was a practitioner in this branch even with very little experience, he must have frequently have observed in children of about six or seven years of age (if the first teeth had not already fallen), large distances between the incisores, which at first were quite close to one another. I have seen hundreds of instances in which the four permanent incisores appeared irregular, but in a short space of time became perfectly regular without any artificial assistance. In a preparation of Dr. Monro's (which he was kind enough to allow me to take a sketch of), the four permanent incisores of the under jaw had appeared, and also the two middle incisores of the upper, and were perfectly regular, though the temporary cuspidati and grinders had remained in the former, and the lateral incisores cuspidati, and grinders in the latter. Surely then these teeth could have gained no room from the difference in size of the grinders and bicuspides; it must therefore be owing to an increase of the arches of the jaws in these parts exactly in proportion to the difference in size of the temporary and permanent incisores. There is still in this case a further necessity for a considerable increase of the arches, on account of the irregular situation of the permanent teeth, as well as because several of them had not as yet arrived at their full size.

The pressure of the front teeth on one another as they rise in the jaw, appears to have some effect in occasioning it to extend at certain parts, or to make the grinders move backwards, to which indeed all the teeth have a tendency. I have a preparation of the upper jaw of an adult, in which the temporary cuspidatus of the right side remained in; the permanent cuspidatus probably from the resistance of the former, penetrated at the internal part of the mouth: in the left side the teeth are all perfectly regular: on comparing the situation of the anterior permanent grinders, I found that of the right side nearer the symphysis than that of the left in proportion to the difference in size, of the temporary and permanent cuspidati. I have met several instances of the permanent cuspidati appearing at first irregular, as they most commonly appear later than the bicuspides, but in ten or twelve months after, the jaw increased sufficiently so as to allow them to become regular. I have met many cases where the arches of the jaws continued to increase, even after the permanent teeth were complete; so that all the front teeth were quite separate from each other; and in one case the middle incisores were nearly half an inch asunder, though there was no defect in the palate.

From what is now said I feel myself justifiable in concluding, that the alveolar arches continue to increase during the entire progress of the formation of the teeth: it is however sufficiently evident, the greatest increase of the jaw is backwards. I do not by any means deny but that we frequently meet with disproportions between the jaws and teeth, and such that the permanent teeth never would become regular without the assistance of art, even in young persons; this may arise from the resistance of the temporary teeth, or from teeth forming so much out of the circle that they have not sufficient power to act on their neighbours and press them back, such as the cuspidati, which are most commonly irregular. Indeed if Mr. Hunter's hypothesis were true, we should never see a regular set of teeth.

Duval concurs with Mr. Blake in considering that the jaws increase in all parts during and before the second dentition, upon which he makes the following observations. After remarking upon the situations taken by the adult teeth he continues. "At this disposition of parts, who is not struck with admiration? but we shall be still more so when we learn that the jaw bone grows transversely, in order to make room for the permanent grinders, which are never shed, not only by increasing in size in that part which lies behind the temporary grinders, as the anatomists have published,* but by developing itself equally in all its points in such a manner that the sockets of the large grinders and these teeth themselves grow and become successively placed from behind

* Duval, page 60.

to before,"* &c. &c. Although the jaws increase proportionably more between the last deciduous tooth and the condyles, yet it must be conceded that during the puerile state, every part of the jaws increase, as do all the other members of the body, the deciduous teeth excepted.

SECTION VII.

ANATOMY OF THE TEETH.†

These organs in the adult are divided into four classes; incisores, cuspidati, bicuspides,‡ and molares. They differ very much in the figure of their bodies, and in the number and shape of their fangs. The cuspidati are of a middle nature between the incisores and the bicuspides; as are the latter between the cuspidati and the molares.

The incisores, or cutting teeth, are situated in the anterior part of the jaw, and form the front of the mouth. In each jaw they are four in number, and are so placed, that the two central stand somewhat more advanced than the lateral.

The bodies of the incisores are broad and rather flat. The anterior surface is convex, the posterior concave; they both go off from the neck of the tooth somewhat sloping. The two surfaces terminate in a cutting edge, which is placed in a direct line with the apex of the fang. When viewed in front, the cutting edge is seen to be the broadest part of the tooth, but gradually becomes smaller as we approach to the

* "See Fox and Hunter." † Fox, chap. 2.

‡ This class is wanting in the infant set.

neck. When viewed laterally the cutting edge is the thinest, and the tooth, to the neck of it, increases in thickness. This gives to the body of the tooth the form of a wedge, which is its true office, it being used to cut or divide soft substances.

The enamel is continued farther, and is thicker on the anterior and posterior surfaces than on the sides; it is even thicker on the forepart than on the back part of the tooth. The fangs are conical, and are shorter than those of the cuspidati.

In the upper jaw the central incisores are much broader and larger than in the lateral; in the lower jaw they are all nearly of the same size, but much smaller than those of the upper jaw.

The cuspidati are four in number, one of them being placed on the outer side of each of the lateral incisores. The shape of the crown of a cuspidatus is like that of an incisor, with its corners rubbed off, so as to end in a point, instead of a broad edge. The fang is thicker and larger and is more depressed at the sides, which causes it to appear considerably larger, when viewed laterally, than when seen in front. The fang, which is the largest of any of the teeth, may be felt with the finger, running up a considerable length, and projecting beyond those of the other teeth.

The cuspidati of the lower jaw very much resemble those of the upper, both in figure and in length. The enamel covers more of the lateral parts of these teeth than of the incisores. When they are first formed they are pointed, but by the friction of each upon the other in mastication, they become rounded, and sometimes acquire a flat edge.

The use of the cuspidati is not like that of the incisores, to cut and divide substances, nor like the molares for mastication, but they are similar to the canine teeth of the carniverous animals, and seem to be designed for the laying hold of and tearing substances.

The bicuspides are situated immediately behind the cuspidati. They were formerly called the first and second grinders, but as they do not possess the true figure of the grinders, and only have an intermediate resemblance between those teeth and the cuspidati, Mr. Hunter considered them as a particular class.

These teeth are very much like each other, and when viewed as they are situated in the mouth, are not unlike the cuspidati. They are eight in number; those belonging to the upper jaw, have the body divided into two points, one external and the other internal. Their fangs appear as if compressed at the sides, and resemble two fangs united, with a depression running between them. Commonly the first bicuspis has two small fangs, the second has seldom more than one, but in this they are subject to variety.

The bicuspides of the under jaw are smaller than those of the upper; the points upon their surfaces are not so distinct, and they have only one fang. The enamel is distributed nearly equally around the crown, and they stand in the jaw almost perpendicularly, and have a slight inclination inwards.

The molares, or grinders, are placed behind the bicuspides; there are three on each side of the jaw, making twelve in the whole. The first and second molares are so much alike in every particular, that the description of one will convey a perfect idea of the other. The third grinder, has several peculiarities, and therefore must be described separately. The molares are the largest teeth; they have a broader base, and furnished with several points, which fits them for their office in grinding food, and they have several fangs.

The molares of the under jaw have an inclination inwards

while those of the upper jaw are placed nearly perpendicularly with respect to the jaw.

The upper grinders have commonly three fangs, two situated on the outer part of the tooth, and one on the inner; the inner fang is very oblique in its direction, and is larger and rounder than the others. Those of the under jaw have two fangs, one placed forwards, the other backwards; they are rather flat, and continue broad all down their length.

Sometimes molares of the upper jaw are met with having four distinct fangs. I have one with five fangs, which is the only one I ever saw.* The molares of the under jaw now and then have three fangs.

The third molaris is called dens sapientiæ; it is smaller than the others, its body is rather rounder, and the fangs are not so regular and distinct. They often appear as if squeezed together, and sometimes there is but one fang. The dentes sapientiæ of the lower jaw often have their fangs curved, and sometimes they are so much inclined inwards, as scarcely to rise above the ridge of the coronoid process.

The incisores of the upper jaw being much broader than the same teeth in the under jaw, cause the other teeth to be placed farther back in the circle, than the corresponding teeth on the lower jaw; hence, in a well formed mouth, when the teeth are shut close, the central incisores of the upper jaw come over the central and half of the lateral incisores of the lower jaw. The lateral incisor of the upper jaw covers the half of the lateral incisor, and more than half of the cuspidatus of the under jaw. The cuspidatus of the upper jaw falls between and projects a little over the cuspidatus and first bicuspis of the under jaw. The first bicuspis of

* Fauchard gives a plate of one having five fangs.

the upper jaw falls partly upon the two bicuspides in the lower jaw. The second bicuspis shuts upon the second bicuspis and the first molaris. The first upper molaris covers two thirds of the first and part of the second molaris of the under jaw. The second upper molaris shuts upon the remainder of the second and part of the third; and the third molaris of the upper jaw, being smaller than that in the under jaw, shuts even upon it. From this mechanism of the teeth, their power in mastication is increased, and if one tooth be extracted, the antagonist tooth does not become useless, since it can in part act upon another.

A tooth is composed of two substances, one of which, called the enamel, is spread over that part which is not covered by the gums. The other substance is bone; it consists of the fang and all the body of the tooth situated within the enamel. The bone of the tooth is formed from the pulp; and the enamel, from the investing membrane. The bony part of the tooth is begun to be formed before the enamel. When the ossification of a tooth is commencing, bone is deposited from the vessels of the pulp upon its extreme points. In the incisores it begins upon the edges, and in the molares upon the points of their grinding surfaces. The ossification usually begins in the incisores in three spots; these increase, soon unite, and produce the cutting edge of the tooth. In the molares it begins in as many spots as there are grinding points, which in the lower jaw are commonly four, and in the upper, five. These soon unite and form one thin layer of bone over the upper surface of the pulp. The ossification soon extends to the sides of the pulp, and a thin shell of bone is spread over its whole surface. If this shell be removed, the pulp, when uncovered, will be found very vascular. This is extremely well seen in the teeth of large animals, when in a state of formation.

Some time ago I had the opportunity of examining the pulps of the teeth of a young elephant, which was dissected by Sir Astley Cooper. Upon removing the ossification which had taken place upon the pulps, I found the vessels to be exceedingly full of blood. There was also a considerable degree of force required to separate the bone from the pulp, and this strength of union between the pulp and the ossified part, I have always found to be in proportion to the size of the tooth.

In the formation of the bone of a tooth the ossific matter is deposited in strata, one within side the other; thus a tooth is formed from the outer part to the inner; and this deposition of bone continues until the tooth becomes complete. When the body of the tooth is formed, the pulp elongates, and takes the form of the fang proper to each particular tooth, and bone is deposited upon it. It then becomes gradually smaller, until it terminates in a point. If a tooth have two or more fangs, the pulp divides, and the ossification proceeds accordingly. The cavity within a tooth, as it is forming, is at first very considerable; it becomes less as the formation advances, until it arrives at a certain point, when a cavity is left in it extending nearly the whole length, and retaining the shape of the tooth.

In the crown of the tooth, the cavity is of the same figure, and it divides into as many canals as there are fangs to the teeth. A canal extends through each fang connected with the cavity in the body of the tooth. Into this cavity the nerves and blood vessels enter and ramify upon a membrane of the pulp, which remains to line the cavity after the formation of the teeth. In this manner the nerves give sensation to the teeth, and the internal parts of them are nourished.

The enamel is situated upon all that part of a tooth which in the healthy state of the gums is not covered by them. This portion of a tooth is called the body or crown. It is formed by the membrane which invests the pulp. When a shell of bone has been formed upon the pulp, this membrane secretes a fluid, from which a very white soft substance is deposited upon the bone; this is at first of a consistence not harder than chalk, for it may be scratched or scraped off by the nail; it however soon grows hard, and seems to undergo a process similar to that of crystalization, for it takes a regular and peculiar form.

The deposition of the enamel continues nearly as long as a tooth is contained within the membrane. It is always most in quantity upon those parts where its formation first began; it is thicker upon the edges and grinding surfaces of the teeth, than upon the sides, and it gradually becomes thinner as it approaches the necks of the teeth. A tooth, when sawn through, shows the arrangement of the enamel; and as it requires more heat to blacken and burn this hardest part of the animal frame than the bony part of the tooth, we can, by exposing it to the effects of fire, obtain a still more distinct exhibition of it. By the time the enamel is completely formed, the tooth has risen so much in the socket, that by its pressure it occasions an absorption of the membrane, which completely prevents any further addition of enamel.

When perfect the enamel of the teeth is so hard, that a file, in cutting it, is soon worn smooth, and when struck with it, sparks of fire will be elicited; an effect I have several times produced with human teeth, and which will be very readily seen, by striking the teeth of large animals with steel, particularly those of the Hippopotamus.

The enamel when broken appears to be composed of a greater number of small fibres, all of which are so arranged as to pass in a direction from the centre to the circumference of the tooth, so as to form a sort of radii round the body of the tooth. This is the crystalized form it acquires some time after its deposit; by this disposition of its fibres, the enamel acquires a great degree of strength, and thus it is not so readily worn down in mastication, nor so easily fractured by violent action of the teeth.

While some eminent physiologists have contended, that the teeth, when they have attained their full growth, are to be considered extraneous bodies, and that they no longer receive nutriment like the other bones of the body, others have supposed, that even the enamel is kept up in future life by continued deposits: but that this cannot be the case will be obvious, when it is considered that the membrane which invested the pulp and produced the enamel, is destroyed before the tooth can appear. When a tooth first appears, the enamel is thicker than at any other period of life, and from that time begins to decrease; this may be remarked in some of the permanent teeth. The incisores, when they first pass through the gum, have their edges notched, the cuspidati are sharp at their points, and the grinding surface of the molares is always irregular. This sharpness of the points of the teeth is occasioned by a larger deposit upon those parts where ossification had first commenced. By the friction of the teeth against each other, and against the food in mastication, the teeth are worn smooth, the notches upon the incisores disappear, the points of the cuspidati are rounded, or in many cases entirely removed, and the surfaces of the molares become much smoother.

The case is quite the reverse with the bony part, for when a tooth is first seen through the gum scarcely more than two thirds of the fangs are formed, but the ossification continues for a considerable time afterwards. The enamel upon some teeth has a very defective formation; instead of being a hard white substance having a smooth polished surface, it is frequently met with of a yellow colour, and having a great number of indentations upon its surfaces. This occasions the teeth to resemble the exterior of a sponge, and gives them what has been termed a honey-combed appearance.

Sometimes this appearance* of the enamel is only met with on the front teeth, near the cutting edge, at others it extends nearly over half of the tooth, the remaining parts being perfect. When the roughness is near the edge, it often wears out in a few years, or at the age of maturity it may be filed out. In some cases one, two, or three indented lines, pass across the front of the teeth.

This defective formation of the enamel is usually confined to the incisores, cuspidati, and first permanent molares; it is rarely met with on the bicuspides, or second and third molares.

The arteries which supply the teeth with blood are called the dental; they are branches of the internal maxillary artery which arises from the external carotid, at that part where it is covered by the parotid gland, and lies behind the middle of the upright plate of the lower jaw where it divides into the condyloid and coronoid processes. It passes first between the jaw and the external pterygoid muscle, and

* This may, and frequently does arise, from some cause that mechanically disturbs the membranes before ossification is completed; for the enamel is exactly of the shape and figure of the membranes from which it is formed.

afterwards runs in a very winding direction towards the back part of the antrum maxillare; it here sends numerous branches to the parts belonging to both jaws, and to the teeth of the upper jaw. It then gives off one branch to the lower jaw, called by some the inferior maxillary, and by others the dental. This enters the jaw bone at the posterior maxillary foramen, passes through the maxillary canal, and gives off branches to the fangs of each tooth, and also supplies the substance of the bone. This vessel having sent a branch to the incisores, passes out at the anterior maxillary foramen; it is distributed to the gums, and communicates upon the chin with branches of the facial artery.

The nerves which are distributed to the teeth arise from the fifth pair, the trigemini. This pair of nerves divides into three branches; the ophthalmic, the superior maxillary, and the inferior maxillary. The ophthalmic branch passes through the foramen lacerum of the orbit, and is distributed to the parts in the neighbourhood of the eye. The superior maxillary nerve goes out at the foramen rotundum of the sphenoid bone, and divides into several branches, being continued to the posterior part of the nose, the palate, velum palati, and contiguous parts. At the posterior part, small filaments of nerves, accompanying branches of arteries, enter the superior maxillary bone by foramina, which lead to the molares and also to the membrane lining the antrum maxillare. The nerve then goes into the canal under the orbit and forms the infra orbitar nerve. Whilst in the canal, it sends off branches to the bicuspides, cuspidati, and incisores; it afterwards passes out at the foramen infra orbitarium, and is distributed upon the cheek, under eyelid, upper lip, and side of the nose.

The inferior maxillary nerve passes through the foramen ovale of the sphenoid bone, and is distributed to the muscles of the lower jaw: it sends off a large branch, the lingual, which goes to the tongue, which is the true gustatory nerve; it then enters the maxillary canal of the lower-jaw, passes through the bone under the alveoli, and gives off branches which, entering the fangs, ramify upon the membrane within the cavities of the teeth; it passes out at the anterior maxillary foramen, and is spent about the chin and lip.

The teeth are fixed in their sockets by that species of articulation called gomphosis. They are attached to the alveolar cavity by a strong periosteum which is extended over the fangs, and which also lines the sockets; it is connected to the gums at the neck of the tooth, and it is vascular like the periosteum in other parts of the body.

SECTION VIII.

OF THE ALVEOLAR PROCESSES.*

We observe the beginning of the alveolar process at a very early period. In a fœtus of three or four months, it is only a longitudinal groove, deeper and narrower forwards, and becoming gradually more shallow and wider backwards. Instead of bony partitions dividing that groove into a number of sockets, there are only slight ridges across the bottom and sides, with intermediate depressions, which mark the future alveoli.†

"In the lower jaw the vessels and nerves run along the

---

* Natural History of the Human Teeth, by John Hunter, London, 1803.

† Page 74, 75—6.

bottom of this alveolar cavity, in a slight groove, which afterwards becomes a complete and distinct bony canal.

The alveolar process grows with the teeth, and for some time keeps the start of them. The ridges which are to make the partitions shoot from the sides across the canal, at the mouth of the cell, forming hollow arches. This change happens first at the anterior part of the jaws. As each cell becomes deeper, its mouth also grows narrower, and at length is almost, but not quite, closed over the contained tooth."

"The disposition for contracting the mouth of the cell, is chiefly in the outer plate of the bone, which occasions the contracted orifices of the cells to be nearer the inner edge of the jaw. The reason, perhaps, why the bone shoots over, and almost covers the tooth, is, that the gum may be firmly supported before the teeth have come through.

The alveoli which belong to the adult grinders, are formed in another manner: in the lower jaw they would seem to be the remains of the root of the coronoid process, for the cells are formed for those teeth in the root of that process; and in proportion as the body of the bone, and the cells already formed, push forwards from under that process, the succeeding cells and their teeth are formed and pushed forward in the same manner."

"In the upper jaw there are cells formed in the tubercles for the young grinders, which at first are very shallow, and become deeper and deeper as the teeth grow; and they grow somewhat faster, so as almost to enclose the whole tooth, before it is ready to push its way through that enclosure and gum. There is a succession of these, till the whole three grinders are formed."

In the adult, the alveoli are usually from one third to two thirds of an inch in depth, being much deeper in the front than on the posterior part of the jaws. They are appendages of the teeth, grow with them, and when they are lost, the alveoli soon disappear. The knowledge of this fact enables us to explain the great changes which take place in the appearance of the features, from the loss of the teeth, and consequent loss of the alveoli : and a knowledge of this circumstance enables us by directing the growth and position of the teeth and alveoli, to prevent and correct deformities from a mal position of these organs.

SECTION IX.

OF THE GUMS.*

The alveolar processes are covered by a red vascular substance, called the gums, which has as many perforations as there are teeth ; and the neck of a tooth is covered by, and fixed to this gum. Thence there are fleshy partitions between the teeth, passing between the external and internal gum, and as it were uniting them ; these partitions are higher than the other parts of the gum, and thence form an arch between every two adjacent teeth. The thickness of that part of the gum which projects beyond the sockets is considerable ; so that when the gum is corroded by disease, by boiling, or otherwise, the teeth appear longer, or less sunk into the jaw. The gum adheres very firmly in a healthful state, both to the alveolar process and to the teeth, but its extreme border is naturally loose all around the teeth.

The gum, in substance, has something of a cartilaginous hardness and elasticity, and is very vascular, but seems not

---

* Natural History of the Human Teeth, by John Hunter. London, 1803, page 66—67.

to have any great degree of sensibility; for though we often wound it in eating, and in picking our teeth, yet we do not feel much pain upon these occasions; and both in infants and old people, where there are no teeth, the gums bear a very considerable pressure, without pain.

The advantage arising from this degree of insensibility in the gums, is obvious; for till the child cuts its teeth, the gums are to do the business of teeth, and are therefore formed for this purpose, having a hard ridge running through their whole length. Old people, who have lost their teeth, have not this ridge. When in a sound state, the gums are not easily irritated by being wounded, and therefore are not so liable to inflammation as other parts, and soon heal.

The teeth being united to the jaw by the periosteum and gum, have some degree of a yielding motion in the living body. This circumstance renders them more secure; it breaks the jar of bony contact, and prevents fractures both of the sockets and of the teeth themselves."

These remarks of Mr. Hunter, considering the gums in a healthy state, are strictly true,—but inflamed and diseased, they become very sensible.

* "The principal use of the gums, is to make the teeth more firm and more permanent in the alveolus, which contains their roots. The gums are the preservers of the teeth; they also contribute to the ornament of the mouth, when they are well figured and shaped in the form of a half crescent, which manifests itself particularly in laughing. They show a vermillion red, which relieves the lustre of the whiteness of the teeth, and which is reciprocally relieved by this same whiteness. This apposition of colour with the order and regularity of the teeth, and edges of the gums, offers to the sight a most gracious object."

---

* Fauchard, page 219.

SECTION X.

OF THE ACTION OF THE TEETH, ARISING FROM THE MOTION OF THE LOWER JAW.*

"The lower jaw may be said to be the only one that has any motion in mastication; for the upper jaw can only move with the other parts of the head. That the upper jaw and head should be raised in the common act of opening the mouth, or chewing, would seem, at first sight, improbable; and from an attentive view of the mechanism of the joints, and muscles of those parts, from experiment and observation, we find that they do not sensibly move. We shall only mention one experiment in proof of this, which seems conclusive. Let a man place himself near some fixed point, and look over it to another distant and immovable object, when he is eating. If his head should rise in the least degree, he would see more of the distant object over the nearest fixed point, which in fact he does not. The nearer the fixed point is, and the more distant the object, the experiment will be more accurate and convincing. The result of the experiment will be the same, if the nearest point has the same motion with the head; as when he looks from under the edge of a hat, or any thing else put upon his head, at some distant fixed object. We may conclude then that the motion is entirely in the lower jaw; and as we have already described both the articulation and the motion of the bone, we shall now explain the action of mastication, and at the same time consider the use of each class of teeth.

With regard to the action of the teeth of both jaws, in

* Natural History of the Human Teeth, by John Hunter, London 1803. Pages 68 to 71.

mastication, we may observe once for all, that their action and re-action must be always equal, and that the teeth of the upper and lower jaw are complete and equal antagonists both in cutting and grinding.

When the lower jaw is depressed, the condyles slide forwards on the eminences; and they return back again into the cavities, when the jaw is completely raised. This simple action produces a grinding motion of the lower jaw backwards on the upper, and is used when we divide any thing with our fore teeth or incisores. For this purpose the incisores are well formed; as they are higher than the others, their edges must come in contact sooner; and as the upper project over the under, we find in dividing any substance with them, that we first bring them opposite to one another, and as they pass through the part to be divided, the lower jaw is brought back, while the incisors of that jaw slide up behind those of the upper jaw, and of course pass by one another. In this way they complete the division like a pair of scissors; and at the same time they sharpen one another. There are exceptions to this, for the teeth in some people meet equally, viz. in those people whose fore teeth do not project further than the gum, or socket, than the back teeth; and such teeth are not so fit for dividing: and in some people the teeth of the lower jaw are so placed, as to come before those of the upper jaw; this situation is as favorable for cutting as when the overlapping of the teeth is the reverse, except for this circumstance, that the lower jaw must be longer, and therefore its action weaker.

The other motion of the lower jaw, viz. when the lateral teeth are used, is somewhat different from the former. In opening the mouth, one condyle slides a little forwards, and the other slides a little further back into its cavity; this throws the jaw a little to that side, just enough to bring the lower teeth directly under their corresponding teeth in the upper jaw ; this is done either in the dividing or holding of substances, and these are the teeth that are generally used in the last mentioned action. When the true grinding motion is to be performed, a greater degree of this last motion takes place ; that is, the condyle of the opposite side is brought farther forwards, and the condyle of the same side is drawn farther back into the cavity of the temporal bone, and the jaw is a little depressed. This is only preparatory for the effect to be produced ; for the moving back of the first mentioned condyle into the socket, is what produces the effect in mastication.

The lateral teeth in both jaws are adapted to this oblique motion ; in the lower they are turned a little inwards, that they may act more in the direction of their axis ; and here the alveolar process is strongest on the outside, being there supported by the ridge of the root of the coronoid process. In the upper jaw the obliquity of the teeth is the reverse, that is, they are turned outwards, for the same reason ; and the longest fang of the grinders is upon the inside, where the socket is strengthened by the bony partition between the antrum and the nose: Hence it is, that the teeth of the lower jaw have their outer edges worn down first ; and vice versa, in the upper jaw."

SECTION XI.

USUS DENTIUM.*

The first and principle of these is for the comminution of the food, whence toothless persons feed only on fluids. It

* Bartholinus' Anatomy Lugduni, Batava, 1686.

was for this reason doubtless that Niceppoorus taught,—if one dream he sees teeth drop out, it portends the death of a friend.*

II. For forming the voice (hence infants do not speak before the mouth is filled with teeth), especially for expressing certain letters the incisive teeth are essential.† Hence toothless persons are unable to pronounce such letters as T and R, where the tongue presses against the front teeth. The loss of the front (incisive) teeth also injures the fulness of the voice, (according to Galenus,) so that the speech becomes slower, less articulate, and attended with effort. Hence persons who have lost these teeth, procure artificial ones firmly set with gold wire.

III. For ornament.—Toothless persons are deformed.‡

IV. For abating garrulity, as Homer thought.||

V. In brutes also for fighting where man uses the hands.§

VI. In brutes also for marking the age, as is well known from the inspection of the mouth of horses.**

* "Primus et primarius, est ad cibos comminuendos. Unde edentuli sorbila tantum horiunt; quam ob causam dejectos dentes videre malum Nicephero, et in somniis vulgo amici casum præsagit."

† Ad vocem formandam (hinc infantes non loquuntur, antequam os dentibus plenum) precipue ad literas quasdam experimendas incisorii conferunt. Hinc edentuli litteras quasdam pronunciare nequeunt, v. g. T. et R. ubi lingua ampliata prioribus dentibus inniti debet. Alioquin incisoriorum amissio lædit vocis explicationem, teste Galeno, ut sermo tardior, et minus clarus facilisque. Hinc edentuli arcte dentes institios sibi procurant, aureo filo vinciendos."

‡ "Ad Ornatum. Edentuli enim deformes sunt."

§ "Homerus putat ad compescendam garrulitatem."

|| "In brutis etiam ad pugnam, ubi homo manibus utiber."

** "Tisdem brutis ad ætatum designandam. Equorum enim ætatem inspectum os prodit.

CHAPTER II.

NATURAL HISTORY THE TEETH.*

"We now proceed in this chapter to a consideration of the Natural History of the Teeth, with a notice of various, physiological and anomalous phenomena connected with them.

The first who gave a description of the teeth was Hippocrates;† Mattheus de Gradibus followed his example;‡ and Castrillo according to the remark of Douglas, wrote a dissertation on dentition, and described the order the teeth follow in their appearance. Celsus has also examined their structure, their number, their position, their differences, and traced the progress of the permanent teeth. Vesalius has described the teeth of the adult, but their development had not attracted his attention, and Ingrassias who was engaged in observing the germination of the teeth, and in describing the vessels which contribute to their growth, admits four dentitions; the first, says he, takes place in the womb of the mother, and the three others at different periods in the course of life."

Fallopius had observed with attention the teeth in the fœtus, and he explains himself thus. "The jaws contain two incomplete rows of teeth; one comes out of their cavities sooner than the other, the anterior before the posterior:

---

* De la Dentition ou du développement des dents, dissertation presentée et soutenue à l'Ecole de Medicine a Paris, 1803.

† In text vii. oper. in fol. Paris 1639, page 5 to 10. par J. Groussét.

‡ De anatomia dentium, in oper. chap. 118, in folio. Paris, 1491.

in coming out they tear the membranous envelopment in which they are enclosed. Eustachius,* is the first who perceived that the the teeth of the first and second dentition were formed in the womb of the mother, that the two sets were placed on the same line, principally of the class of incisors, canine and first molar teeth, and that their production could not be sensibly perceived until after birth; after two months, there are found in each dental arch four superior incisors, two canine, and three molares, above and below, shut up in their follicles, and surrounded by a gelatino-mucus liquor, and each tooth is contained in its socket; he gives a description of the teeth of the adult, examines in order the structure and composition of the first teeth, explains the manner in which they are produced, and points out the time when they fall out of their sockets, their varieties, their diseases, and their uses: it is a complete treatise on dentition, which merits to be used as a model."

Hemard has made the same researches as Eustachius and Fallopius, but he did not carry them so far as those two anatomists.†

Until the time of Duverney, little attention was paid to this important part of anatomy and physiology; it was reserved for this celebrated anatomist to extend the knowledge of Eustachius, and to explain the particular structure of the teeth at different periods of life;(*a*) Delahire his cotemporary and his friend pursued in some degree the same course,(*b*) and Winslow profited by the knowledge of these

---

* Opuscula anatomica tractatus de dentibus. Lugduni Batavorum, 1707.

† Recherches de la vraie anatomie des dents, nature et propriètè d'icelles. Lyon, 1582.

(*a*) Mem. de l'Acad. des Sciences, an. 1689. (*b*) Do. do. do. an. 1699.

two learned men.(*c*) Albinus(*d*) described with the utmost exactness the production and appearance of the teeth, examined the follicles which contained them, and explained the wrong positions to which they are subject when they make their appearance. Haller,(*e*) Fauchard,(*f*) Jourdain,(*g*) have observed with much attention the progress of different dentitions. Lassonne(*h*) and Herissant,(*i*) analyzed the teeth at different epochs, to discover their constituent parts, and the last has given a new explanation of the formation of the teeth. Betin(*j*) has treated also on the structure and production of these parts, and has observed several accidents which accompany their appearance; the greater part of anatomists and physiologists who have written since his time, have copied him, and the celebrated Albinus, without acknowledging themselves indebted to them for their profound knowledge.

Hunter pursued the course of these celebrated men, and has given a work which has been translated into Latin and French,(*k*) and Blake sustained at the University of Edinburg(*l*) a thesis upon the formation and structure of the teeth, &c.

(*c*) Exposition anatomique, page 43, in 4to.

(*d*) Annotationum Academicarum; liber secundus, cap. 1, page 3, in 4to. Leydæ, 1755.

(*e*) Elementa Physiologiæ corporis humani, lib. xviii. p. 19, tom. vi. in 4to. Bernæ, 1764.

(*f*) Le Chirugien Dentiste, ou traité des dents, tome 1, Paris, 1786.

(*g*) Essai sur la formation des dents.

(*h*) Mem. de l'Acad. des Sciences, an. 1752.

(*i*) Idem. do. an. 1754.

(*j*) Traitè dósteologie, tome 2, p. 238.

(*k*) Historiæ naturalis dentium humanorum.

(*l*) Disputatio de dentium formatione et structura in homine, etc. 1798.

SECTION I.

OF THE FORMATION OF THE TEMPORARY SET OF TEETH.*

When the fœtus has advanced so far in the organization of its different parts, as to take some determinate form or figure ; we may perceive a considerable progress in the preparatory steps for the formation of the teeth.

As soon as the ossific deposit commences in the cartilaginous part of the embryo, both jaws are filled with small membranous, and, in the anterior parts, we may perceive the rudiments of the alveolar processes.

In a fœtus of about four months, the jaw bones are distinctly formed ; but at this time they only consist of thin grooved bones, having a cavity, extending through their whole length.† In the under jaw, anteriorly, this cavity is narrower and deeper ; but, posteriorly, it becomes wider and more shallow. At this time, if the membranous parts be removed, small processes of bone may be perceived, shooting across from each side, which as the fœtus increases in growth, gradually acquire more distinctness, and at length form separate sockets for the teeth.

During the fœtal state, and also for some months after birth, the blood vessels and nerves belonging to the teeth, run along at the bottom of this cavity, immediately below the pulps of the teeth ; but afterwards, a distinct canal is formed, through which the principal vessels and nerves pass ; separate filaments being sent off to the several teeth.

* Fox, 1st to 5th page, first part.

† The description of what takes place in one jaw, will completely exhibit what concerns the formation of the teeth in both, therefore in order to avoid confusion, I shall refer to the under jaw only.

When the gum which covers the alveolar groove of a fœtus of the age above mentioned, is stript off from the bone, small processes or elongations from the inner surface of the gums may be distinctly perceived; these are the first appearances of the pulps from which the teeth are formed.

The alveolar processes soon become perfectly distinct; for, the bony partitions which divide the longitudinal cavity in the jaw, rise to the upper margin; and thus those membranous processes, now enlarged and become more evolved, begin to be contained in separate cells.

In a fœtus of about four months old, the rudiments of the teeth may be distinctly seen; upon examining those substances found in the jaws, they are seen to be soft or pulpy bodies, bearing a resemblance to the figure of the body of the tooth to be formed, and each of them is contained in a membrane proper to itself.

For sometime during the formation of the teeth, the alveoli grow much faster than the teeth themselves, which are consequently but loosely contained within them. At the time of birth, the alveolar processes have increased so much, that they almost enclose or cover the teeth; thus a firm support is given to the gums, and the infant is enabled to make considerable pressure in sucking, &c., without injury to the progress which is going on underneath.

The ossification of the teeth begins to take place very early; it is first visible upon the tips of the incisores. In a fœtus of about five or six months, ossification has commenced upon the pulps of the incisores and cuspidati, and on the points of the molares; this gradually advances and extends itself over the pulp, down to the neck of the tooth, from the cutting edges of the highest points, where it had first commenced.

At the time of birth, the bodies of ten teeth are distinctly formed in each jaw; these are the teeth designed to serve during the years of childhood, and are commonly called the temporary, shedding, or milk-teeth.

These temporary teeth, which constitute the first set, are twenty in number, and are divided into three classes, incisores, cuspidati, and molares, and the teeth on one side of the mouth, correspond in figure with those of the other, so that they are situated in pairs.

Besides these twenty teeth, there are in a very early stage of their formation, the rudiments of some other teeth, which are to form part of the permanent or adult set. After birth, as the ossification goes on, the teeth become too long to be contained within the alveolar cavity, they therefore begin to make pressure upon those parts which cover them; this produces the process of absorption, which proceeds with the enlargement of the tooth, first removing the membranes which enveloped the teeth, and afterwards the thick gum which covered them, this gradually becoming thinner and thinner, till at length the teeth are suffered to pass through.

There is considerable variety as to the precise time when the teeth begin to make their appearance. This frequently seems to depend upon the health and vigour of the child; for sometimes the first tooth comes as early as four or five months; while, on the contrary, in those of more delicate and weakly constitutions, no tooth makes its appearance until the child is ten or twelve months old; and it is not very uncommon for a child to be turned of fourteen months before any tooth appears.

SECTION II.

OF THE COMMENCEMENT AND FORMATION OF THE PERMANENT TEETH.*

Having now fully traced the temporary teeth from their origin to their perfect state, that I may be better understood, I shall follow nearly a similar plan, with respect to the permanent. I think it unnecessary to dwell on the ingenious hypotheses of Vesalius, Diemerbrock and others who supposed that the bodies of the permanent teeth were produced from the old roots of the temporary. Diemerbrock adduces in support of his doctrine an instance of the stag, who changes his horns every year, or year and a half, when as he supposed from their old roots, new horns arose; but a full account and refutation of these opinions may be seen in the works of the learned Albinus.† Fallopius supposed that a certain latent seed in the jaws produced a new range of teeth.‡ But Eustachius explained much more clearly what takes place, than any of his predecessors, and indeed, comes very near the truth, in the following words.|| "On dissecting a child immediately after birth, both jaws being laid open, the incisores, canini, and three grinders appeared, partly gelatinous, partly bony, of no small size, and completely surrounded by their sockets; but having carefully removed the incisores and canini, I observed a very thin interstice, scarcely converted into bone, which being removed with equal care, I discovered the like number of incisores,

* Blake, Essay on the Teeth in Man, page 26 to 27.

† Acad. Anat. lib. 11, page 3.

‡ Observat. Anatom.

|| Opuscul. de Dentil, page 46.

and canini, almost gelatinous and of a smaller size, which lying behind the former ones, and in their proper cavities, were placed directly opposite to one another. I confess I did not see any trace of the grinders and jaw teeth which appear about the seventh year, and often much later."

Urbain Hemard, an ingenious French anatomist, makes use of nearly the same words, when treating on this subject.* "He had dissected in presence of his friends, capable of understanding this demonstration, several infants three or four days old, others just born; he says that the incisores, the canini and some molares on each side of the jaws, were in part bony, and in part mucilaginous, of middling size, and surrounded by their little cases or sockets; that after having removed the first incisores and canine teeth, he observed a bony partition; and that after having likewise removed this, he met under it, as many new incisores and canine teeth, as there were of the first, almost entirely mucilaginous. But as to the great molares, which at seven or eight years old, or a long time after, begin to appear through the gum, he confesses, he never found any trace or beginning of them." It appears that Urbain Hemard was not acquainted with Eustachius's work, so that he is entitled to an equal share of merit; and although the celebrated Albinus confirms the description of these parts, as related by Eustachius, yet Dr. Nesbitt thought them imaginary and says,† "There is not at birth, as Eustachius imagined, the least appearance that I could ever find of the layer or row of teeth, by which the first is afterwards usually thrust out." Since so great an anatomist as Dr. Nesbitt did not credit the demonstrations of Eustachius, though supported as I have already

---

* Fauchard Chirugien Dentiste, page 37, &c.

† Hum. Osteogony, page 98.

mentioned by Albinus, because similar appearances did not occur to him, and finding such an imperfect description of their origin in Mr. Hunter's work; I have dissected a great number of infants to ascertain this point, which I think of the greatest importance.

I have already mentioned that in the youngest fœtus I examined, I observed the rudiments of the four anterior permanent grinders, though I could not discover the slightest appearance of any of the other permanent teeth. But in a fœtus about the eight month, I found the commencement of the sacs of the incisores and cuspidati; they were not placed under the temporary teeth, nor indeed so deep in the jaw, but within side of them, that is to say, in contact with their inner surface, lying between that and the internal plate of the alveolar process, and as Albinus remarks, they were contained in the same sockets with the temporary. In a fœtus between the eighth and ninth months, these sacs were all perfectly distinct, and the pulps of the middle incisores were tolerably advanced, they were elongated a little in the sockets, and the jaws happened to be so far advanced, that the upper surface of the sockets of the middle permanent incisores were ossified, the lower part remaining still membranous; the other sockets were less perfect, and exactly in that state as described by the accurate Eustachius. In children somewhat farther advanced, I found them nearly as Hemard mentions, and I confess I did not observe in such young subjects the slightest vestige of those that succeed the temporary grinders, or any appearance of the middle permanent ones.

Having fully shewn that the assertions of Eustachius, Hemard and Albinus are true, I come now to treat more at large, of the relative situation and connexion of the rudiments of the permanent with the temporary teeth, which have been hitherto unaccountably overlooked. By the writings of those great men we are informed, that a certain number of the permanent teeth begin to be formed previous to birth, but we are still perfectly ignorant respecting the manner of their formation or connexion; and have nothing to guide us but imaginary conjectures, respecting the teeth which appear at a more advanced period of life. I think it unnecessary to say any thing on the hypothetical suppositions of Hippocrates, Fallopius, Eustachius, &c. but will dwell on the facts which I have discovered, and which I mentioned to a few celebrated anatomists, five years since in London.

When the rudiments of the temporary teeth are tolerably advanced, the internal part of the gum, or rather the upper part of each membrane destined to form one of the temporary teeth, sends off a new sac. These sacs, situated as just now described, are each at first contained in the socket of the one to which it is to succeed; and are so intimately connected with the membranes of the temporary teeth, that they cannot be separated without tearing one or both, and may be torn along with the first sacs out of the sockets. This circumstance might have misled Dr. Nesbitt, but it is strange he did not observe the commencement of the permanent sockets, which are very evident in every subject I examined, just before or at birth. These sacs were observed by the ingenious Mr. Hunter, for he says,* "There is another pulpy substance opposite to that which we have described; it adheres to the inside of the capsula, where the gum is joined to it, and its opposite surface lies in contact with the basis of the above described pulp, and afterwards

* Nat. Hist. pages 94 and 95.

with the new formed basis of the tooth; whatever eminences or cavities the one has, the other has the same, but reversed, so that they are moulded exactly to each other.

"In the incisores it lies in contact not with the sharper cutting edge of the pulp, or tooth, but against the hollowed inside of the tooth; and in the molares it is placed directly against their base, like a tooth of the opposite jaw. It is thinner than the other pulp, and decreases in proportion as the teeth advance. It does not seem to be very vascular. The best time for examining it is in a fœtus of seven or eight months old.

"The enamel appears to be secreted from the pulp above described, and perhaps from the capsula which encloses the body of the tooth. That it is from the pulp and capsula, seems evident in the horse, ass, ox, sheep, &c. therefore we have little reason to doubt of it in the human species."

Now whether we are to understand, by the words "the pulp above described," that which he speaks of as connected to the membrane of the first pulp, or the first pulp itself, he has left us quite at a loss to determine. At all events with the nature, use, and formation of this second pulp he seems to be utterly unacquainted; for he first leaves us, as beforesaid, in doubt, whether its use be to form the cortes striatus of the first teeth, a thing next to impossible; and again he says, that in proportion as the teeth advance, it becomes thinner, which is actually the very reverse of what really happens. I need hardly add, that there are no such pulps as he describes to be found on the bases of the temporary grinders, (another inaccurracy which he has strangely fallen into,) but merely a thickening of their proper membranes.

As the sacs of the permanent teeth advance, the sockets of the temporary ones become enlarged, and little niches are formed in the internal plate of the alveolar processes answering to each socket, which are situated rather laterally, that is to say, at a greater distance from the symphysis of the jaw, than the centre of each respective temporary socket. These niches do not penetrate so deep as to the bottom of the temporary sockets, but increase in proportion with the size of the permanent sacs, and gradually form a distinct socket round each of them. There is, however, an opening left immediately under the gum, through which the membranes of both sets of teeth continue to be connected. The pulps of the incisores in general are so far advanced at birth, that soon after ossification commences on them. In a child about six or seven months old, I found their shells much more advanced than, a priori, I could have expected, and those of the cuspidati also had begun to ossify. The sacs of the bicuspides which succeed the anterior grinders had appeared, yet I did not remark those which were to succeed the posterior grinders, although those of the middle permanent grinders had already commenced.

In a child about four years old, the bodies of some of the permanent teeth were very much advanced, ossification had commenced on the bicuspides, all the points of ossification of the middle grinders were united, and the membranes of the posterior grinders or wisdom-teeth were forming. I have examined a number of children's jaws about this age, and found in general a similarity of appearance with respect to the number of teeth which were then formed, and also those which were forming. So that I may safely say there are more teeth formed and forming at this, than at any other period of life, that is twenty-six teeth, in each jaw.

Soon after the sacs of the permanent teeth have commenced, a very curious and beautiful process takes place, for they retain their situation at the bottom of the jaws, whilst at the same time, the temporary teeth rise and appear through the gum. The alveolar processes become enlarged, or seem to rise in proportion to the elongation of the roots of the temporary teeth. The situation as well as connexion of both sets of teeth, can be easily understood from the representations, &c. Albinus was perfectly acquainted with the foramina through which the connecting membranes passed, and concerning which he makes use of the following words. "The sockets in which the permanent incisores are contained, extend to the margin of the jaw; not far from it gradually becoming more contracted, and at length terminating in a small hole: the hole which belongs to the socket of the first incisor, is placed behind the first of the deciduous incisores, in the interval between it and the second; that which belongs to the second, in like manner is placed behind the second of the deciduous incisores, in the interval between it and the canine tooth. The socket of the new canine tooth, extending only a little beyond the bottom of the socket, in which the deciduous canine tooth is contained, thence terminating in a narrow little canal, before it terminates in this canal, it gradually becomes more contracted. The sockets of the new jaw teeth, (the bicuspides) do not extend by any hole to the margin of the jaw. I find these penetrate into the bottom of the deciduous sockets, and first indeed into the internal part of its roots."* Nothing can be more accurate than this description, but it has been taken from dried jaws, otherwise he certainly would have discovered the connecting membranes.

We have seen the membrane of the posterior temporary grinder, and that of the anterior permanent grinder intimately connected together and contained in the same socket, but

---

* Acad. Annotat. lib. 11, pages 13, 14 and 15.

as the permanent grinder advances and the jaw increases in length, a process is sent backwards from the upper part of its membrane, which at first is contained in the same socket. This process gradually swells into a sac, in which is contained the pulp, whence the middle grinder is to be formed; and as ossification advances, the parts become separated by a bony partition: the connection however is still kept up. When the membrane of the middle grinder is tolerably advanced, it sends off a process in a similar manner, to form the sac of the posterior grinder or wisdom-tooth.

I think it absolutely necessary to point out in this place some of the very great oversights and anatomical errors of Mr. John Hunter; as his highly respected authority has frequently misled the inexperienced practitioner: he says,* "The pulp of the first adult incisor, and of the first adult molaris, begin to appear in a fœtus of seven or eight months; and five or six months after birth the ossification begins in them; soon after birth the pulp of the second incisor and cuspidatus begin to be formed, and about eight or nine months afterwards they begin to ossify; about the fifth or sixth year the first bicuspis appears; about the sixth or seventh the second bicuspis, and the second molaris; and about the twelfth, the third molaris or dens sapientis." It is evident that this description is entirely theoretical; and not deduced from anatomical observation; for not a single point of it will agree with what I have already demonstrated. However, he has arranged his plates in such a manner as to make them correspond in some degree with his doctrine; for instance in Tab. ix. Fig. 6.† the teeth of a child six or seven months old are represented, some of the temporary incisores,

* Nat. Hist. pages 82 and 83.

† Nat. Hist.

were so far advanced as to have nearly cut the gum; the shells of the permanent incisores, cuspidati and anterior grinders were a little advanced, but the cuspidati had not commenced in the upper jaw, yet he says they are the teeth of a child eight or nine years of age. This error must surely be attributed to the printer.

But in plate x. Fig. 1. the teeth of a child he says of five or six years of age are represented, only the anterior bicuspides of the upper jaw had commenced, the middle grinders had not. In the same plate, Fig. 2, the teeth of one side of both jaws of a child of seven years of age are represented; all the succeeding teeth had commenced, but even at this period the middle permanent grinders had not. He mentions this as "an age in which there are more teeth formed and forming than at any other time of life," though the entire number by his calculation amount to but forty four. When I come to treat on the shedding of the temporary teeth, we shall find that some of the permanent incisores appear through the gum before seven years; or that the roots of some of the temporary teeth, instead of being perfect as Mr. Hunter has represented them, are entirely wasted. Again in plate xi. fig. 2, similar mistakes have been committed; for he says, in a youth about eleven or twelve years old, the first two molares of the second set, were so much advanced that they had cut the gums. Now these teeth in general appear about the sixth or seventh year; and in the same plate he represents the bodies of the middle and posterior grinders only as slightly formed.

It is unnecessary to recapitulate what I have demonstrated in the beginning of this chapter. Indeed it appears as an established law of nature, that there should be more teeth formed and forming at four or five years of age, than at any period of life, that is, in all fifty two. Yet Mr. Hunter has represented at seven years only forty four, and at nine years forty eight, excepting that at the latter period the middle temporary incisores of the under jaw had been shed. Although I omitted saying any thing particularly respecting the formation of the permanent teeth, when treating of the ossification on the pulp of the temporary; I think however from the observations then made, a few words more will now suffice.

The incisores and cuspidati resemble their predecessors but are much larger, but those which succeed the temporary grinders differ very much from them, in size and shape, being about one third smaller. Ossification commences on them in general by two points, the shells formed round each of these gradually unite, and ossification goes on then for some time as in the incisores and cuspidati, until the greater part of the root is formed, which commonly divides in the upper jaw into two processes near the extremity. I have met sometimes two distinct roots proceeding from the neck; in the under jaw in general they have but one root. Now the grinders which they succeed have four or five points on their grinding surface, and in the upper jaw they have commonly three distinct roots; in the under jaw two. Nor, according to the celebrated Albinus, do they differ only in their number of points, but in their entire figure, by which we can readily distinguish one from the other. Although the accurate Eustachius remarks, those of the under jaw in general want the internal point, I think the term bicuspides, which Mr. Hunter has given, is sufficiently applicable, as it at once distinguishes them from the temporary grinders; on which account I retain it, particularly as it has been the term made use of in practice for some years since.

As to the permanent grinders, the anterior have each five points, the middle grinders four, sometimes five points, and the posterior or wisdom-teeth three or four. In other respects their formation is exactly similar to that of the temporary grinders, but they are much larger. In the under jaw they have in general two roots, in the upper three, but the posterior, though they have sometimes two, three, or even four distinct roots, seem most commonly to have but one.

SECTION III.

OF THE PULP, AND FORMATION OF THE BONY PART OF A TOOTH.*

The pulp seems intended for a purpose similar to that of the cartilaginous matter of the other bones, though the process of its ossification is conducted in a different manner. A tooth is formed from without inwards, the first part formed being the outermost layer, which is as large, and probably as perfect at first, as at any subsequent period of life. I allude here to that part only of the outermost layer, on which the fibres of the cortex striatus are afterwards to be arranged.

Ossification commences on the highest or most prominent point of what is afterwards to be the cutting edge or grinding surface of the tooth; as also, on as many points as there are eminences on the pulp. The bony matter being first deposited on these points, it necessarily becomes hollowed towards the pulp, and gradually augmenting, at length forms over it small elastic shells.

On the incisores and cuspidati, whose formation is more

---

* Blake, Essay on the Teeth, in Man, Pages 5 to 15.

simple than that of the others, there is in general only one shell formed, but on the grinders several of them appear. On the anterior or small grinders, there are four shells formed, sometimes however but two. On the posterior or large grinders there are in general five shells, of which, in the under jaw, three are placed externally or next the cheek, and two internally. In the upper jaw, they are so situated that their eminences are adapted to the hollows of the opposite teeth in the under jaw. As ossification advances, the bases of these shells come in contact, and at length unite, so as to form one shell, after which ossification proceeds for some time, as in the incisores and cuspidati, gradually extending over the greater part of the pulp; and when so far advanced as to form the body of the tooth, it begins to contract from without, thus shaping the neck, from which the root or roots are to commence.

As the bone of the tooth increases in thickness, the pulp is proportionally diminished, and seems as it were converted into bone; its connexion however with the bony part is very slight, except at its extreme elastic edge, so that when the membrane surrounding the tooth is cut open, the shell can be taken from off the pulp, without any apparent violence; indeed without altering the shape of the pulp, or scarcely its connexion with the vessels. When the shell is removed, the pulp appears covered with a very delicate membrane, on which the vessels form a net-work. This seems to be a propagation of the periosteum which enters the cavity of the jaw, along with the vessels, and probably from whence are derived the bony lamellæ of which a tooth consists. Though this membrane is so slightly connected with the internal part of the shell, I cannot think Mr. Hunter's assertion warrantable, when he says, "nor are there any vessels going from the one to the other.* He might as well have denied the existence of vessels in the crystaline lens; as it more readily slips out of its capsula, than this pulp from its shell.

As the pulp has originally no process answering to the root or roots, it has been supposed that it is lengthened, or squeezed out so as to form them, according as the cavity in the body of the tooth is filled up by the ossification.† I have already mentioned that the pulp at first assumes little more than the size of the upper part of the body of the tooth, which is to be afterwards formed upon it; but it is deposited and extends in proportion, as ossification advances. It is the pulp and its vessels which give a determinate shape and size to the body of the tooth, and it will in its proper place be shown that its processes determined the size and shape of the roots. How it is possible that the simple filling up of the cavity in the shell of a grinder, could occasion the pulp to lengthen out into two, three, and sometimes four roots?

Of those teeth which are to have but one root, the pulp increases in length as I have described, becoming more and more contracted towards the point; and as ossification advances, the bone forms on it a kind of conical tube. But, in those teeth which are to have more than one root, a beautiful process is carried on. In the grinders of the lower jaw, which in general have but two roots, the pulp is divided into so many processes a little below the neck: at this period there is but one general opening in the shell, from the opposite sides of the edge of which, osseous fibres or little bars shoot across, through the division of the pulp; these meet and unite in the middle, and so divide the cavity of the shell into two openings, forming over it a little arch. In the grind-

---

* Nat. Hist. page 89. † Nat. Hist. page 90.

ers of the upper jaw, which have in general three roots, the pulp is divided into as many processes, and the osseous bars shooting through them, from as many different points in the margin of the shell, and uniting in the middle, divide the cavity into three openings, two of which are placed externally, and one internally. Sometimes an osseous point is deposited in the centre of these processes, and fibres shooting across from the margin of the shell join it, which answers the same purpose.* From these openings, the processes of the pulp commonly become more and more divergent and ossification extending on them forms a conical or flatted tube on each, as in teeth which have but single roots. Sometimes the pulp is divided at the neck only into two processes ; ossification goes on for some time as usual, but one tooth or both of these become divided again, and so three or four roots are formed. I have met a few of the permanent grinders, in which the pulp did not divide into processes, so that only one root was formed. The pulp continues to advance faster than the ossification, until each process has acquired its proper length and shape ; then the pulp except where the vessels and nerves enter, becomes entirely surrounded with bone.

Mr. Hunter mentions,† " by the observations which I have made in unravelling the texture of the teeth when softened by an acid, and from observing the disposition of the red parts in the tooth of growing animals, interruptedly fed with madder, I find that the bony part of a tooth is formed of lamellæ, placed one within another. The outer lamella is the first formed, and is the shortest : the more internal lamellæ lengthen gradually towards the fang, by which means in

---

* Albin. Acad. Annot. Lib II. P. 17.

† Nat. Hist. page 92.

proportion as the tooth grows longer, its cavity grows smaller, and its sides grow thicker." Now, from my observations, the fact is directly the reverse; the outer lamella, which is the first formed is longest, the internal lamellæ become shorter and shorter, and the last formed is the shortest. Hence in teeth with single roots, the cavity of the shell is not only diminished, but it recedes from the apex or cutting edge of the tooth, whilst a conical tube is left for the admission of vessels, &c. the base of which ending in the body of the tooth, has its opening or point nearly in the extremity of the root. The lamellæ of a grinder, are distributed more irregularly than those of any other tooth, on account of the protuberances of its pulp. As its external lamella advances very slowly, a great number of the internal ones are advancing, at the time that the external lamella has got so far as to form the neck. So that the cavity of a grinder recedes from the grinding surface, more rapidly than that of any other tooth. After the roots commence, the cavity is soon diminished, the ossification going on at the same time at both the upper and under parts of it. As many conical or flatted tubes are left leading to the cavity, as there are roots; and as many hollows or depressions in the superior part of the cavity, as there are protuberances on the grinding surface. The pulp, though very much diminished, still retains nearly its original shape.

It may appear singular, that the pulp should not be entirely obliterated, and the ossification completed, without any remaining cavity; it however affords this advantage, that the vessels and nerves distributed on the soft membrane of the pulp may have free action and not be compressed; by which means the internal bony part of the tooth may be more readily nourished.

It is asserted by a celebrated anatomist that he has constantly found two holes near the point of each root, for the admission of vessels, not only of the incisores and cuspidati, but also of those of the grinders; which he supposes to have been established by nature, in order to guard against accident, lest if one vessel were injured or destroyed, the other might continue to nourish the pulp. I confess I was never so fortunate as to meet a single instance of this kind, even in the incisores of large animals; except in such cases as Eustachius mentions, where he says, (speaking of the roots of the permanent grinders,) " Many of these roots (s. c. roots,) being flattened, their sides thus approach; so that, instead of a circular opening, an oblong one is formed, the central points of whose sides coming into contact, leave at either end a small canal." In such roots, however, I have frequently found but one opening externally, for the admission of vessels, &c. but after their entrance each divided into two branches. Haver mentions, * that in a tooth which had but one root, he met two passages, one at each side. This must have been formed in the manner Eustachius describes. I have seen a few of the permanent incisores with almost two distinct roots, the cuspidati with two, sometimes with three roots, and the grinders with four and even five roots, and of course as many openings as roots.

---

* Ostreologia, page 79.

SECTION IV.

OF THE GRADUAL WASTE OF THE MEMBRANE WHICH SURROUNDS THE BODY OF A TOOTH, AND THE PERIOD AT WHICH THE TEMPORARY TEETH IN GENERAL APPEAR.*

The membrane which deposits the earthy matter of the cortex striatus, does not adhere to, but closely surrounds the body of the tooth; but as soon as the neck is formed, the margin of the membrane adheres to it so firmly at that part, that it cannot be separated from it, without lacerating several vessels which pass from it to the bone. The membrane becomes much thinner at this part, and I could not separate it at any period into two lamellæ.

As ossification advances on the root or roots, the body of the tooth rises in the socket, and of course the investing membrane rises with it. The cortex striatus is first perfected or crystalized on the cutting edges or protuberances of the tooth, and proceeds gradually from thence to the neck where it terminates; and in proportion as the first part of the cortex striatus is crystalized, that portion of the membrane which formed it becomes thinner, less vascular, and at length, having performed the particular function for which it was designed, is totally wasted or absorbed. The gums also partake of this tendency to waste, and the tooth gradually appears through it; part of the membrane still remains on the body of the tooth, this however is wasted as the cortex striatus covered by it, attains to perfection. So that all that portion of the membrane, which loosely surrounded the

---

* Blake, pages 16 to 26.

body of the tooth, is destroyed, when the tooth has risen to its proper height.

De La Sonne,* and other physiologists, attempt to assign a cause why the teeth rise and pass through the gum, by saying that as roots are added, the bodies of the teeth are pushed or forced up through the gum, this being softer than the bottom of the sockets. But when we come to consider the appearance of the permanent teeth, we shall be fully sensible how inadequate such a theory is.

It has been mentioned by most authors, who have written on dentition, that the membrane which surrounds the body of a tooth is stretched, bruised, and even lacerated by the increased size of the tooth. Dr. Underwood supposes it to be strong and nervous, and adds, "The most painful part of dentition, and that in which children are most exposed to convulsions, is usually from the teeth cutting through the periosteum, (or nervous membrane mentioned above,) that covers the teeth." Van Swieten although he did not believe the temporary teeth had roots, says, "These rudiments of the teeth are placed in the sockets of the jaws; but the opening from each of these sockets, is covered by a thick coriaceous membrane, which must be bruised, or even torn by the tooth in bursting out, so that after the tooth had burst out, the ragged edges of this membrane have been observed by the accurate Herissant. These edges becoming dry fall away spontaneously. Therefore the tooth in endeavouring to make its way out, must exert a considerable force in order to break through this membrane."†

It appears rather strange that Van Swieten could imagine that the temporary teeth, which in another part of his work,

* Acad des Scien, in 4to. L'an. 1752. Mem. p, 168.

† Comment. Vol. xiv. page 743.

he observes have no roots, could perform all these violent efforts, so as to burst through this membrane. Even Mr. Hunter says,* "When the tooth cuts the gum, this membrane or capsula is likewise perforated, after which it begins to waste." Others are of opinion, that the membrane being lacerated, the body of the tooth passes up through it, and that it afterwards becomes the periosteum of the root. From what I have already said, the impossibility of a tooth bursting or rising through its membrane will be readily perceived, for as it is firmly united to the neck of the tooth, it must take of the same precise motion with the tooth, and therefore must, after such motion of the tooth, retain the same relative position towards it as before. So that the disappearance of the membrane is not owing to a rupture of it, but to a wasting or absorption of it, in proportion as it has perfected the cortex striatus.

This fact will be more fully explained, when we come to speak of the teeth of animals in general. I have seen the ragged edges of the membrane, appearing above the level of the gum; a similar appearance was no doubt observed by Herissant, though he attributed it to a wrong cause.

Galen, Eustachius, and others, were of opinion that the upper teeth appeared sooner than the under; they were fully aware, however, that they appear irregularly and at different periods. Mr. Hunter describes their appearance in the following words.† "The incisores begin to cut or pass through the gums; first, generally, in the lower jaw; but the cuspidatus and molares of the fœtus, are not formed so fast as the incisores; they generally all appear nearly about the same time, viz. about the twentieth or twenty-fourth month;

* Natural History, page 87. † Natural History, page 78.

however, the first grinder is often more advanced within the socket than the cuspidatus, and most commonly appears before it." Chirurgical writers in general, give us a most curious jumble, respecting the appearance during dentition; and most of the strenuous advocates for cutting and hacking the gums of children, seem perfectly ignorant of the order in which the teeth appear. Dr. Underwood says, "The two front teeth in the lower jaw are usually cut the first, and it is commonly a few weeks longer, before the corresponding ones in the upper jaw make their appearance. After which it is frequently a considerable time before the next under teeth come out; but sometimes, though not often, six or eight are cut in a hasty succession. Children sometimes cut their teeth irregularly, or cross, as it is called, both by the teeth appearing first in the upper jaw, and also at a distance, instead of being contiguous to each other: this is accounted, and with some reason, an indication of painful or difficult dentition." It is unnecessary at present, to enter more fully into the inaccuracies of these authors, or to say any thing respecting their operations, (which are blindly, and I may say, very often rashly performed, for want of anatomical knowledge of these parts,) as I intend to enlarge considerably on this subject, when I come to treat on dentition.

As ossification does not commence on all the pulps at the same time, in general those on which it first commenced are soonest perfect, and of course they appear through the gum first. I have observed on examining the teeth of a number of children, that the bodies of the middle incisores of both jaws were most perfect; the lateral incisores and the small grinders next, and the cuspidati and small grinders least perfect. In general the teeth begin to appear about the sixth, seventh, or eight month after birth; but there are some exceptions to this rule, owing to the rapid progress of ossification in some children, and the slowness of it in others. There are a few instances of children at birth having one or two of the incisorés already cut, and in such cases it is often necessary to remove them immediately; on the contrary, in children apparently healthy, they have not begun to appear till the first, second, or even the third year. They for the most part appear in pairs, or the two corresponding with each other, nearly at the same time. The first are the middle incisores of the under jaw; in a few weeks after the middle incisores of the upper; in a month or six weeks after, we have reason to expect the lateral incisores of the under jaw, and in a short time after those of the upper; about the twelfth or fourteenth month, the anterior or small grinders of the under jaw appear, and frequently about the same time those of the upper; about the sixteenth or twentieth month the cuspidati appear first in the lower jaw, and from the twentieth to the thirtieth month the posterior or large grinders appear in the same order: so that in general about the second or third year, the twenty temporary teeth are complete. We must not expect however to find the teeth always appear in the precise order I have just now mentioned. I have frequently met with some irregularities, such as one tooth appearing a considerable time before its fellow; all the incisores of the under jaw appearing before any of the upper; and the reverse, though very seldom, has sometimes taken place: the anterior grinders sometimes appear sooner than the lateral incisores, and the lateral incisores of the upper jaw, sooner than those of the under. I have sometimes observed the posterior grinders appear earlier than the cuspidati; but I never saw an instance of the cuspidati appearing previous to the small grinders; sometimes three or four teeth appear nearly at the same period, but I never met an instance of the cuspidati and grinders appearing in such rapid succession as Mr. Hunter and Dr. Underwood mention. Dr. Armstrong says * that he met with two cases, where the small grinders appeared first of all; I have lately met a similar case; however, by carefully examining the gums of a child, we can seldom mistake what tooth is about to appear, as the gum is frequently somewhat higher over it, than elsewhere, or it becomes so thin, that through it the shape of the tooth can be perceived.

SECTION V.

OF THE SHEDDING OF THE TEMPORARY TEETH AND OF THE PERIOD AT WHICH THE PERMANENT TEETH APPEAR.†

We meet with such strange opinions in the works of a celebrated author, (Van Swieten,) respecting the temporary teeth, that I think it worth while to insert some extracts from them: He says, "I have taken out and examined several of the first teeth when they begin to loosen, and in most of them I did not observe the slightest appearance of a root. This surprised many surgeons, who, in the treatment of disorders of the teeth, were esteemed exceedingly skilful. They were of opinion that the teeth which are usually shed about the seventh year have had roots, but when they took out those that were already loose they found no roots. To account for this, they said that the second tooth while it rises, rubs away the roots of the first and so reduces them to the most minute powder, which, being so very fine, en-

---

* Diseases of Children, page 82.

† Blake. Essay on the Teeth, &c. pages 55 to 70.

tirely disappears, for no body could ever perceive it. But could the action of the second tooth, gently rising, whilst it moves the first out of its place, be so great as to reduce the roots of them to powder? Bourdet, celebrated for his skill in this branch of surgery, asserts, that the first teeth before they loosen, have roots nearly as strong and hard, as the second are observed to have. And whilst he refutes the opinion of Bunon, who supposed the roots of the first were destroyed by the friction of the second teeth when rising, he refers to those which are found in the jaws of fresh subjects, at that period when the second teeth are forming, and the first (called milk-teeth) are still in their sockets; whether they are still firm, or are more or less loose; for it seems that the second tooth whilst it rises, remains enclosed in its proper membrane, until it is about to appear. Therefore a membrane is interposed between the roots of the milk-tooth and the second tooth. However the roots of the milk-teeth are destroyed before the second tooth can touch them. Besides a small space is observed between the first and second teeth, from whence Bourdet concludes, that the roots of the milk-teeth are destroyed by some other cause, and not by the friction of the succeeding teeth. He therefore thought that some acrid humour was secreted from the neighbouring parts, which might consume their roots. I confess it appears to me much more probable that the milk-teeth are without roots. Nevertheless some observations seem to show that the milk-teeth, if they are not shed, at the proper period, or, when loose are not taken out, are capable of protruding roots from their body, by means of which they often remain fixed in the jaws through life."*

---

* Comment. Vol. xiv. page 743, &c.

It is almost superfluous to mention that the temporary teeth have as perfectly formed roots as the permanent, indeed as far as I recollect, Van Swieten is the only person who at all doubted the fact.

Mr. Hunter ingeniously observes, * "that the first set of teeth are pushed out by the second; this, however is very far from being the case: and were it so, it would be attended with a very obvious inconvenience; for were a tooth pushed out by one underneath, that tooth must rise in proportion to the growth of the succeeding one, and stand in the same proportion above the rest." Mr. Hunter, however, does not seem to be acquainted with the writings of the very accurate Albinus; if he were, he would be induced to give a very different description of what takes place, with respect to the wasting of the roots of the temporary teeth and the appearance of the permanent, as will appear from the following quotations. Mr. Hunter says, † "it would be very natural to suppose that this wasting was owing to a constant pressure from the rising teeth against the fangs or sockets of the first set: but it is not so, for the new alveoli rise with the new teeth, and the old alveoli decay in proportion as the fangs of the old teeth decay, and when the first set falls out, the succeeding teeth are so far from having destroyed, by their pressure, the parts against which they might be supposed to push, that they are still enclosed, and covered by a complete bony socket. From this we see that the change is not produced by a mechanical pressure, but is a particular process in the animal economy." And page 100 he makes use of the following words, "when the incisores and cuspidati of the new set are a little advanced, but long before they appear through their bony sockets, there

---

* Nat. Hist. page 98. † Nat. Hist. pages 98 and 99.

are small holes leading to them on the inside, or behind the temporary sockets and teeth, and these holes grow larger and larger, till at last the body of the tooth passes quite through them. Mr. Hunter supports this theory still farther in page 90 &c. " As the body of the tooth is pushed out, the socket at the same time contracts at its bottom, and grasps the neck, or beginning fang, adheres to it, and rises with it, which contraction is continued through the whole length of the socket as the fang rises; or the socket which contained the body of the tooth, being too large for the fang, is wasted, or absorbed into the constitution, and a new alveolar portion is raised with the fang." The observations of the ingenious Mr. Hunter are however entirely hypothetical and do not accord with anatomical truth; indeed they entirely overturn some of his former opinions. For if, as he affirms, the permanent teeth were formed at the internal part of the jaw and in a new series of alveolar processes, it is evident that they must necessarily be placed in a smaller circle than the temporary teeth. As if the processes and sockets of the temporary teeth, as Mr. Hunter asserts, were absorbed or totally destroyed, the permanent sockets should extend to the anterior part of the jaw, accommodate themselves to the teeth, and thus form a segment of a larger circle.

Albinus however comes very near the truth, for when speaking of the holes by which the connexion between the membranes of the permanent and temporary teeth were preserved, he says, " as the new teeth increase, the contracted part of the sockets is gradually dilated, and afterwards in like manner the little opening, and thus they appear. But if previous to the formation of the new teeth, the temporary had fallen out, or were loosened in consequence of their roots being wasted, then the socket of the temporary tooth is gradually destroyed, while that of the other being dilated anteriorly, the new tooth passes into its place, so that the root of the new tooth is contained in a socket formed partly of that in which it was before, and partly of the socket which belonged to the temporary tooth. But if contrary to what commonly happens, the tooth which ought to be shed, is not shed, then the permanent tooth appears behind it, and remains similar to it fixed in its own appropriate socket."*

Had Albinus been acquainted with the use of the small holes leading to the permanent teeth, he would immediately have discovered what usually takes place.

I have already shewn that the temporary and permanent teeth were about the fourth year separated from each other by a bony partition, each root being at this period contained in a distinct socket. Now according as the permanent teeth rise, they have a natural tendency to come more and more to the anterior part of the jaw; whilst in consequence of the pressing forward of the rising tooth, a change is induced in the mode of action of the surrounding vessels, such, that that portion of the bony partition immediately pressed upon, as well as the root of the temporary tooth, with the adjacent parts, become fit to be absorbed, and actually are absorbed.

In some cases part of the roots of the neighbouring temporary teeth are absorbed, particularly where the jaw does not increase as rapidly as the permanent teeth. So that in proportion as this absorption takes place, the permanent tooth passes partly into the socket of the temporary tooth proper to it, and partly into the sockets of the neighbouring temporary teeth. And as Albinus justly remarks, a socket is formed for the reception of the root of the new tooth, in part by its own appropriate socket, and in part by the temporary socket of the tooth with which it was originally con-

* Acad. Annat. lib. II. pages 14 and 15.

nected, and sometimes in part by the neighbouring temporary sockets. When the permanent teeth pass into the cavities which surrounded their membranes, they are always very irregular, and appear as Albinus remarks at the inside of the temporary teeth, which frequently remain in their situations. This irregularity however is seldom the case, unless where the temporary teeth retain their roots, and resist the influence of the permanent. In some cases they appear more internally than the cavities through which the connecting membranes passed. It is worth remarking that when the temporary teeth fall out, if we examine their bodies, we find them quite excavated, and the bony part reduced nearly to its former pulpy state.

Mr. Hunter, in support of his theory, has represented the wasting of the roots of the temporary teeth, as it were, proceeding from the point gradually upwards to the neck.* This, however, is seldom or never the case, for the part first affected is considerably above the point; how this takes place will be easily understood by viewing plate ii. fig. 5, and plate iv. figs. 26, 27, and 28. This circumstance Albinus was fully aware of, and has given drawings to illustrate it.†

With respect to the appearance of the permanent teeth, Dr. H., in a letter he wrote to me at Edinburg, judiciously remarks, "the time of shedding is very various, happening a year or two, or three, earlier or later in some than others; and in many subjects some of them remaining to adult or even old age; and this is so common, that almost every day I meet with them from one to three or four, or double the number in the same person. I have seen two instances where scarcely any of them fell, and such I may affirm must

---

* Nat. Hist. plate xv. † Acad. Annat. lib. II. Tab 2.

have been those historic facts, handed down to us, of a third set appearing in the old age of heaven-favoured mortals where it could be nothing else than the then matured second set. Such I have met with, but never any thing like a third set, at least, which I was convinced was such." It appears from the foregoing observations, that the permanent teeth, whilst they are rising in the jaw, have considerable influence with respect to the wasting of the temporary roots; for while they are at rest, the roots of the temporary teeth are not wasted. However it does not appear to me, that the wasting of the temporary roots, is in any degree the effect of mechanical trituration, as Mr. Bunon and other authors would affirm.

In general, children begin to shed their teeth about six or seven years of age, and the permanent teeth appear nearly in the following order. First, the middle incisores of the under jaw, soon after, those of the upper; then the lateral incisores of the under jaw, and nearly at the same time the anterior grinders; then the lateral incisores of the upper jaw appear, though some time elapses between their appearance and that of the former: the anterior bicuspides appear about the ninth year, the posterior about the tenth or eleventh, and the cuspidati and middle grinders nearly at the same time, that is, about the twelfth or fourteenth year, and finally, the posterior grinders or wisdom-teeth from the sixteenth to the twenty-fifth year. Though Dr. H. remarks, there are many exceptions to this general rule, yet I do not think it necessary to dwell so much on the order or period of their appearance, as I have done with respect to the temporary.

The anterior permanent grinders frequently appear a considerable time before any of the temporary teeth are shed, and there are many varieties with respect to the wisdom-teeth, for in some cases they do not appear until a very late period of life; sometimes they appear in one jaw and not in the other, and sometimes it has been observed that in extreme old age they have not perforated the sockets. It is certainly a curious fact, how very long some of the permanent teeth remain within the jaws without appearing; and if there ever was a third set of teeth, it is sufficiently evident, that their rudiments must have been deposited, previous to the appearance of the second set through the gum.

In the preceding remarks of Dr. Blake I can readily concur as to their general application. With respect to the tardy appearance of the adult teeth it is an occurrence frequently observed. We often notice the retention of the infant teeth to the fifteenth, twentieth, twenty fifth and even thirtieth year. A lady aged about twenty seven called upon me last November, for the purpose of having some operations performed upon her teeth, and upon examining them I found she had never shed the infant molares, and as the permanent molares appear behind the infant molar teeth, if she had not have lost some of these last, her rows of teeth would have presented the novelty of twenty instead, as usual, of twelve molares. I am acquainted with a gentleman in whom one of the infant lateral incisores is retained, and as the permanent incisores have appeared and are perfect, he has five instead of four incisores. Great aberrations from what we have described as the usual order of nature are occasionally noticed in regard to the appearance, numbers, renewal of the teeth, &c.

Cases have been noticed when the teeth have been entirely wanting. Mr. Murphy observes,* "A few instances have occurred of persons who never had any teeth. One case was communicated to me by a lady on whose veracity I

* Page 48.

place the highest dependence. It is very well known to his numerous private friends, as well as to the gentlemen of the faculty in Lincoln, and its vicinity, that the late Mr. Bromhead of the above place never had any teeth." The bicuspides are often wanting as I have noticed in several instances. Duval observes—*"We read in the Ephémérides des Curieux de la Nature, that a magistrate and a surgeon of Frederick-stadt had never any teeth but the grinders, and were left entirely without the incisores and canine. But what appears very surprising is the fact of several persons having been totally destitute of teeth from their birth; several examples of which are given by authors. Boxelli reports in his Medical Centuries that a woman had never any teeth, who nevertheless lived to the age of sixty years, and M. Baumes knew an hussar, who had never cut a tooth. It may happen that some of the milk-teeth may never be cut, but only the secondary ones as I witnessed in 1790, in the son of a Russian nobleman. By an inverted order nature sometimes preserves the milk-teeth, and withholds the permanent ones; this observation is very important as it may tend to render us cautious in having the temporary teeth extracted, unless there be a necessity for it. In other cases nature is more prodigal and gives much more than the ordinary number, many such examples have been furnished by anatomists: these teeth which should be regarded as supernumerary are not always well formed nor well arranged as I have had occasion to observe: sometimes they are conical and are placed either betwixt the incisores or before or behind the spaces which separate these teeth, at other times they are regular and properly arranged; sometimes we find these supernumerary teeth on the outside of the large grinders:

---

* Dentiste Jeunesse, pages 56—57—58—59.

but to see two rows of teeth as in the son of Mithradatus or three as in Hercules, must excite our astonishment: perhaps we might be tempted to doubt these facts if in a collection of observations published at Brusland in 1772 and dedicated to the celebrated Haller Arnold had not reported that he had seen a child, aged fourteen years, who had seventy-two teeth, thirty-two for each jaw, which were healthy and well placed in two rows, except the front ones, which were slightly irregular. The number of the teeth is generally fixed but it is not exempt from those sports of nature which sometimes produce six fingers on each hand."

A highly respectable physician of New York, informed me that he had in his anatomical museum, the lower jaw of an adult negro, procured in the Southern States, in which were twenty-seven teeth. Whether this number arose from not having lost all the deciduous teeth it is difficult to say without a particular examination. A great many more instances of this kind might be adduced, but I deem it unnecessary.

In many instances the teeth are reported to have been renewed the third time but from the fact that the deciduous teeth may be retained for many years and after this the germs of the second be brought forward, the reports of third dentition have been generally considered as fabulous. However, I am rather persuaded that a third dentition may have taken place in some very rare cases. A highly respectable gentleman, and remarkable for probity of character, with whom I am well acquainted, has assured me that he has thrice renewed the front incisores of the upper jaw, the second set having been lost by accident. It is said by the celebrated Lord Francis Bacon,* that the Countess of Des-

* Retrospective Review.

mond with whom he was very intimate, and who died at the age of 140 years thrice changed her teeth. It is also said by Alexander Benedictus that there was a lady of his acquaintance, who at the age of fourscore years, had a complete new set of teeth.*

Mentzelius a German Physician assures us that he saw at Cleves an old man, aged 120 years who two years before had renewed his double teeth.† He likewise saw, at the Hague, an Englishman, who renewed a complete row of teeth at the age of 118 years.

I subjoin a case of this kind from the Dentiste Observateur by Coustois, and which bears every mark of authenticity.

‡. "A Lady aged from 50 to 52 years, had three artificial teeth in the upper jaw for the space of twelve years, and which I renewed from time to time. Some months after I had put in the last, she sent for me to show me that these teeth were neither so good, nor solid as they were accustomed to be. Not being able at once to comprehend why these teeth were so bad, I cut the wires by which they were attached to the neighhouring teeth. I searched to no purpose to discover the defects of the artificial piece. I at length turned my attention to the side of the jaw of this lady: In examining her gums, I perceived some slight eminences that inclined me to judge that they were the only obstacles which opposed the solidity of the artificial teeth. These eminences which I saw for the first time, made me examine it with much more attention. I found that two large incisors had nearly divided the gum: my surprise was still greater since

* Retrospective Review.

† Traite d'orotalgie par Pierre Auzébi Chirurgion Dentiste à Lyon, 1771, page 81.

‡ Le Dentiste Observateure, pages 198 to 200. Paris, 1775.

I did not know that the teeth of this lady had been renewed by a second germ, and had been privy to it only by accident. This lady, still more astonished than myself that at her age she should cut teeth, could not be convinced of the truth of what I told her, until her eyes persuaded her. These teeth grew up, but they were neither so long nor so strong as the others, they became in the mean time fast enough to preclude her any more from having artificial teeth."

Is it not astonishing that at so advanced an age, these two large incisors had neither the same strength, nor the same solidity which might be expected at 30 years or under; the nourishing liquid is not furnished so abundantly at this age as it is in youth. Besides the sanguineous vessels obliterate; from whence comes a less abundant nutrition and a defect on the part of nature, which appears to stop at the time when she operates at the formation of the different parts of which we are constituted."

Instances more recent may be mentioned. I am acquainted with an old lady resident in this city who renewed several teeth, after she was 50 years of age. The following instance is mentioned in one of our daily papers for August 19th, 1828. "It is stated that a Mrs. Galusha of Monmouth Maine now 88 years of age, has had, within the last three years, an entire set of new teeth, a new head of hair, and her sight, of which she had been for some time deprived has been so perfectly restored that she is now able to read the finest print without the aid of spectacles." *U. S. Gazette.*

In some cases a bony union is said to have taken place between the jaw and the fangs of the teeth, so that the alveoli and roots of the teeth, formed one inseparable bone: As has been reported in part of Pyrries king of Epyrus, and a son of the King of Bythinia. Courtois mentions a case of this kind which involved the teeth of both jaws and with which I close the present section, without any longer detaining the reader with a detail of anomalies with which, to say the least, we very rarely meet. Courtois observes;—

"My brother being at the Hotel-Dieu, where he lived in quality of Surgeon, furnished me with the following observations. 'A man of about thirty or thirty-five years of age being dead in the said Hospital, was brought to the Amphitheatre to undergo the different operations practised by M. Moreau, for the instruction of the young students of this house. This dead man having very fine teeth, my brother wished to extract them, particularly the incisors and canine which the dentists occasionally want. All his teeth broke off when cautiously seized hold of them by the pincers to draw them out of their sockets. The two jaws being stripped of all the flesh with which they were covered, were sawed through; and it was observed with much surprise that not a single trace of the alveolar partition nor any difference of the spongy substance could be distinguished, of which the maxillary bones, together with the substance of the roots of the teeth are so commonly composed. The bones of the jaw and teeth of this man were composed but of one substance; the germs of the teeth were so much confounded with the osseous juice of the maxillary bones, that it was impossible to recognise the least trace of the teeth in the alveolar region, whilst on the exterior the teeth were seen well formed and arranged in the most regular order.'" M. Petit a celebrated anatomist reports in his course of anatomy a similar case. I will ask a question rather than any other should ask of me. Had this man ever any milk-teeth? This problem as difficult as it appears to resolve, is in the mean while susceptible of some conjectures, it is very likely that in the subject of whom I speak, the teeth were cut but once only;

from whence the teeth of this man cannot be regarded as milk-teeth, since they never fell out, during dentition; the germs of the teeth were so much amalgamated and confounded with the osseous juice of the maxillary bones, that it made but one and the same body; it could not have been possible that a second germ, supposing that it existed, would have made its way through, and not been checked by the presence of a body as hard and as compact as the combination of the teeth with the maxillary bones.

I have omitted to mention many cases of endentula or toothlessness with which I have become acquainted, either by personal observation or the observation of my friends. I know one gentleman in whom the bicuspid teeth of the lower jaw, have never appeared. It is but a few days since a highly respectable lady of this city showed me the teeth of her daughter, a young lady of about eleven years of age, in whom the lateral incisores of the upper jaw had never appeared, and she informed me that this was the case with every member of her family. There is at present resident in Charleston, South Carolina, a family of whom several individuals have never had any teeth, and this has been remarked for several generations.

SECTION VI.

OF SUPERNUMERARY TEETH, &c.*

When we consider the formation of the teeth, and the contiguity and intimate connection subsisting between their ru-

---

† Blake. Essay on the Teeth in Man, pages 110 to 116.

diments, we cannot be surprised to meet with such frequent deformities and varieties as occur amongst them. Though deviations in the shape or size of their bodies seldom occur, yet their roots vary considerably, some being much larger than those commonly met with, others curved in different directions, or exceeding their usual number.

Eustachius, Jussieux, Fauchard, and other writers, mention some instances remarkable for the singular position of the teeth in the jaws. They also speak of having met with a few cases where two or three of the front teeth, and as many even of the grinders, were completely joined together by ossification. I have met with more than a dozen cases somewhat similar for instance, the bodies and roots of the lateral temporary incisores and cuspidati joined together, and among the permanent teeth, the middle and lateral incisores, as also the lateral incisores and cuspidati. Here it is evident that both pulps must have been contained in the same investing membrane or sac, for their ossification is in general so complete, that one hole serves to both for the admission of vessels, &c. In those cases the body of each of the teeth so conjoined commonly retains its own appropriate form, though both are completely surrounded by the cortex striatus.

Among the permanent teeth however I have met with one instance, where one of the middle and lateral incisores were so intimately united, that on viewing them externally, they appeared as one large middle incisor, no trace being left of their having originally two distinct bodies; but on the internal surface there is a very marked difference, and each retained nearly its proper shape. Excrescences of the cortex striatus are very seldom met with; one singular instance of it occurred to me, in a patient about seventeen or eighteen years of age. The right permanent cuspidatus in this person did not appear through the gum until the sixteenth year, on the side of it next the lateral incisor there was a bulbous protuberance of the cortex striatus, with a hollow or depression in the middle; this protuberance did not, however, extend to the apex of the tooth. Between the bulbous part and the perfectly formed body of the tooth, there was also a deep groove, which perhaps retained part of the investing membrane longer than usual, or the external lamella of the membrane was not wasted, for there was a substance somewhat similar to the Crusta Petrosa of graminivorous animals deposited round the protuberance of the cortex striatus, and even on a considerable portion of the root. This substance stuck out and formed a sharp hook under the lip, which was very troublesome to the person, and as there was not sufficient room for the tooth in the arch of the jaw, it was of course advisable to have it removed. This is the only instance I have met with, or even heard of, where a Crusta Petrosa was deposited on a human tooth.

With respect to the uncommon situation of the teeth in the jaw, by far the most curious case is related by Albinus of an adult in whom he found "two teeth, one on each side of the nose, between it and the orbits of the eyes, enclosed in the roots of those processes, which extend from the maxillary bones to the eminence of the nose. They were long and remarkably thick, similar to the canine teeth, and seem to have been these very teeth which had not in this case appeared. But there were, besides these, other canine teeth, unusually small and short, placed in their proper sockets. The former seem therefore to have been the new canini which had not penetrated their sockets, on the contrary they were situated where the new ones usually are observed to be in children. But what is still more strange, the points of their bodies were turned towards the eyes, as if they had been the new canine teeth inverted, convex on the posterior part, concave on the anterior, the reverse of what generally happens." This case fully shews the great accuracy of Albinus: he did not mistake those singularly situated canini for supernumerary teeth though he was aware that such frequently occur.

Mr. Hunter mentions his having met with a case somewhat similar, and gives* "a sketch of the upper jaw of a child, where the cuspidatus was inverted, so that its point was turned up against the jaw, and the growing mouth of its cavity towards the gum."

Amongst the temporary teeth supernumerary ones are seldom observed. Dr. H. however has met with a few instances of this kind; they are much more frequently found amongst the permanent teeth, and especially in the upper jaw. Their shape in general resembles the cuspidati. He further observes, "They are not confined to the front of the mouth. I have found them in every part of the jaw, between the middle incisores, between the middle and lateral, between the lateral and cuspidati, &c., among the large grinders, on the outside or inside of them, and in the palate. I have also ten or twelve times found teeth beyond the dentes sapientiæ superiores. They were all small, the enamelled part shaped like the adult grinders, but never with more than one fang. I call them second wisdom-teeth, and always compliment my patient on the probability of possessing a double portion of sagacity."

How supernumerary teeth are formed we can easily conceive, but how teeth could be inverted as Albinus and Mr. Hunter have shewn, is much more difficult to be accounted for. I have sometimes observed a supernumerary tooth, firmly attached to a grinder; Fauchard has noticed similar

* Nat. Hist. explanat. of Tab. VIII. Fig. 9.

appearances and also mentioned his having met with two grinders joined together, and a supernumerary tooth likewise connected with them.* However I do not think it necessary to dwell on this subject, particularly as it is a subject of curiosity more than of importance.

Mr. James Gardette of this city has mentioned to me having seen and extracted a considerable number of supernumerary teeth, situated in different parts of the jaw. I have met with one instance of this kind; the tooth was situated on the outside of the dens sapientia, was small, round, and had but one fang. Mr. Gardette mentioned to me that he had seen complete and perfect supernumerary bicuspid teeth, situated in apposition to and on the inside of the natural and perfect bicuspids.

SECTION VII.

OF THE IRREGULARITY OF THE TEETH.†

During the shedding of the teeth there are several circumstances which prevent the permanent teeth from acquiring a regular position, and often give rise to very great irregularity in their arrangement.

The most frequent cause is a want of simultaneous action between the increase of the permanent teeth and the decrease of the temporary ones, by the absorption of their fangs. It rarely happens that so much of the fang of a temporary tooth is absorbed as to permit its removal by the efforts of the child, before the permanent tooth is ready to

---

* Tom. 11, Planche 27, Fig. 16.

† Fox, Part First, pages 45 to 51.

pass through: on which account the new tooth takes an improper direction, and generally comes through on the inside.

Cases are very frequent in which scarcely any absorption of the fangs of the temporary teeth have taken place, previous to the appearance of several of the permanent teeth; and it often happens, that upon the removal of the shedding teeth to give room for the permanent ones, that no absorption of the fangs of the temporary teeth has taken place. Irregularity of the permanent teeth is most commonly occasioned by the resistance made by the nearest temporary teeth; this is always the case if the temporary teeth are small and close set, for, as the permanent incisores are much larger than the temporary, they require more room; but as the space left by the shedding of the temporary teeth is too small for the regular position of the permanent; they are exposed to the pressure of the next tooth, and hence are frequently turned out of their right direction.

Another cause of the irregularity of the teeth arises from the permanent teeth being too large for the space occupied by the temporary ones; those parts of the jaws not being sufficiently extended to permit a regular position of the new teeth. In this case the irregularity is considerable, and occasions great deformity in the appearance of the mouth. The incisores and cuspidati being much larger than those of the child, require more room, for want of which they are turned out of their proper positions. The central incisores over lap each other, the lateral incisores are either placed obliquely, with their edges turned forwards, or they are pushed back, and stand between and behind the central incisores and the cuspidati; the cuspidati are projected, occasioning the lip to stand out with considerable prominence, and the bicuspides are placed very irregularly.

It will be proper in this place to observe the manner in which the jaw bones grow, (the under one being taken as an example,) and to point out the difference between the temporary and permanent teeth.

After a child has obtained all the temporary teeth, the jaw, in general, grows very little, in the part which they occupy. In those children who are an exception to this rule, the temporary teeth become a good deal separated from each other, and these are the cases in which the shedding of the teeth is effected without the assistance of art. When the jaw of a child is compared with that of an adult, a very striking difference is observed; that of a child forms nearly the half of a circle, while that of an adult is the half of a long ellipsis. This comparison clearly points the part in which the jaw receives its greatest increase, to be between the second temporary molaris and the coronoid process; and this lengthened part of the jaw is destined to be the situation of the permanent molares.

By the elongation of the jaw, a great change in the form of the face is produced; that of a child is round, the cheeks are plump and the chin flat; in the adult the face is more prominent with a flatness of cheek and a considerable length of chin.

The temporary incisores and cuspidati are much smaller than the permanent, while the molares of the temporary set are larger than the bicuspides which succeed them. Hence it is that the incisores and cuspidati are so frequently irregular, and they never could be otherwise, were it not that some space were gained from the molares, in consequence of the bicuspides being much smaller. This circumstance is rendered intelligible, by examining jaws at various ages, and observing in what particulars they differ from each other.

Until about twelve months after birth, the jaw grows uniformly in all its parts, and at that time as far as the teeth extend, it approaches nearly to a semi-circle; at about three years of age, when all the temporary teeth have appeared, it begins to lose its semi-circular form, and become somewhat elongated; an extension takes place between the last temporary molaris and the coronoid process; and in that part in an advanced state of formation, the first permanent molaris will be found.

At about seven or eight years of age, the jaw is more extended, the first permanent molaris has grown up, and the second is advancing in formation. At about eleven or twelve years of age, it will be found still longer; the second molaris is ready to come through the gum, and the third molaris has begun to form.

The jaw acquires its full proportion, at about eighteen or twenty years of age, when the third molaris makes its appearance, and the teeth are seen in the figure of their arrangement to form part of an ellipsis.

The growth of the jaw being nearly confined to the part situated behind the temporary teeth, where the permanent molares are placed, the anterior part of the jaw undergoes little more than an alteration in form; it adapts itself to the permanent teeth there situated, and scarcely receives any increase of size.

The same comparison of jaws exhibits the cause of irregularity in the permanent incisores and cuspidati. When a child is about to shed its teeth, the first permanent molares come through the gums behind the temporary molares, and therefore the teeth which are situated anteriorly to the permanent molares can obtain no additional space.

The permanent incisores occupy the space of the temporary incisores, and half of that of the cuspidati. It commonly happens that the bicuspides are earlier in their appearance than the cuspidati; therefore, when the first temporary molares are shed, a little room is gained, as the teeth which succeed them are smaller. When the second molares are shed, still more room is gained; the two bicuspides go back against the first permanent molares, and thereby give sufficient room for the cuspidati. Thus by the change of the molares of the child which are large, for the bicuspides of the adult which are small, room is obtained for the increased size of the permanent incisores and cuspidati.

This change of small teeth for larger, and of larger for smaller, points out the necessity of giving some assistance to nature in one of her processes, viz. that of throwing out the temporary teeth before the permanent teeth appear; if this be done at a proper time, the teeth will always take a regular position, and every deformity arising from irregularity be prevented.

During the progress of the second dentition, an opportunity presents itself for effecting this desirable object; but every thing depends upon a correct knowledge of the time when a tooth requires to be extracted, and also of the particular tooth; for often more injury is occasioned by the removal of a tooth too early, than if it be left a little too long; because a new tooth, which has too much room long before it is required, will sometimes take a direction more difficult to alter than an irregularity occasioned by an obstruction of short duration. If an improper tooth be extracted, irreparable mischief will ensue; as in the case where young permanent teeth have been removed, instead of the obstructing temporary ones, which I have several times known to have been done. As regards the growth of the jaws, &c. I think Mr. Hunter is a little too restricted in his views. *See observations of Duval on this subject, before mentioned.*

SECTION VIII.

ANALYSIS OF THE TEETH, &c.*

Analysis of the Enamel.

One hundred grains of the enamel of human teeth, (carefully rasped,) were placed in 600 grains of nitric acid of the specific gravity of 1.12. Slight effervescence ensued, and after twelve hours 200 grains more of the acid were added. Allowing for the loss by evaporation in a corresponding vessel, after thirty-six hours it was found to have lost four grains and an half. It was then diluted with four ounces of distilled water precipitated by pure ammonia, and then filtered.

The precipitate obtained being dried in a water bath, at 212°, weighed 102 grains. It was then ignited, after which it was found to weigh 78 grains. The filtered solution was then precipitated by carbonate of ammonia in solution and filtered.

The separated precipitate being dried in a heat of 212° weighed six grains. Enamel then consists of,

Phosphate of lime, - - - - -	78
Carbonate of lime, - - - -	6
	84
Water of composition and loss,	16
	100

A loss of 16 grains here takes place which is easily accounted for, from the impossibility of directly ascertaining

* By Wm. H. Pepys, jun. Fox, First Part, pages 96 to 100.

the state of dryness in, which the ingredients existed originally in the enamel; for we have seen, that by drying the phosphate of lime in a heat of 212°, (after which it had the appearance of being as dry as possible,) it yet contained so much moisture as to yield a gain of 8 grains in the analysis. On the other hand, when ignited, its state is driven to the opposite extreme, and there is a loss of 16 grains. It is impossible, however, that the materials could exist in the teeth, in a state of dryness to be compared with that produced by exposing them to such a high temperature. And it appears but reasonable to conclude, that the real quantity of moisture lies nearer to that given by the heat of 212°, than to that given by ignition, and consequently that the 16 grains lost by exposure to such a high temperature were chiefly water.

Bone or roots of teeth, yielded by analysis, in 100 grains,

Phosphate of lime - - - - -	58
Carbonate of lime, - - - -	4
Gelatine, - - - - - -	28
	90
Water of composition and loss -	10
	100

The teeth of adults yielded on analysis, in 100 grains,

Phosphate of lime, - - - - -	64
Carbonate of lime, - - - -	6
Gelatine, - - - - - -	20
	90
Water of composition and loss,	10
	100
Specific gravity of adults teeth, -	2.2727

The shedding or primary teeth of children yielded on analysis, in 100 grains,

Phosphate of lime, - - - - -	62
Carbonate of lime, - - - - -	6
Gelatine, - - - - -	20
	88
Water of composition and loss, - .	12
	100

Specific gravity of children's teeth, 2.0833

In these analyses, as in the former, the phosphate of lime was also exposed to a red heat, and consequently was reduced to a greater degree of dryness than that in which it existed in the tooth. In all of them the carbonate of lime was dried in a heat of 212°, above which it would have been liable to decomposition, and the gelatine of the three last in the same temperature.

*Analysis of the Small Bones of the Teeth of Man.**

One hundred parts of these small bones, calcined in a small platina crucible, left a white residuum weighing 59. 5.

The loss of weight occasioned by the animal matter which was burnt therefore out of it 40.5.

The 59. 5, of the remainder, on which was poured weak nitric acid, dissolved entirely with a slight effervescence.

The solution was precipitated by ammonia; the precipitate, white, gelatinous, taken and washed in warm water, then dried and calcined, weighed 38; it appeared, from the examination which was made, like phosphate of lime.

The fluid which was precipitated by this phosphate of lime, mixed with a solutiou of the sub-carbonate of soda, gave a

* L. F. E. Rousseau, page 34.

white precipitate which, after having been washed and dried, weighed 21. 5. This precipitate treated with sulphuric acid, was altogether changed into the sulphate of lime; from whence it might be concluded it was the carbonate of lime.

The same process was employed in the analysis of each of the articles comprised in the following table. I ought to acknowledge here that I am indebted for the details of this procedure, and the results presented by this table, to M. Lassaigne, my friend, and chemist to the veterinary school at Alfort.

A TABLE,

*Presenting the results obtained by the Chemical Analysis of the Human Teeth, and of each one in particular.**

DESIGNATION OF THE OBJECTS SUBMITTED TO ANALYSIS.	Of 100 parts of each was obtained.		
	Animal matter.	Phosphate of Lime.	Carbonate of lime.
Teeth of a man of eighty years	33	66	1
Teeth of an adult	29	61	10
Teeth of a child of six years	28.571	60.009	11.420
Teeth of a child of two years } Teeth of 1st dentition	23	67	10
Teeth of a child of two years } Teeth of 2d dentition	17.5	65	17.5
Teeth of a child of one day	35	51	14
Teeth of a mummy of Egypt	29	55.5	15.5
Enamel of the teeth of a man	20	72	8
Cartilaginous matter of the teeth of an infant of one day	86.7	11.3	2
Pulp or ganglion of the teeth of an infant of one day	77	23	
Dental sac of an infant of one day . . .	57	37	6
Matter of the caries of the teeth	40.5	38	21.5

* L. F. E. Rousseau, page 35.

SECTION IX.

SENSIBILITY OF THE OSSEOUS SUBSTANCE OF THE TEETH.

We now proceed to the notice of an interesting and much controverted point in a physiological consideration of the Teeth.

Is their osseous structure* organized, and does it possess sensibility? The limits of this work will not allow of my entering into a lengthy discussion of this subject, but as it is one that involves some of the most important principles of Dental Surgery, I feel myself bound to lay before the reader some of the principal authorities and arguments in the negative and affirmative of these questions, reminding him that it is only in the general that we can examine the opposing answers. From the fact, that without pain, the Cortex Striatus or Enamel could be operated on with cutting and rasping instruments, it was inferred by some that the whole osseous structure of the teeth was likewise insensible. This has led to the practice, in many instances, of destroying the nerves of the teeth, on the supposition that they were of little or no use after the teeth were fully formed. A difference of opinion upon this subject appears to have been entertained at an early period. Benjamin Martin, in speaking of it, says:† "I am bold yet in saying, that the osseous substance of the teeth, has sensibility by the animal spirit, which the nerve distributes and carries to it, or, physically speaking,

* By which is meant the bony substance, with the exception of the cortex striatus.

† B. Martin, pages 6 to 8.

in its spiritual substance, which is infiltrated through the whole extent of the tooth; for without this it would be lost to the osseous part, that subsists but by this means, after the same manner, that we see trees, and other vegetating things, subsisting by means of the sap. For it may be said, that the tooth vegetates and grows, and when its root is changed, and this spiritual substance begins to degenerate, and is no longer communicated, it becomes dry and black; and after having lost its natural colour, eventually perishes."

Fauchard appears to have unequivocally considered the osseous structure of the teeth as possessing sensibility, for he says:*

"Those who have treated of the teeth, have found partizans on the subject of the sensibility of these parts. Some have thought that the teeth were insensible; others have maintained the contrary. It is true, that considering the teeth simply like the bones, it might be said they were insensible: but if they are considered as organized parts, covered and furnished with membranes, vessels, and nerves, they ought not to be denied the property of being sensible, as well as all the other parts of the body.

It is easy to perceive that this different way of considering the teeth, conciliates with much facility these two opinions, which appear so opposite to one another: nevertheless, I believe it is better to think like the last, for the reason which I have just mentioned, and which is confirmed by daily experience, which proves that the diseases by which the teeth are attacked, cause pain, and of course, the teeth are endowed with feeling."

To understand better the sensibility of the teeth, it must

* Fauchard, On the Sensibility of the Teeth, pages 135, 136.

be remembered that which I have established at the beginning of this treatise touching the different parts of which the teeth are composed; that supposes, I believe that their sensibility is of two kinds in general, and may he thus distinguished: one was comprised under the name of fixed and permanent pain; that which is generally understood when one says he has the tooth-ache: and the other, that of their being set on edge or passing pain. I believe that this disagreeable sensation resembles, and may be compared to, what is experienced when the hand is passed upon certain things, as on a hat, or when certain instruments are attempted to be ground in a certain way, one against the other, &c.

Conjectures* so very similar have given me room to conclude that the teeth are sensible, not only on account of the membrane in which their roots are enclosed, but more on account of the nervous and membranous threads which are expanded over all the body of the tooth. The only thing that ought to be remarked, is, that the sensibility is much less at the enamel than the rest of the tooth; because its tissue being very compact, and its pores very close, nothing can easily penetrate it. From whence it is impossible, that the same causes can occasion on the enamelled part, a sensation as sharp and as painful as that which can be felt on the rest of the tooth. The particular manner in which the nervous threads are found in the enamel of the tooth, might in the meanwhile make us conjecture, that it is the only seat of their being set on edge.

This will be the place here to explain more or less this kind of disagreeable sensation which I have arranged with setting

* Fauchard, On the Sensibility and setting on edge of the Teeth, page 142.

on edge, and which is felt very sensibly by the incisor and canine teeth, when the hand is passed on the body of a hat, or on other similar bodies, or when certain instruments are heard clashing against each other at a certain distance; but as these are things for which the aid of the dentist is not commonly wanted, and the explanations also that have been given on this subject, appear to me very uncertain, I like better to spare the reader the trouble of reading parallel conjectures, and confine myself to the limits my profession prescribes me."

Mr. Robert Blake, who examined the various phenomena of healthy and diseased, and of living and dead teeth, was a warm advocate in favour of the position, that both in their osseous and vascular portions, the teeth are truly organized bodies, and possessed of sensibility. He was also strongly opposed to Mr. Hunter's views of this subject, and remarks: "Having repeatedly injected and examined the jaws of young subjects, I observed blood-vessels passing from the gum to the membranes destined to form the cortex striatus. It was natural enough, then, to conclude, that, as the investing membranes were derived from the gum, their nourishment too, did originate from the same source, and that the use of the vessels which entered the proper foramina of the jaws, was only to form the pulp and bony part of the tooth. Further consideration of the subject, however, urged me to relinquish this opinion: it would by no means hold good on comparing it with what takes place in the jaws of large animals, for (as mentioned in chapter eight, page 83) the cortex striatus continues to be formed on the external plates of

* Blake, Essay on the Teeth in Man, pages 117 to 122.

their teeth, even after the upper part of them has appeared through the gum."

As frequent opportunity occurred in the course of this essay to mention the vessels and nerves of the teeth, I would not have allotted them a distinct chapter, were it not that Mr. Hunter asserts that the teeth are nearly inorganic, and also, that "we can actually transplant a tooth from one person to another"* Although transplanting teeth was for some time practised, yet the dreadful consequences which so frequently ensued, as well as the bad success which commonly attended this operation, induced its most strenuous advocates (I trust for ever) to lay it aside.

Mr. Hunter in support of his doctrine, asserts, "he could never trace the nerves distinctly even to the beginning of the cavity."† Yet Eustachius seems to have been much more fortunate in his dissections of man as well as other animals, which appears from the following quotation: "When we pass from the grinders to the small teeth, the nerve with its concomitant artery is divided into two branches, one of which passes out through the hole in the jaw near the lower lip; the other branch proceeds on to the roots of the incisores, and sends each a twig, one portion of which is expanded on the external membrane of the root, but the other, and that the most delicate, passes into the internal cavity. This fact, indeed, can be easily observed, even in the human body, by those who are engaged in accurate dissections. But it is truly wonderful, and seems almost inconsistent with the laws of nature, that the incisores and canine teeth, which are small and have only one root, possess large and conspicuous branches of nerves and vessels, whilst the grinders, which

* Nat. Hist. pages 38 and 126. See also part II. pages 94, 95, &c.
† Nat. Hist. page 42.

are much larger, and have three, and sometimes four roots, are supplied by branches proceeding to each root, nearly as small as hairs."

Doctor Munro has several preparations in his museum, in which the nerves and vessels were traced by him into the roots of the teeth, and also into the pulp, which appears sufficiently evident in Tab. I. Fig. 4, &c.*

Mr. Hunter observes, "a strong circumstance in support of the teeth having no circulation in them, is, that they never change by age, and seem never to undergo any alteration, when completely formed, but by abrasion; they do not grow softer like the other bones, as we find in some cases, where the whole earthy matter of the bones has been taken into the constitution. From the foregoing experiments it would seem that the teeth are without absorbents as well as other vessels, and are to be considered as extraneous bodies, with respect to a circulation through their substance."

These remarks of Mr. Hunter are by no means just, for the bony part of a tooth undergoes changes by age, as well as any other part of the body. Indeed, if by chance the vessels which enter the roots and are distributed on the pulp, be torn or destroyed, the body of the tooth becomes discoloured, sometimes nearly black, the external membrane which surrounds the roots not being sufficient to supply it with nourishment, so that the bony part acts as a foil to the cortex striatus. I have frequently observed their roots changed nearly to a cartilaginous substance, and rendered perfectly transparent by the absorption of the bony matter. The roots of the grinders have been so frequently observed joined together by exostosis, that its occurrence was well known to Eustachius. nay, even to Hippocrates.† However,

---

* Nat. Hist. page 39.

† Opuscul. De Dentih. page 97.

an incontestible proof of the presence of vessels, both circulatory and absorbent, and consequeatly of nerves, may be deduced from the progressive or continued growth of the incisores, in the squirrel tribe, and the colouring of the teeth of all animals from feeding on food mixed with madder, and the subsequent loss of the acquired colour from discontinuing the use of madder.

Mr. Fox is equally positive, and observes,* "It is very extraordinary that Mr. Hunter should have considered the teeth as devoid of internal circulation, and destitute of the living principle. The structure of the teeth is similar to that of any other bone, and differs only in having a covering which is called enamel, for the exposed surface, and the bony part being more dense. There are several parts of the body in which we cannot by injections demonstrate the existence of blood-vessels, of the vascularity of which no one can entertain a doubt; and as bones in general are continually receiving nourishment from the vessels which enter into their substance, it may be justly inferred, that the blood sent to the teeth affords a similar supply, especially as a considerable portion of animal matter enters into their composition.

A large quantity of blood is distributed to the teeth; this may frequently be seen in performing some operations. In cutting off the crown of a tooth, in which the caries had not spread to the fang, for the purpose of engrafting a new tooth, I have several times seen a discharge of blood from the internal cavity. This blood came from the vessels of the membrane in the cavity, which I have also several times seen injected. Blood carries with it the basis of nutrition, and is sent to those parts only where renovation is necessary. For what other reason then, but to impart some principle of nu-

---

* Fox, History of the Teeth, pages 33, 34.

trition, can so much blood flow into the teeth? If the teeth, after their first formation, receive no supply from vessels, or did not require any nourishment, it would have been better if they had been destitute of an internal cavity, and of regular organization."

*It is always observed, that as persons advance in life, their teeth loose that whiteness which they possessed in the time of youth. This change in the appearance of the teeth seems to depend upon one which takes place in their cavities, by which the vessels entering them are gradually destroyed, and the supply of blood is proportionally diminished. In the teeth of persons advanced in years, the cavity is very frequently obliterated, in consequence of a deposit of bony matter, which entirely destroys the internal organization. When this happens, the teeth always lose their colour, and become very yellow, their texture also becomes more brittle, and they acquire a horny transparency.

When a tooth has become loosened by a blow, and has afterwards fastened in the socket, a great alteration in its colour is the consequence; it gradually loses its whiteness, and acquires a darker hue; this proceeds from the vessels which enter the teeth, being destroyed, and the teeth consequently losing their supply of blood.

The teeth being constructed like common bones, are governed by the same laws, and are liable to be affected with similar diseases; like them they are affected with the various causes of inflammation, and have the same diseased appearances produced upon them.

In bones the power of resisting the effects of disease is in an inverse proportion to their density. The living principle is always less in the close textured cylindrical bones, and

---

* Fox, History of the Teeth, Part I, Pages 35, 36.

greater in those which are flat and spongy. The teeth being the most dense bones in the body, have the least power of resisting disease, and in them the general termination of inflammation is in mortification.

In the second part of his justly celebrated work, published some years after the first, from which we have taken his foregoing opinions, Mr. Fox again recurs to the vitality of the teeth with increased confidence, and observes,* "In the former part, I endeavoured to prove that the teeth are organized in a similar manner to other bones, and that as possessing *life*, they are connected with, and form an integral part of the system." I have now the satisfaction to find that the same opinion is entertained by almost all the enlightened members of the surgical profession. Mr. Hunter, who made many experiments by feeding animals with madder, in order to ascertain the effect it would produce in colouring the different bones of the body, having observed that the teeth did not become tinged so speedily as the other bones, or when tinged, that they retained their colour longer, hence concluded, that "they are to be considered as extraneous bodies, with respect to a circulation through their substance.

The consequence of having formed this opinion was, that he could not, in any satisfactory manner, assign a cause for the different diseases of the teeth. It must however, appear extraordinary, that Mr. Hunter, who was so accurate an observer of the phenomena of nature, should have published this opinion, when he immediately added, that "they (the teeth) have most certainly a living principle, by which means they make part of the body, and are capable of uniting with any part of a living body.

* Fox, Part II, pages 1, 2.

Mr. Duval, in reference to this subject, remarks:* "We cannot be surprised, that men who have not studied the laws of the animal economy, should have regarded the teeth as inorganic bodies, without life, and consequently capable of resisting the most destructive causes; from this circumstance arose, no doubt, the ingenious fable, which represents Cadmus as giving birth to men, by sawing the teeth of the dragon which he had slain.

The sensibility of the teeth ought never to have permitted a doubt of their being organized; whether they be composed of a peculiar bony substance, as may be observed by inspecting their internal parts and roots, or whether the crown is enveloped in a transparent covering, as if vitrified, called enamel; the hardness of which is such, that it resists the action of fire, more than the osseous substance which it covers, and from which one might even draw sparks, either by striking it with steel, or filing it in the dark.

The growth of the teeth, and their piercing the gums, could not take place without this vitality, which is peculiar to them, and which continues during life; for even when the alveolus or socket is destroyed, they are still attached to the gums by certain fibres. This vitality, which is in connexion with that of the whole frame, is not confined solely to that soft and very sensible follicle contained in the cavity of the teeth, which extends from the centre of the crown to the extremity of the fangs: the hard parts also partake of it, though in a much less degree: and in both cases it is supplied by the arteries, veins, and nerves; these vessels, being distributed over all the face, and communicating with each other, keep up a constant and admirable sympathy.

---

* Duval, Dentiste de la Jeunesse, pages 23, 24.

Mr. Hertz says:* "Though from their very condensed structure it is impossible to demonstrate the vascularity of teeth in a great degree, yet the circumstances which attend their diseased state clearly show their possession of circulation, sensibility, and absorption, the same as prevails in the soft parts.

Mr. Audibran gives an opinion affirmatively of this question, and uses as strong language as any writer I have seen. In reference to it, he says:† "The circulation of the blood takes place in the interior of our teeth as in other parts of the body, by means of ramifications which penetrate all their bony structure, inasmuch if a tooth is broken, the blood may be seen oozing from the middle of the bone."

Mr. Koecker strenuously contends for the affirmative of these opinions, and speaking of the internal membrane of the teeth, observes:‡ "This membrane consists of a nerve, an artery, a vein, and, most probably, of some absorbent vessels. This nerve seems to be particularly intended for an internal protection to the tooth against general morbid influences, and for this reason it appears to be possessed of the most exquisite sensibility.

By means of these nervous branches, the teeth are connected immediately with the fifth pair of nerves, and through it with the whole nervous system.

The lining membrane of the teeth distributes its arterial fibres throughout the whole of their bony structure, and thus becomes the immediate means of nutriment to them, as the nerves are of sensibility.

The health and vitality of the teeth depend almost alto-

---

* Hertz, on the Structure and Diseases of the Teeth, page 3.

† Audibran, page 80.

‡ Koecker, Principles of Dental Surgery, page 39.

gether upon their membrane, and if the life of this membrane be destroyed, the tooth will become not only extraneous, but a noxious body."

"Notwithstanding, therefore, that the teeth consist of the hardest and most solid bony texture, they are, nevertheless, organized, vascular, and interwoven with nervous and arterial fibres."

Mr. Hunter, from not having an intimate and practical acquaintance with the dental organs, and from several considerations which I will presently give in his own words, came to a conclusion, that in their osseous structure the teeth possessed neither circulation nor sensibility, and even that they were bodies almost "extraneous" to the system. He says,* "the following considerations would seem to show that the teeth are not vascular. First, I never saw them injected in any preparation, nor could I ever succeed in any attempt to inject them, either in young or old subjects; and therefore believe that there must have been some fallacy in the cases where they have been said to be injected. Secondly, we are not able to trace any vessels going from the pulp into the substance of the new formed tooth; and whatever part of a tooth is formed, it is always completely formed; which is not the case with other bones. But what is a more convincing proof, is, reasoning from the analogy between them and other bones, when the animal has been fed with madder. Take a young animal, viz. a pig, and feed it with madder for three or four weeks, then kill the animal, and, upon examination, you will find the following appearance: first, if this animal had some parts of its teeth formed before the feeding with madder, those parts will be known by their remaining of this natural colour; but such parts of the teeth

* Hunter, Natural History of the Human Teeth, pages 37 to 39.

as were formed while the animal was taking the madder, will be found to be of a red colour. This shews, that it is only those parts that were forming while the animal was taking the madder, that are dyed; for what were already formed will not be found in the least tinged. This is different in all other bones; for we know that any part of a bone which is already formed, is capable of being dyed with madder, though not so fast as the part that is forming; therefore, as we know that all other bones, when formed, are vascular, and are thence susceptible of the dye, we may readily suppose that the teeth are not vascular, because they are not susceptible of it after being once formed. But we shall carry this still farther; if you feed a pig with madder for some time, and then leave it off for a considerable time before you kill the animal, you will find the above appearances still subsisting, with this addition, that all the parts of the teeth which were formed, after leaving off feeding with the madder, will be white. Here then, in some teeth, we shall have white, then red, and then white again; and so we shall have the red and white colour alternately through the whole tooth.

"This experiment shews, that the tooth once tinged, does not lose its colour: now, as all other bones that have been once tinged, lose their colour in time, when the animal leaves off feeding with madder, (though very slowly,) and as that dye must be taken into the constitution by the absorbents, it would seem that the teeth are without absorbents, as well as other vessels."

* This shews that the growth of the teeth, is very different from that of the other bones. Bones begin at a point, and shoot out at their surface; and the part that seems al-

* Hunter. Nat. Hist. of the Human Teeth, page 39.

ready formed, is not in reality so, for it is forming every day by having new matter thrown into it, till the whole substance is complete; and even then it is constantly changing its matter.

Another circumstance in which teeth seem different from bone, and a strong circumstance of their having no circulation in them, is, that they never change by age, and seem never to undergo any alteration, when completely formed, but by abrasion; they do not grow softer, like the other bones, as we find in some cases, where the whole earthy matter of the bones has been taken into the constitution."

* "From these experiments it would appear, that the teeth are to be considered as extraneous bodies, with respect to a circulation through their substance."

Had Mr. Hunter been a practical dentist, there is hardly a doubt but what more scrutinizing and accurate observations would have wrought an entire change in his opinions upon this subject; and indeed, as it was, his accurrate knowledge of the animal economy, forced him to the conclusion, that the teeth in order to unite with living parts, must possess a degree of vitality; for he well knew that dead and living bodies, cannot by any process whatever, be made to unite with each other; for subsequently, to what I have already quoted from his book, he remarks,† "From these experiments it would appear that the teeth, are to be considered as extraneous bodies, with respect to a circulation through their substance; but they have most certainly a *living principle*, by which means they make part of the body, and are capable of uniting with any part of a living body." If Mr. Hunter could have operated upon the bony structure of the teeth, in some states of disease he would certainly have per-

* Hunter. Nat. Hist. of the Human Teeth. page 39. † Pages 39, 40.

ceived that in many instances they possess a high degree of sensibility. It is well known that in the phenomena of living organs, their sensibility increases in a ratio inverse to their density, and hence some structures in a state of health appear quite insensible; but when diseased, are the seat of most acute pain, because disease usually increases their vascularity. These observations apply not only to the osseous substance of the teeth, but to the tendons, ligaments, and cartilages. In some instances the enamel is removed from a portion of the tooth, and an inflammation of the exposed bony structure takes place. In these cases the touch of a tooth-pick, of a tooth-brush, or even the slightest impression, will cause the most acute pain. This state of things we often find on the necks of the teeth, and on their lateral surfaces. Some of those who advocate Mr. Hunters opinions, on the extraneous nature of the bony substance of the teeth, explain this, as they say, apparent sensibility in that part, by supposing that any substance which touches the exposed part communicates a vibratory and painful impression to the nervous pulp within the tooth, and in this way they suppose that all the uneasy sensations, which are so often complained of by persons having diseased teeth arise; that is, by an impression conveyed through the bone to the nerve and membrane, lining the internal cavity, and that the osseous structure itself is not susceptible of pain. What seems entirely to controvert this opinion is, that if this diseased portion of the tooth is entirely and carefully removed, so as to leave the bone free from any diseased part, the tenderness and pain are entirely removed; and although the bony part is left much nearer the nerve than before the diseased portion was excised, still no painful sensation is experienced as before, by the impression of a brush, tooth pick, or any thing of the kind. It follows a matter of course, as certainly as any demonstration in the

Euclid, that if the reasonings of these gentlemen are correct, the nearer we approach the nerve, the greater will be the pain, and the greater will be the liability to it; but the fact is otherwise, for after the complete removal of the diseased portion, the tenderness and pain are also removed; nor are they again perceived unless the bone becomes diseased. I have noticed these facts in repeated instances, and on these principles, I have often excised diseased portions of teeth, to the uniform relief of the patient, and often entirely arresting the disposition to disease. A reason which Mr. Hunter urges against the idea of circulation through the osseous portion, is because he was "never able to inject it." This argument loses all its consequence, when we consider that the tendons, ligaments and cartilages, and the chrystaline lines of the eye cannot be injected; and yet it is seldom contended that these parts are not vascular and possessed of vitality. If the osseous portion of the teeth cannot be injected by art, I am certain that in the higher grades of inflammatory fever in some instances, no blood passes into the bony structure so as to be perceptible to the observation of the physician, and likewise to be so after death. I have at this time five teeth taken from the jaws of a very plethoric woman, aged 27 years, who died of a violently inflammatory fever, which appear to be completely and beautifully injected with red blood: their enamel is perfectly natural, whilst the bony structure is of a deep red, and this red colour is proved not to proceed from the injected vessels within, for after sawing off the fangs, and drilling out the nerve and vessels, the same appearance remains. I hardly need pursue this subject any farther, after what has now been said upon it, and the observations of the eminent and learned dentists already quoted; nor should I have said as much as I have, if it was not a practice with some persons who favour Mr. Hunter's opinions, to drill out and destroy the nerves of some of the teeth when diseased, and fill the cavity with a metallic stopping, when in a vast majority of cases, a more judicious practice would have perfectly restored the teeth to health, and preserved their vitality. The difference in the appearance of those teeth in which the nerve, blood-vessels, and membrane of the internal cavity are destroyed, and those in which they are healthy, is great and as striking as between the appearance of a dead and living tree in the vernal season; and although like the dead tree, it may, from the density of its structure, for a time preserve its form, and from the vigour and firmness of its roots maintain its position, yet sooner or later it will crumble to pieces. A great deal more might be said upon this subject, but the limits of this work will not allow me to extend the discussion any farther, save only, in conclusion, I would ask the candid enquirer after truth, to peruse the observations, arguments, and opinions of Martin, Fauchard, Blake, Fox, Duval and Koecker, and what I have advanced upon this subject, consider that they were practical dentists, and some of them very learned men; then compare these observations, &c. with the hesitating manner in which Mr. Hunter, who was not a practical dentist, speaks of the subject, and reflect upon the analogy which is observed between the dental organs and other dense structures, and I think all will conclude with me, that in proportion to its density, the osseous substance of the teeth is endowed with as much vitality, as any other organ in the animal system.

SECTION X.

OF THE PHYSIOGNOMY OF THE TEETH.*

The effect of the teeth in giving character and expression to the human countenance, has been remarked by most physiognomists, ancient as well as modern, and both have attributed certain dispositions of mind to certain kinds of teeth. That the teeth have a great effect upon the expression of a countenance, is unquestionable; but I will venture to assert, that the theory of physiognomy, as far as it relates to the teeth, and in most instances to the projecting chin is extremely fallible: the conclusions drawn from physiognomical remarks upon the expression of both must, of consequence, be unjust.

The often repeated indulgence of any particular passion, may give to a countenance a cast or expression of that passion; but no action or disposition of the mind can have the least tendency to make the teeth long or short, to regulate their order, or to render them sound and beautiful.

The learned and scientific Lavater insists much on the characteristics of the teeth and chin. His ingenious and beautiful system has many favourers. It is foreign to my purpose to consider either the truth or the fallacy of his general system of physiognomy, nor is it my intention to derogate from its merits; but as his argument upon the characteristics of the teeth, and of the projecting chin, are certainly founded in error; and, as in the exercise of my profession, I have daily proofs of the injustice of attributing certain pas-

---

*Murphy, pages 143 to 155.

sions and dispositions of mind, to persons possessing certain kinds of teeth, I feel it a duty to endeavour to rescue many worthy and amiable people, who have bad or irregular teeth, from the unjust odium cast upon them by the disciples of Lavater.

I shall here give some of the principal of his observations upon this subject, and then hope to show that they are erroneous.

"Nothing is more certain, more striking, or continually visible, than the characteristics of the teeth, and the manner in which they display themselves.

"Small, short teeth, which have generally been held by old physiognomists to denote weakness, I have remarked in adults of extraordinary strength, but they seldom were of pure white.

"Long teeth, certain signs of weakness and pusillanimity. White, clean, well arranged teeth, visible as soon as the mouth opens, but not projecting, nor always entirely seen, I have never met with in adults, except in good, acute, honest candid, faithful men.

"I have also met foul, uneven and ugly teeth, in persons of the above good character; but it was always either sickness or some mental imperfection, which gave this deformity.

"Short, broad teeth, standing close to each other, shew tranquil, firm strength.

"Melancholy persons have seldom, well arranged, clean and white teeth."

There is no doubt that the above appearances excited in the mind of Lavater the ideas of the mental qualities he ascribes to them, and that they make the same impressions on other readers of the human countenance; but those who study the history of the teeth will know that the unworthy and profligate may possess those external marks which Lavater attributes to the good, acute, honest, candid, and faithful disposition of the mind, in common with those who really possess the amiable qualities of which they are the symbols.

Foul, uneven, ugly teeth, are also as frequently seen with persons of the most amiable disposition, who have no mental imperfection, nor any malady except that which may arise from the state of the teeth.

Foul teeth are certainly ugly, and those who make no attempt to keep their teeth clean undoubtedly betray great negligence of character; and may, without injustice, be suspected of not possessing a taste for cleanliness or delicacy.

Well arranged teeth are justly esteemed a beauty, and irregular teeth a deformity; but it is a deformity which is produced by physical and not by mental causes.

The general causes of the irregularities of the teeth have already been pointed out in the chapter on that subject; it would, therefore, be superfluous to repeat them.

It has also been remarked that the size of the teeth depends on the ossific matter deposited for their formation; their size must consequently be determined long before the actions of the passions of the mind begin to develope themselves; and hence it is evident that the mind cannot influence the length or breadth of the teeth. The size and shape of the teeth cannot therefore, be a more just criterion by which to judge of the mental qualities of individuals, than the variations of personal height or circumference.

In the glowing pages of the philosophic Herder are many observations upon the physiognomy of the teeth; but they are founded as much in error as those of Lavater. Neither Lavater, Herder, nor any of the physiognomists, seem to have been acquainted with the physiology of the teeth; their observations should however, by no means, be disregarded; they tend to prove the importance of good, clean, and even teeth; and it is also certain from them that foul, bad, and irregular teeth, give to a countenance an effect so peculiarly unpleasing as to lead an observer to suspect something wrong in the mind.

Those kinds of teeth which are held by physiognomists to be indicative of the character of different nations, may all be observed in different individuals of the same country. For example: the well arranged teeth of the Spaniards; the long separated teeth of the Tartars; and the extremely white teeth of the Hottentots, are all to be found with the natives of Great Britain. The appearance of the teeth cannot, therefore, be a more true mark of national than of individual character.

Most civilized nations agree in considering soundness, whiteness, and regularity, essential to beautiful teeth. There are some nations however of a different opinion, and think that in order to be beautiful, the teeth cannot be too black. The ladies of the Marian Islands blacken their teeth. The Tonquinese and Siamese employ every art for the same purpose. The inhabitants of Sumatra and Malacca also blacken their teeth. Father Tachard says that these people blacken their teeth from an idea that man ought not to have white teeth like brutes.

The married women of Java dye their teeth black, which we may suppose is intended as a mark of distinction. In some other of the East India Islands the inhabitants gild the too front incisores of the upper jaw, and blacken the adjoining teeth. Many savage tribes have modes peculiar to themselves of ornamenting their teeth; and some offer their front teeth as a sacrifice to their gods.

The Abyssinian Negroes take off the corners of their front teeth, and make them spear pointed. The Malay Indians make a groove across the incisores of the upper jaw; they also grind the cutting edges of their teeth with a stone till they all become of an equal length.

The natives of Hindostan, the Bramins in particular, are extremely delicate in every point relating to the teeth; every morning when they rise, they rub them for upwards of an hour together with a twig of the raeemiferous fig-tree, at the same time addressing their prayers to the sun, and calling down the blessing of heaven on themselves and their families. As this practice is prescribed in their most ancient books of law and divinity, we imagine it coeval with the date of their religion and government. It exhibits a curious proof of the regard which this polished and scientific people had for the purity and beauty of the mouth when so simple a practice is inculcated as a law and rendered indispensable as a religious duty. The reddish cast which the constant use of the betel and areca nut gives to the teeth of both sexes in India, though now considered as a beauty, does not seem to have been always regarded as such, since in their poetical works, the lover, enumerating the charms of his mistress, never fails to notice, as a principal attraction the whiteness and regularity of her teeth.

"The cunda blossom yields to the whiteness of the teeth."

"Speak but one mild word, and the rays of thy sparkling teeth will dispel the gloom of my fears."*

Such images as these frequently occur in the Indian Poets.

A very whimsical custom with respect to the mouth is practised by the inhabitants of Prince William's Sound. These people appear at first sight to have two mouths. They make an incision in the upper lip, parallel with the mouth, sufficiently large to admit the tongue through. When the

---

*Gitagovinda.

sides of the incision are healed they have very much the appearance of lips. In this artificial mouth they wear a shell, which is cut to resemble a row of teeth.

These different customs prove that the most polished and the most savage nations agree in attaching a high degree of importance to the teeth, which is evinced by some considering their preservation and cleanliness as a religious duty, and others offering some of their principal teeth as a sacrifice to their deities.

Lavater extends his physiognomical remarks on teeth, even to those of brutes. Of the river horse Behemoth, he says: "How stupidly savage and inexorable! How irregular are the position and figure of the teeth. How peculiar the character of satanic, but foolish self destructive malignity."

"The crocodile proves how very physiognomical teeth are."

Of the teeth "There is as little wildness in the line of the mouth, as in the form and position of the teeth."

It is certain that the "countenance is the theatre on which the soul exhibits itself;" but it is the action of the muscles of the face which gives to it the expression of the inward workings of the mind, and not the size, form, or position of the teeth. The same countenance may one moment express the ferocity of the tiger, or the most inexorable, savage stupidity, and the next, exhibit the meekness of the lamb, and this without any alteration in the teeth. How then are the teeth so very physiognomical? How unreasonable, how uncharitable as well as unjust, would it be to suspect all those, who have irregular teeth, of possessing the horrid disposition attributed to the river-horse; or to bar our doors against those who have long and separated teeth, lest they should prove robbers, like the Tartars. The case is different with respect to beauty and deformity: no countenance, I believe can be beautiful, with foul, unsound, or irregular teeth. Nothing indeed can be more disgusting than the laugh of a person who on opening the mouth, exhibits foulness and deformity. It will ever be the happy lot of a beautiful or a pleasing countenance, to conciliate affection, and to impress an idea of perfection of mind on the beholder; whilst on the contrary, deformity and personal neglect, as surely alienate the affections, and create however unjustly, a suspicion, at least, of equal deformity of mind. It is most undoubtedly a duty we owe to ourselves, and to society, to render our persons as agreeable as possible.

The justness of the following assertion of Lavater will not, I think, be disputed; it is evidently made from observations on the personal habits of mankind.

"As are the teeth of man, that is to say their form, position, and cleanliness, (so far as the latter depends upon himself,) so is his taste."

CHAPTER III.

Having passed over the anatomy and natural history of the teeth and their appendages, we shall proceed in the following chapter to consider the diseases of those organs, and shall endeavour to point out the most obvious causes of those diseases, and their most successful and rational modes of cure and prevention.

DISEASES OF THE TEETH.

Mr. Fox* mentions the following affections and diseases of the teeth; to wit:

---

* Fox, History of the Teeth, &c. Part II, pages 7—42, 50, 52, 54, 57, 58.

Firstly, Caries: which signifies a decay of some part of the substance of the tooth.

Secondly, Exostosis of the Fangs: by which is meant a growth or deposition of bone upon them, and, consequently, they are rendered larger, and press against the internal sides of the socket, occasioning great pain to the patient, and rendering the loss of the tooth inevitable.

Thirdly, Necrosis: by which is meant the death of some part of the fang of a tooth.

Fourthly, Spina Ventosa: by which is meant a disease of the membrane lining the internal part of the fang, accompanied with a discharge of matter.

Fifthly, Removal of the enamel by the denuding process.

Sixthly, Fractures of the teeth.

Seventhly, Wearing down of the teeth in mastication. The diseases of the soft parts will be taken up after considering the diseases of the teeth.

SECTION I.

CARIES.

It was well observed by *Monton, "that caries and tartar were the two grand agents that give business to the Dentists. At the head of these is caries, one of the most common and most formidable diseases to which the teeth are subject; indeed so little are they liable to any other affections, that if it were not for caries they would be among the most healthy organs of the system

---

* Essai d'Ontotechnique, page 26.

Caries signifies a decay of the teeth, by which a part or all of their substance is lost. This is divided by most authors into superficial and deep-seated caries, and into simple and complicated.

By the first they mean a decay of the tooth, commencing on the outside, and proceeding gradually to the internal part.

By deep-seated, they mean a decay of the tooth, commencing within its substance between the enamel and the lining membrane of the tooth. Simple caries is applied to the state of caries before it has progressed so far as to expose the nerve, and complicated, when the nerve is exposed.

Messrs. Hunter,* Fox,† and Koecker,‡ agree in saying, that decay of the teeth does commence sometimes in the substance of the tooth, between the enamel and the lining membrane, and even before the tooth has passed through the gum.

Mr. Hunter says, it does commence then, but very early.

Mr. Fox speaks of caries usually commencing within the substance of the tooth.

Mr. Koecker says, he thinks it commences rather oftener on the outside, than in the substance of the tooth,

From the manner in which Messrs. Fox and Koecker speak of the subject, we might be led to infer, that caries, commencing in the substance of the tooth was of very common occurrence.

If the observations of the two latter gentlemen are true, I must acknowledge, that the sphere of usefulness on the part of the Surgeon Dentist in preventing the decay of the teeth, is, to say the least, extremely limited. For if their observations are true, this disease in its commencement, in one half of the cases, is entirely out of the reach of medical aid,

---

* Page 137. † Part II, Page 7. ‡ Page 222.

and a most powerful incentive on the part of the patient, is partially taken away; to wit, the assurance that if his mouth and teeth are kept perfectly clean, the latter will seldom be liable to decay.

I have paid the most anxious attention to this subject, and have examined the teeth of many persons, and have noted the effect of early and constant cleanliness upon them, and my observations have led me always to observe, that those persons who were constant in keeping their teeth clean, had far, and beyond comparison, better teeth, than those who were dirty and slovenly with them.

This remark we have seen verified in persons of the same family; for it is not to be denied, that some families, and individuals, and classes of men, have naturally better teeth than others.

Another remark which we have been led to make, and which is indirectly concurred in, by all writers upon the subject, is, that caries, in almost every instance, makes its appearance where the enamel has been removed by art, or accident, or where it is naturally thinnest. For instance, in the small cavities upon the crowns of the teeth, about their necks, just where the enamel becomes much attenuated, or entirely disappears, and on those parts of the teeth which come in partial contact with each other.

These remarks explain the reason why those persons whose jaws are well developed, and possess a considerable rotundity, instead of being pointed or narrow at the anterior part, and thereby compressing the teeth, and those whose teeth are not crowded together, which allows them to be well developed, and the enamel to be equally thick and strong over the body of the tooth, have so much better teeth than persons under contrary circumstances. This also explains to us a reason, and one which I have been repeatedly asked, why the negroes nave so much better teeth, as a general rule, than the white inhabitants. Behind their thick lips, they conceal a peculiar rotundity of the jaw which is very favourable to the perfect developement of the teeth; and for the same reason, and some others, men in general, have better teeth than women. To prove that cleanliness has a great effect in preserving the teeth from decay, we have only to notice the difference in the disposition to decay in the different teeth of the same individual. As an example, whilst we notice decay to have commenced in the front upper incisors, and in the grinding teeth of both jaws, we often, and most generally notice, that the front under incisors are perfectly sound, and I never saw the under incisors diseased, and the upper in health, and I believe it is the experience of every dentist, that he has occasion to operate upon, and to replace a vast many more upper than under incisors, and the reason of this demonstrates my first positions; and it is, that these teeth are kept clean by mastication, and they seldom crowd upon each other, except at their very upper points, and, therefore, they are kept free from, and enabled to resist those agents, in a great many instances, which produce the decay of the other teeth.

I will not deny, and firmly believe, that in some instances, from constitutional or local causes, decay does commence within the substance of the tooth, but I must say, with Mr. Hunter, whose acumen as to matters of observation has been seldom surpassed, that this commencement of decay occurs very rarely.*

Having spoken of what Messrs. Hunter, Fox, and Koecker define to be deep-seated caries, and having given an opinion,

---

* See Hunter, Part II, page 137.

that it was comparatively of rare occurrence, we now proceed to speak of

Superficial Caries.

This is defined to be a decay of the tooth, commencing on the outside, and thence proceeding inwardly, until it reaches the cavity of the tooth. Mr. Koecker* distinguishes two states of this caries, the one before the decay has extended to the nerve of the tooth, and the other after the decay has exposed the nerve. There is a material difference in the practice for the relief and cure of these two states of disease in the teeth.

The causes of superficial caries may be reduced to the following general ones:

First, A vitiated state of the saliva.

Secondly, Foreign or extraneous matter lodged upon the teeth; and

Thirdly, Any thing, which, either chemically or mechanically, injures or destroys the enamel of the teeth.

It cannot be denied, that in common with all the other organs of the system, the teeth suffer by general and constitutional diseases, and yet I must believe, that caries will seldom directly take place from constitutional causes, but only indirectly, by the teeth being weakened in their vital powers, by which they are rendered less able to resist some one of the above classes of causes of decay.

We will now take a separate view of each of the foregoing classes of causes which produce decay of the teeth; and here I feel myself at home: for I can easily conceive of causes acting upon the teeth externally, to produce their de-

---

* See his article, Caries, Part II.

cay, and of constitutional and local causes which affect their living powers and organization internally. But to conceive of a latent cause which acts upon the substance of the bone of the tooth, without relation either to its nerve or blood-vessels, or lining membrane on the inside, or to any deleterious influence on the outside, is a stretch of conception which I can hardly form; still I will not deny but what it may be. If so, why are not the fangs as often affected as the crowns of the teeth. The only answer I can make, is, that those who advocate the first idea, as a common principle, have either mistaken themselves in their statements, or they have mistaken the subject in its true pathology. It would far exceed the limits of this work to enter into all the relations of this very important and interesting subject; but I must again assert, that it is to external causes we must revert to explain satisfactorily the reason of most instances of decayed teeth.

The First General Cause of External Caries

We proceed to notice, is a vitiated state of the saliva or liquor of the mouth. When I consider that lead, tin, copper, &c. are very soon dissolved in the liquor of the mouth; that even silver should be eroded and dissolved, as is sometimes the case with silver springs and plates when put in the mouth, and this is most commonly the case; that even gold, which is scarcely acted upon by aqua fortis (nitric acid) should become tarnished in the mouth, and that the firmest and best ivory is there subject to decay, I am not at a loss to conceive that under some states of the saliva, it is capable of acting upon the teeth with the most pernicious influence, and causing a rapid decay of these organs.

I will now enumerate some of the causes which affect the

liquor of the mouth, and prove thereby indirect causes of decayed teeth. Every degree of uncleanness with respect to the mouth, is ready to vitiate its juices. Bits of animal food, and many articles of diet, sticking between the teeth, and allowed to remain there for any length of time, become exceedingly offensive and injurious. All decayed teeth, and decayed and dead stumps of teeth, not only create an offensive state of the breath, but vitiate the saliva, so as to prove a most active cause of decay in the teeth. Various kinds of medicines seem to affect the liquor of the mouth, so as to prove to the teeth a source of disease. Mercurial medicines given so as to excite salivation, often vitiate the saliva, so as greatly to injure the teeth. Certain febrile states of the system appear to affect the mouth, producing a furred tongue, and a nauseous taste, may have a bad effect upon the teeth. Water-brash, improper artificial teeth, often vitiate the saliva to a great degree, greatly affecting the teeth, and so much so, that in this way, two or three bad artificial teeth ruin all the others in the mouth, And, in fine, whatever vitiates the saliva, whether of constitutional or local origin, tends to produce external caries of the teeth.

A diseased state of the gums often vitiates the saliva, and thereby produces superficial caries.

The Second General Cause of External Caries.

We now go on to notice what we have considered as the second general cause of external caries, or superficial caries, which was, extraneous or foreign matter adhering to the teeth.

Upon the bodies of the teeth, generally just where the gum begins to cover them, we often notice a peculiar substance adhering to them, of a consistence like hardened mortar. Many persons, upon scaling off pieces of it, consider that they have broken off pieces of their teeth. It discolors the teeth, giving them a black appearance. This substance is called the tartar of the teeth. It is said by Mr. Koecker to act chemically upon the teeth, and thereby proves a cause of superficial caries, &c. and it likewise proves a common cause of soreness and even ulceration of the gums. A peculiar kind of greenish tartar is often observed, oftenest on the fore part of the upper incisores. I have thought that this was more apt to occasion caries, than the mortar-like-tartar, which is found about the roots of the teeth. There is no doubt but that the tartar often occasions superficial caries, especially the last variety.

I should not so strongly insist upon the principle that caries of the teeth, arises in nearly all cases from external causes, were I not certain of its truth, and were it not of such great practical utility. It encourages both the surgeon dentist and the patient to persevere in their efforts, to keep the teeth perfectly clean, and to detect and relieve the first appearance of disease. But the former principle will lead the patient to believe, that one half the causes of diseased teeth are out of the reach of art to prevent.

The Third Genexal Cause of Superficial Caries

Which we proposed to notice, was, any cause that in any way attenuates, weakens, or injures, or destroys the enamel of the teeth.

When we notice that the enamel is the part of the tooth first formed, or nearly so, that even before the young organ has passed the gums, it is firmly encased by a coat of mail, if I may use the expression, and when we consider that this coat is one of the most dense, hard and impenetrable animal substances known, that it is so hard as to give fire with the steel, we must consider that the wise author of nature, formed the tooth more for resisting great external violence, both chemical and mechanical, than for internal disease; and this with me is a strong argument in favor of the idea, that the causes of external caries are far more common in occurrence than those of internal.

Of these causes we notice all the strong acids which are sometimes very improperly used in cleaning the teeth, with a view of dissolving the tartar, and which are sometimes exhibited for medical purposes; these last should always be taken through a small tube, carried back so as to pass the teeth.

We should remark that all the strong acids act chemically upon the teeth, by corroding the enamel. All substances taken excessively hot or cold, may injure the teeth by impairing their vitality. The teeth by growing in a very crowded manner so as to overlap and press upon and against each other, and from this cause preventing the growth of the enamel, are rendered much more liable to be acted upon by the vitiated saliva, than those teeth which have free space to grow, and whose enamel is thick and strong.

I believe it is a common idea that separating the teeth with a file, is nearly as well as if they grew separate; but no greater mistake on the subject can be formed. Of this I shall speak more particularly hereafter.

All injudicious operations upon the teeth by the dentist, prove a most fruitful source of destruction to them. Such as improper filing, scraping, &c. of which I shall speak more particularly in another place. Improper ligatures used in fastening the teeth, or in confining artificial ones, often occasion caries of those teeth to which they are applied.

Improper or gritty dentifirices act upon the teeth, in weakening the enamel, and subjecting them to the action of the more immediate causes of superficial caries.

Too hard or improper tooth-brushes in some cases, seem to injure the teeth, especially young teeth. And in fine, all chemical and mechanical causes which act upon the teeth, so as to destroy their substance, enamel, &c. prove a cause indirectly of caries of the teeth, by rendering them much more liable to be acted upon by vitiated juices of the mouth.

The appearances of superficial caries are very various, both as regards its shape, colour and situation.

At times, the decay is confined to a small point, at others, it spreads superficially, like an irregular patch.

Often we notice a large internal cavity, with a small hole through the enamel; the reason of this is, that the bone of the tooth is much more liable to decay than the enamel, and after the caries has penetrated the enamel, it proceeds much more rapidly within the tooth than on the enamel.

Sometimes the front of the upper incisores and canine teeth, appear as if scooped out, as it were, by the process of decay, and also the sides of the jaw teeth, are often affected in the same manner.

Very often caries commences at those parts where the teeth are in contact with each other, because foreign matters are most easily retained there; and the enamel is much the thinnest, and for the same reason, it appears often in small cavities of the crowns of the grinding teeth, and near the necks of the teeth where the enamel becomes attenuated.

The various colours of caries make no practical difference in the practice for their cure, &c.

Internal caries, says Mr. Hunter, is detected by a peculiar shining black appearance from the dark caries being seen through the enamel, before it has proceeded so far as to break out of the external part of the tooth, as it is said always to do before it affects the nerve of the tooth.*

Inflammation and suppuration of the lining membrane do in some rare cases take place, of which some cases will be given; and when the tooth appears perfectly sound externally, the excessive pain occasioned by the matter collected in the cavity of the tooth, compels us to extract it to relieve the patient. It was proposed by Mr. Fox,† to bore into the tooth and discharge the matter; others deny its utility. The teeth are said in some cases to have been carious before they have passed through the gum. *See Koecker, page* 231.

The Proximate and Exciting Causes of Caries.

Having taken some notice of the commencement of caries, and of some of its remote and exciting causes, we will proceed into a more minute investigation of its proximate and exciting causes.

Mr. Fox observes,‡ "that the proximate cause of caries, appears to be an inflammation in the bone of the crown of the tooth, which on account of its peculiar structure, terminates in mortification."

Mr. Koecker observes,‖ that "Caries in fact, is that state of the tooth in which mortification has taken place in one part, and inflammation in the part contiguous to it; the former originally produced by the latter, and the latter kept up by continual contact with the former." This is so until the whole tooth has lost its vitality.

---

* See Hunter, page 137.
† See Fox, Part II. page 12.
‡ See Fox, Part II. page 12.
‖ See Koecker, page 210.

The reader will recollect with what assiduity, I have before endeavored to defend the doctrine of sensibility in the bony structure of the teeth; we now see how beautifully on those principles, the process and causes of caries are exposed and explained. In the remarks of Messrs. Fox and Koecker, I fully coincide, and am certain that caries of the teeth, is the result of inflammation in their bony structure, terminating in mortification. This is the pivot upon which all turns. To this all other causes are subordinate. The secretions of the mouth when in a vitiated state, are the grand and prominent causes of caries. They chemically dissolve and remove the enamel of the teeth, inflame the bony part which consequently mortifies in most cases, and is then dissolved by the same vitiated liquor. In some cases the dead part is not dissolved, and then the caries remains stationary, and does not progress with much rapidity, and in this state has been denominated by nearly all the old French writers,* "carie seche," and has been called by the vulgar among the English "Dry Rot." In many cases the mortified part is readily dissolved, or allows the vitiated juices to penetrate its texture, so as to keep up a constant irritation and inflamtion of the bony structure, and thereby the progress of the disease is greatly accelerated. The foregoing remarks lead us to the following conclusions upon this subject. First, any thing which prevents a perfect organization of the teeth in their growth, will render them much more susceptible of the exciting causes of caries, than if perfectly developed and perfectly organized; and hence we learn, why in many subjects, a crowded state of the teeth is often followed by caries. Secondly, any thing that weakens the vital powers of the teeth, renders them much more susceptible to the ex-

---

* See Fauchard, vol. i. page 146.

citing causes of caries, because slight irritation will induce inflammation, and this much more readily followed by mortication. Under this class we may rank all cases of hereditary carious affections of the teeth, that is as we often notice, the parents may have bad teeth, and those of their children will be notoriously so. It is well known to all physiologists and pathologists, that organic weakness may be transmitted from parents to their offspring; hence all the train of hereditary diseases which generally baffle medical aid.

Thirdly, all those agents which vitiate the secretions, or induce an irritable or inflammatory state of the system, will either become powerfully exciting causes of caries, or render the teeth greatly susceptible of deleterious impressions from all the exciting causes of caries. In this third class we find all gross and high livers, and especially the dispeptic, habitually affected by slow fever, which furs the tongue and vitiates the secretions of the stomach and mouth. As this state is almost peculiar to the refined and luxurious states of society, it is here we find caries most prevalent. Seldom is it noticed among the uncivilized societies of men, or those who have little access to all those articles of diet which vitiate the secretions and induce an inflammatory state of the system. It is but a few weeks since that I saw the family of an Oneida Chief at Saratoga. Upon inquiring into the state of their teeth I found that they were very much diseased in several individuals, and the wife of the chief informed me that diseased teeth were frequently met with among their people, but observed that it was not so with their ancestors; that her mother died at 90 years of age, and had never lost any of her second teeth. These facts are easily explained upon our foregoing principles. The ancient Indians of North America lived upon the most simple diet and used a great deal of exercise; war and hunting being their principal and almost only employment, whilst their diet, beside a few vegetables and maize, consisted of the precarious articles afforded by the chase. This state of society is, and ever has been highly conducive to health, or at least to the absence of febrile and dispeptic affections. The succeeding generations of these indians have become much less active, living upon a much more luxurious diet. They spend a great deal of their time in perfect indolence, and more especially indulging in the use of ardent spirits, which tend to produce disease in their tribes. I have been more particular in mentioning this instance, as its parallel is found with all the American people. Our ancestors enjoyed far better health than we do. Their diet, as a general rule, was much more simple, and with them there was an absence of nearly all the predisposing and exciting causes of caries. It is at this time a common observation that among the mass of the people in this country the teeth were much better 50 years ago than at present. This was not the case in Europe, as luxurious habits were formed there long before the settlement of this country. Fauchard says, that in his time it was rare to meet those who preserved their teeth to an advanced age.* On these principles we understand why, as persons advance in life, and the irritability of all the organs diminishes, that the teeth likewise feel the salutary change and are much less liable to become affected by caries. Mr. Hunter clearly expresses this fact in his remark† that " this disease," (caries) " and its consequences seem to be peculiar to youth and middle age; the shedding teeth are as subject to it, if not more so, than those intended to last through life: and we seldom or ever see

---

*Fauchard's preface, page 7. †See Hunter, Part II. page 141.

any person whose teeth begin to rot after the age of fifty years." In a ratio inverse to the age of the teeth are they affected by the predisposing, and susceptible to the exciting causes of caries: because, as they advance in age, the proportion of animal matter becomes less, and, consequently, the irritability of their bony structure is diminished. From this fact and our previous principles we understand why caries proceeds so rapidly in the teeth of children, so as often to destroy them in a few months. In this city we notice a vast many instances of diseased teeth in children, often nearly all their deciduous teeth are found carious; for this reason: that in general, their diet is gross, consisting of a great proportion of animal food, pastry, and all the thousand condiments used in our luxurious cookery. This usually generates, in nearly all children, an inflammatory diathesis. They are often attacked by febrile diseases. Their secretions are vitiated; mercurial medicines, which generally induce an inflammatory and irritable state of the system, are frequently exhibited, and finally, as if to complete the climax of causes, the teeth are neglected, and suffered, in a vast many cases, to be unclean, and the gums allowed to become diseased, inflamed, and often in a state of ulceration. All these constitutional and local causes, operating as we have before explained, act with tenfold violence upon the teeth at this tender age. All the causes, direct and indirect, of caries in the teeth of children, will be found to affect those of the youth and adult in the same ratio that we have before remarked. An inflammatory diathesis, accompanied with a vitiated state of the secretions, we have considered as forming at once a predisposing and exciting cause of caries. Hence we learn why pregnancy, by always, or nearly so, inducing an inflammatory and febrile state of the system, should be a period when the teeth of the female are extremely liable to be attacked by caries; or, if previously carious, that this should proceed with redoubled violence. Hence we understand why persons possessing a sickly and irritable state of their systems should be extremely liable to caries of their teeth.† I will not deny that many persons possessing good constitutions have bad teeth; yet in these cases we shall find some- of our before-mentioned causes acting locally upon the teeth and causing their destruction. On the other hand we sometimes notice persons having sickly constitutions, whose teeth are good, in these cases we shall find some of the exciting causes obviated, and the disease prevented. *Exceptió probat Regulam.* Caries itself, once commenced, is to a certain extent contagious, and proves a powerful excitant of caries. Upon our foregoing principles, we immediately learn why frequent attacks by acute or chronic febrile diseases, render the teeth liable to be affected by caries, and why frequent salivations, by inducing a general or local inflammatory state of the system, or of the mouth, and by vitiating the secretions of every part, are so apt to induce caries. On the contrary, we learn why a good constitution, with a perfect organization and developement of every part, why a plain, simple, and wholesome diet, free exercise in the open air, and an absence of febrile diseases, &c. &c. conduce so powerfully to render the teeth free from caries, and place the mouth in a healty state. The child of our luxurious citizens, may have bad teeth, yet it is not so with the chimney-sweepers' child who rarely tastes of any thing beyond a piece of bread, and whose clean and shining white teeth, form a striking contrast with his sooty face; and what confirms our doctrine to its fullest extent, is that coloured children, placed in the houses of the luxurious citizens, and living

---

†See Koecker, page 53, and following.

on a variety of rich food, are soon apt to have bad teeth, and grow up with their teeth, in a great many cases, as bad or worse than those of their masters' children. It is generally thought that our coloured population, have very fine and healthy teeth. The teeth of the negro are usually extremely well developed, and if by exercise and simple diet they preserve their systems in a healthy condition, free from febrile symptoms and a vitiated state of the secretions, these organs will be preserved in the greatest perfection. But, on the contrary, if their diet is gross, and they indulge in indolent or luxurious habits, and especially neglect cleaning the teeth, they in a vast many instances become diseased, and are often lost at an early age. I find that I am extending this subject much farther than I at first intended, but I consider that a correct knowledge of the manner in which caries takes place, and its predisposing and exciting causes, forms a key to Dental Surgery, and without which, all our conceptions of the diseases of the teeth, will be confused and unsatisfactory. I beg permission of the reader to recapitulate for one moment, the principal points upon which we have insisted in this section.

External Caries.

Proximate Cause.—Inflammation of the bony part of the tooth terminating in mortification, the enamel being previously removed by chemical or mechanical agents, or if it takes place where there is no enamel, then the gum removed by disease or mechanical agents.

Exciting Causes.—A vitiated state of the liquor of the mouth caused by vitiated secretions—a diseased state of the gums and soft parts—by caries of the teeth—by dead teeth and stumps—by a febrile state of the system—by the exhibition of mercurial medicines—by bad artificial teeth—by allowing the mouth and teeth to remain in an uncleanly state —by the presence of tartar.

Predisposing Causes.—An imperfect organization of the teeth, by which their perfect development is prevented, and the vital powers of their organic structure is weakened—a febrile and irritable state of the system—exhibition of mercurial medicines—attacks of inflammatory and nervous fevers—injudicious operations upon the teeth, as filing, scraping, &c.

In the detail of these causes, I have omitted the consideration of many particulars, but I know of none that may not be clearly explained upon our foregoing principles.

*Of External or Superficial Caries.**

External caries differs considerably from internal caries, particularly in its origin and remote causes. Each will therefore require a separate consideration.

Although external caries may be slower in its progress than the other, it is not less certain of producing ultimate destruction, and I am inclined to consider it of more frequent occurrence than internal caries, and consequently a source of at least, as serious apprehension.

All the teeth are quite as liable to this variety of caries, as they are to the other; but this not only extends its morbid action, like the former, to the crown, but also to the neck and roots of the teeth, whenever exposed to the ordinary causes of the disease. Although all parts of the crown and of the body of the teeth are liable to this disease, yet it is apt most frequently to commence at those sides which are in contact with the neighbouring teeth.

---

* Koecker, pages 219 to 222.

It never affects the extreme ends of the roots, but it is most frequently seen in them near the neck; and it generally attacks both the roots and the neck on those sides of the tooth which form the semicircle or arch of the jaw.

When it makes its first appearance on the surface of any part of the crown of the tooth which is covered with enamel, it generally presents itself as a very small speck, though sometimes as a large, round, or irregular spot.

After the removal of this irregular, broad, or round spot of caries with the file, it will be generally observed to have extended superficially only, and to have penetrated in this manner through a part of the whole enamel. It will next exhibit on the surface of the bony structure a small spot, similar to that sometimes observed on the enamel: whence in either case, it almost invariably proceeds, in a dircet line, towards the cavity of the tooth. This spot appears in some cases not larger than a point, although it may already have penetrated a third or even half of the bony structure of the affected side of the tooth.

On such parts as are not covered with enamel, the neck and roots of the tooth, for instance, the spot generally appears irregular, and extending across a considerable portion of the surface of the neck, having the appearance of a notch of an oblong form. The colour of carious spots may be white, grey, yellow, brown, or black; the specific appearance being presumed to depend upon the chemical influence of the external fluids on the diseased parts.

Sometimes the disease of the crown penetrates very nearly to the lining membrane of the tooth, before the mortified bony structure becomes sufficiently soft to allow the escape of the diseased matter, so as to form a cavity; but this is more rarely the case in the roots or neck, which are generally of a softer or more easily corroded nature. This state greatly depends upon the different proportion of the animal and earthy constituents of the bony structure of the tooth; and also on the chemical state of the saliva, which is naturally much influenced by the state of the other teeth and parts of the mouth, as well as by the general state of the health of the individual.

As the carious matter increases in its corrosive qualities, and the affected part becomes softer, the disease causes a cavity in the crown of the tooth, similar to that produced by internal caries; excepting that the cavity produced by the latter is generally large and round, whilst that produced by superficial caries is frequently narrow, like a tube.

When seated in the necks and roots of the teeth, caries rarely forms such a cavity, but extends itself on the surface, and becomes broad and more irregular in its progress, and sometimes in the neck of the tooth it has the appearance of undermining the enamel towards the crown, so as to form an oval or oblong cavity, ending in a point at each extremity, such as might be cut into it artificially, by a triangular file.

After the disease has penetrated through the enamel, its progress and effects, as well as symptoms, are precisely like those of deep-seated caries. It is subject to all the same general and local influences, with this difference, however, that such teeth as are affected by external caries being of a stronger original construction than such as are affected with deep-seated caries, they are acted upon more slowly than the latter; consequently, if we suppose that the diseased action of deep-seated caries requires from one to five years to penetrate through the bony structure of the tooth, and to destroy the life of its lining membrane, superficial caries may require from four to ten years: and the chemical destruction of a tooth, the death of which has been effected by the latter disease, will occupy a much longer time than that of the former.

This kind of caries sometimes advances so slowly in an originally strong tooth, and extends itself so little on the surface, that its progress may appear to be altogether arrested. Entire suspension of the malady, however, is impossible, as long as dead matter is allowed to remain in contact with the living structure ; although it may proceed so very slowly as to make its progress imperceptible for some time, it will, however, in the event, never fail to become evident on the accession of symptomatic inflammation, or of any other sufficient cause of irritation.

*Of the Symptoms of Simple Caries.**

The symptoms produced by simple caries, whether external or internal, depend upon the stage of the disease, and on the general and local causes by which the disease is disturbed and aggravated.

Caries, in its first stages, produces hardly any pain or inconvenience ; it is generally in the latter period only of its progress, when it has penetrated almost the whole side of a tooth, and nearly reached its nerve, that the bony part of the tooth becomes tender, and productive of some slight uneasiness.

The inconvenience, however, is so trifling, that it is disregarded, unless when exasperated by some cause of general or local irritation, which might produce symptomatic inflammation in the bony structure, through the medium of the lining membrane of the tooth. This state of more than ordi-

---

* Koecker, pages 227, 228.

nary irritation, however, always subsides after the removal of the temporary irritating cause.

Even at the time when the disease has penetrated the whole bony structure, and has exposed the nerve to many additional general and local causes of irritation, this delicate membrane may sometimes remain in that state for a considerable time, without producing any great inconvenience.

These symptoms, however, are often much aggravated by certain general and local causes, such as general diseases, especially inflammatory fevers of any kind, sudden and frequent changes of temperature from extreme heat to extreme cold, abuses in the application of active internal and external medicines, such as mercury, opium, acids, improper tooth-powders and tinctures, &c. as well as dental operations, such as filing, cutting, and stopping the teeth, &c.

*Of Internal or Deep-Seated Caries.**

Internal caries generally affects the parts between the enamel and lining membrane, but somewhat nearer to the former part of the tooth, on the surface of which, it is first observed from its giving the tooth a bluish hue. It becomes more evident by presenting the appearance of a blue mark, and afterwards a brown spot, till it shall have penetrated through the whole external bony structure and enamel, and become a cavity, either on the grinding or on one of the lateral surfaces.

The orifice of this cavity is at first very narrow; but it increases in time externally, in the same proportion as the caries extends itself in the cavity. This disease as far as my

---

* Koecker, page 222 to 227.

experience has enabled me to judge, always attacks the crown of the tooth, and never the neck or the root.

As the disease is more actively resisted by the greater vascularity, and consequent activity of the internal bony structure, than by the harder and less vital external parts of the tooth, it never proceeds so far towards the cavity containing the nerve, as to render this membrane altogether unprotected by the bony structure, before it has penetrated through the external osseous part including the enamel, and has thus formed a natural outlet for the bony abscess.

Mr. Fox and other writers assert, that they have seen caries sometimes produce idiopathic inflammation in the living membrane, and the death of the tooth, before the disease has penetrated through the external surface of the crown; but I am perfectly assured of the contrary, because it is in opposition to the principles of that chemical action, to which the tooth is exposed, when affected by this disease, and against all accurate observation and experience. *See Fox's. Nat. Hist. &c. Part II. page* 14.

The cases which have given rise to this opinion, have not been considered with sufficient accuracy; this has arisen either from the difficulty of discovering the carious cavity, or from erroneously attributing the death of the tooth to the effect of caries, when it has been produced, perhaps by some mechanical irritation, an accidental blow, clumsy operation, or great irregularity in the situation of a tooth, &c.; in consequence of which, an inflammation and mortification of the membrane has taken place before its extraction.

I have already explained the great difference in the effect produced by the chemical influence of dead or carious matter upon the living bony structure, and that upon a tooth already destitute of life; a fact, however, totally disregarded, and therefore productive of the most injurious mal-practices in the treatment of this disease.

Putrefaction acting upon a dead tooth, destroys the bone by immediate chemical action, and produces a direct change from a state of mortification to that of putrefaction. It therefore naturally finds the greatest resistance in the hardest and least vascular parts of the tooth.

But putrefaction in the form of caries of a living tooth, destroys the bony parts, with which it is placed in immediate contact, in an indirect manner, producing by its chemical irritation, in the first place, inflammation, and afterwards mortification. It is in this instance, therefore, much more actively resisted in its destructive influence by the vascular than by the hard parts of the tooth. Consequently as the bony structure of the tooth is more vascular the nearer it is to the lining membrane, and harder and more compact the nearer it is to the enamel; and, therefore, endued in proportion to its vascularity, with a greater or less power of resisting inflammation; the diseased action of caries, will proceed more rapidly towards the exterior, than towards the interior of a tooth, and invariably produce an outlet at some part of its surface, before it can come in contact with its lining membrane.

Although the enamel of the tooth, from its not being organized, is not subject to the immediate influence of inflammation; and although, from its crystaline nature, it is also most admirably calculated to resist putrefaction and other chemical influences; it is nevertheless, from its peculiar structure, easily destroyed by mechanical causes when once deprived of the support of its bony structure; consequently, where caries has destroyed that support, it is soon removed by mastication, and an external orifice to the carious cavity is thus produced.

When the disease has thus made itself an outlet, through

the bony structure and enamel, its progress towards the lining membrane, is at this time somewhat-retarded by the free evaporation of the putrid vapour, and the partial discharge and separation of the dead matter; it is however soon afterwards exasperated by other exciting causes, viz. the additional external chemical and mechanical influences.

The caries now proceeds towards the cavity, more or less speedily according to the constitutional strength of the tooth, and violence of the general and local causes; until, at last, the disease penetrates through the whole bony structure, and produces considerable irritation upon the lining membrane, so as to involve that important and exquisitely sensible structure in idiopathic inflammation. At this period the disease may properly be called complicated caries.

The degree of rapidity of the destructive progress of deep-seated caries, depends upon the constitutional strength of the affected tooth, and on the degree of violence of the general and local exciting causes, which act simultaneously in aggravating the disease.

Internal caries, however, proceeds much more rapidly than external; and it may be said to be generally from one to five years from the commencement of its corroding process, to penetrate through the whole bony structure, and from three to twenty-four months afterwards, before the destruction of the vitality of the lining membrane of the tooth is totally affected; putrefaction and absorption however may still require from seven to fifteen years, to complete the entire destruction and removal of the dead parts.

Simple caries, in each of its forms, differs in its effect on the temporary teeth, from that on the permanent set, only in proportion to their less dense and less durable construction, and requires no separate consideration, except in the surgical treatment.

*Of Complicated Caries, or Caries accompanied by Disease in the Lining Membrane of the Tooth.**

When either external or internal caries has penetrated the bony structure as far as the natural cavity of the tooth, the lining membrane becomes inflamed and diseased. In this state the disease may be called complicated caries, as the tooth is affected not only by the caries of the bony structure, but also by inflammation of the lining membrane.

Instead of being resisted in its progress by the healthy action of this membrane, the caries is now aggravated by its diseased state; and this caries by its greater extent, becomes a greater exciting cause of inflammation in the nerve. The tooth being thus subjected to the influence of these two distinct diseases, which are rapidly advancing to their final crisis, viz. suppuration of the internal membrane, now soon loses its vitality.

For a just understanding and a judicious treatment of complicated caries, this disease requires to be minutely observed during its progress in every stage, and its different causes and effects, as well as symptoms and appearances very perfectly understood. In this state the disease differs somewhat in appearance from simple caries; the tooth so affected has generally an opaque appearance all over the surface of the enamel. This however is not easily distinguished, except by the very experienced dentist.

When the disease in its first stage has penetrated into the interior, and destroyed the vitality of the bony structure, the osseous parts although dead retain their hard and dry state for a long time. Although the lining membrane is then slight-

* Koecker, pages 236 to 239.

ly irritated by the contagion of these dead parts, yet it is at the same time protected by them from several irritating causes; and although some increased action may be produced in this membrane, yet it remains sometimes apparently free from disease for a long period; and may be considered as only in a state of mordid predisposition.

In the second stage when the disease has produced a greater extension of the carious cavity, and consequently the admission of a greater quantity of corroding matter, the dead bony parts in the neighbourhood of the nerve gradually become softer, and this membrane is more irritated, and rendered more liable to inflammation from the application of any chemical, mechanical, or other cause.

Still, in this state, the living membrane may frequently recover from such inflammation, and resist the local irritation arising from the contact of the dead bony matter, exposure to the saliva, or atmospheric changes for a considerable time, if the disease is not aggravated by causes of extraordinary violence.

But when the disease has reached its third stage by the great violence and long continuance of the influence of the general and local causes, and the repeated return of the inflammation and suppuration of the nerve, the disease is fast approaching its fatal termination, namely, the total destruction of the lining membrane, and consequent loss of vitality of the tooth itself; the dead bony structure of which is then left to be destroyed either by chemical solution, putrefaction, or absorption.

The rapidity, therefore, of the transition from one stage to another in complicated caries, depends greatly on the degree of violence of its causes, and its progress is not always so rapid as is generally supposed, for a period from three to twenty-four months is required by it to destroy the vitality of the lining membrane and bony structure of the tooth, although this progress is much more rapid in the temporary, than in the permanent teeth, and may sometimes be greatly accelerated by accidental or artificial causes; such as, falls, blows, acids, caustics, the actual cautery, and surgical operations; all of which might be considered as likely to be no less violent in their future morbid effects, than they are rapid in destroying the vitality of the tooth.

*Of the Symptoms of Complicated Caries.**

The symptoms of complicated caries, like those of simple caries, differ according to the state of the malady, and the violence of the local and general causes by which the nerve of the tooth is irritated.

In its first stage the disease seldom produces so much inflammation in the lining membrane as to render it very painful, and its effect is generally no more than a slight irritation or hard pressure, on exposure to heat or cold, as real toothache is very rarely found to result from the disease in this stage.

The symptoms of the second stage differ from those of the first only in the degree of their violence and frequency. The pressure of a blunt probe will produce more or less pain, and the slightest external or general irritation, arising, for instance, from heat or cold, or acids, or indigestion, or a little more wine than usual, may bring on a violent fit of the toothache; but when the inflammation in the lining membrane

* Koecker, pages 240 to 245.

subsides, the tooth-ache generally ceases, and the tooth will be quite free from pain or uneasiness, until the inflammation is produced again by the same, or similar causes.

When the disease has arrived at its third and last stage, that is, when the whole lining membrane is inflamed and proceeding to suppuration, it is exquisitely painful, and the symptoms are then very violent, and sometimes very alarming.

Inflammation now increases in one, and suppuration follows in the other part of the nerve of the tooth, and the pain and morbid action are constantly excited, not only by the previous causes but also by the suppurated matter of the diseased parts; which as it cannot be discharged like that formed in other soft parts, so as to afford relief, continues a constant cause of irritation and rapid destruction.

The disease, therefore, proceeds, constantly changing from acute to chronic inflammation, and vice versa, accompanied by more or less pain in the whole affected tooth.

At this period, the teeth nearest to the diseased tooth, and sometimes those of one or both sides of the same jaw, are symptomatically affected, and rendered almost as painful as the one primarily diseased.

The symptomatic inflammation frequently extends not only to the gums, periosteum, alveoli, and maxillary bones, but also to parts more or less distant; such as the eyes, ears, and throat, and sometimes the digestive organs, as well as the whole nervous system, are symptomatically affected; the latter to such a degree, as almost to produce madness, on which account the French have given the acute state of tooth-ache the appropriate term of "une rage de dens."

When the disease has continued to rage in this manner for some time, and the suppuration has carried off the principal part of the lining membrane, its powers become partly exhausted, and it returns into the chronic state, without interruption of the diseased action, and with little pain, until it has destroyed the principal part of the lining membrane, and afterwards the small fibres which pass through the root. The tooth is then deprived of all its vital principles, and the death of the bony structure follows.

The symptoms, however, which have been just described, are not always present, and some teeth are more subject to them than others.

The upper cutting teeth, for example, may be observed to be under the influence of simple and complicated caries in all their different stages, without being in the least painful; and the incisors and cuspidati of both jaws may be considered in general, to be less subject to the above painful symptoms, than the bicuspidati and the molares; and even in these last these symptoms may also never appear, in consequence of the disease remaining in an uninterrupted chronic state. The pain may also be prevented by the sudden death of the lining membrane of the tooth from some accidental or artificial cause, as has been before mentioned.

Hence it frequently happens that one or more teeth may, lose their vitality by the ravages of complicated caries without giving the individuals any warning of their perilous state; whilst in other cases the most painful and alarming symptoms are experienced. Though this fact may seem very surprising, it may, nevertheless, be well accounted for in every instance, by a particular inquiry into the nature of the disease.

If caries, for instance, is left entirely to its own course and natural influences, and not aggravated by general and local causes, its progress is generally regular and chronic.

During its progress through the bony structure, it produces by its ordinary chemical action, a constant change from chronic inflammation to mortification, until it comes in contact with the living membrane, when the same regular diseased action produces that gradual chronic inflammation and almost imperceptible suppuration, which gradually destroys the soft parts, without any particularly painful symptoms.

When, at a later period, many teeth are carious at the same time, and the other parts of the mouth are in a more or less diseased state; or when, by accident or injudicious treatment, many diseases are produced in the teeth and their relative parts, it also frequently happens that no tooth-ache is produced, although perhaps one tooth is lost very soon after another; and thus, by the constant counter irritation which is produced by one diseased part upon another, all are kept in a state of constant disease of a chronic kind; while at the same time the tender state of all parts of the mouth obliges the patient to be perpetually on his guard, to avoid accidental irritations, which might produce acute inflammation.

And even if it should happen that acute inflammation should arise from some temporary exciting cause, such as fever, derangement of the digestive organs, pregnancy, or suckling, cold, or other external irritation, it will frequently be of short duration, and both the inflammation and the pain will be confined either to one tooth only, or, as is most frequently the case, to the parts more or less related to the teeth; and the general state of the mouth will soon change to its chronic state again, and the. tooth-ache or pain will cease.

In consequence of this long duration and slow progress of these chronic maladies, and the apparently small inconveniences produced by the diseased nerve, or lining membrane of the tooth, complicated caries is, frequently, altogether overlooked; the pain being considered as a symptom of general disease, or of some remote morbid cause; and the temporary exciting causes of the change from the chronic to the acute state of the disease, such as have been just mentioned, are frequently considered the original and proximate causes of the painful symptoms.

This mistaken notion frequently leads to an entire neglect, not only of the proper treatment, but also of the necessary regular attention to cleanliness.

The individual, supposing the teeth to be secondarily affected only, under a constant apprehension of disturbing them too soon, puts off this attention until the tender state of his mouth shall have been cured by the removal of the mistaken cause. In consequence of this removal not being effected, the disease, together with the tenderness of the affected tooth is constanly increasing; much tartar is deposited, and a diseased state of the gums is produced, by which the breath is rendered very offensive; effects productive of no little inconvenience, and excitement of the diseased action in the parts affected, as well as of the general system.

This morbid state of the mouth, which would be more distressing, were it to seize upon the patient suddenly, is, from its supposed insignificant origin and slow progress, sometimes supported by habit, and even left altogether unobserved; and often while the individual considers himself in a state of tolerable local and general health, he is under the influence of many disgusting diseases, which are not only destroying the teeth, but impairing the constitution: and which, with any other unexpected general disease are likely to become the means of a premature death.

Surgical Treatment of Caries.

Having now considered, in a very brief manner, the most common phenomena of caries, and having briefly mentioned its causes and symptoms, we now proceed to a particular consideration of the surgical treatment necessary and proper for its cure, whilst the treatment of sound teeth, and the means of preventing their decay, and the means proper for preserving them in a healthy state, will be the subject of a separate chapter. First,

The Treatment of Simple Caries.

This we defined to be a decay of the teeth, commencing externally and gradually, proceeding to the internal cavity of the tooth. In its progress discolouring the tooth, producing a mortification of the affected part, by which means the substance of the tooth, in some degree, is removed, and continues to be so, until the lining membrane becomes affected, and finally inflammation of it takes place in a great many instances; producing that most distressing affection, the tooth-ache, called emphatically by the French, "une rage de dens." If the disease itself does not produce the tooth-ache, still it exposes the tooth to be acted upon by external causes which do produce it.

If the teeth are not extracted during the inflammation of the membrane, in consequence of the patient not being able or willing to endure the pain of their extraction, then, I say, the inflammation changes from the acute to the chronic form, and in this state the tooth may remain for some time, until by repeated changes from acute to chronic inflammation, and vice versa, the lining membrane and nerve lose their vitality, the crown of the tooth changes its colour from a yellowish white to a peculiar dark bluish, while all the internal cavity of the tooth usually becomes entirely decayed.

The enamel resists the process longest, and is often seen a mere shell and form of a tooth, having an opening when the caries first commenced until, at last, by some slight accident in mastication, the remaining shell of the tooth is broken, and the fang or fangs of it are left in their sockets. As the fangs of the teeth are nourished by the blood-vessels of the gums externally, and the blood-vessels of the lining membrane internally, if support from the last is lost, still if the gums are in a healthy state, the fangs will often live many years; but if the gums are in a diseased state, the stumps of the teeth soon die, and become a source of great injury to the other teeth, if any remain. In the progress of this disease, from the first commencement of caries until the tooth is destroyed, we notice, for the sake of clearly understanding the surgical treatment, four stages of the disease, which require distinct treatment and a separate notice.

First, The simple abrasion and decay of some part of the enamel, and often a destruction of a small portion of the substance of the tooth beneath the decayed portion of the enamel.

A perfect cure of the tooth in this stage of the disease, may be made by skilfully filing away all the diseased portion of the tooth, so that not the least vestige of decay shall be left. This operation is one of no small importance, and should be skilfully and effectually performed to be of service to the diseased tooth, for if any part of the decay is left, it usually proceeds until the tooth is destroyed, or farther operations for its cure are rendered necessary. I could, in this case, mention many cases, both from the works of others and my own experience, of the perfect success and great utility of this operation, when well performed, but of this I shall speak particularly when I come to notice the operation of filing the teeth, its utility, and the indications for its performance, and the great injury of its injudicious performance, which will be considered in a separate section hereafter.

The second stage in the progress of superficial caries, is after the decay has passed through the enamel, and has produced some destruction in the bony substance of the tooth, between the lining membrane and the enamel, but not so far as to affect or implicate the lining membrane. The surgical treatment and cure, in this case, consists in cleaning or cutting out all the decayed portion of the tooth, and filling the cavity with some metallic substance, as gold, silver, tin, or lead, and a complete cure in this way may be obtained. This operation, if well done, and the cavity filled with a suitable substance, I believe I may venture to assert, is one of the most effectual ever performed in surgery. The cure obtained by it, if properly done, &c. is perfect, and the tooth becomes as sound as it ever was, with the exception of the loss of some part of its substance.

The proper manner of performing this operation, and the substance most proper for filling the cavity of the tooth caused by the decay, and its great utility, if well done, will form the subject of a separate section in the operative part of this work.

The third stage in the progress of simple caries which we notice, is when it has proceeded so far as to implicate the lining membrane and nerve of the tooth, in many instances producing the tooth-ache, by exposing the nerve to the action of those irritating causes which bring on inflammation of the lining membrane. I shall not, in this chapter, take up the consideration of odontalgia, (tooth-ache) but continue the consideration of the diseased tooth and its membrane, and leave the consideration of odontalgia hereafter.

After caries has proceeded so far as to expose the lining membrane, before the surgeon dentist is required to operate upon the tooth, we need not despair of curing the tooth, but in most cases we shall most probably succeed, if proper means are used.

We can always ascertain that the tooth is carious, and the situation of the caries, by examination.

Of the Treatment of complicated caries, or the third stage in the progress of caries.

Nothing can be more unsurgical in the treatment of decayed teeth in this stage, than that proposed by Mr. Hunter, who says, if pain comes on, the tooth, and especially the grinders, may be extracted and boiled, and then returned to the socket; when, he says, it will sometimes grow and be useful, being a more certain way of killing the tooth than to burn the nerve.* Mr. Fox mentions no correct surgical treatment of the tooth in this situation, save that, if the cavity is merely irritable it may be washed with a solution of lunar caustic, and then plugged; this often, I think, will save the tooth. Mr. Koecker† recommends covering the nerve with a plate of lead, and then filling the cavity with gold; this may answer in some cases, but in many, I believe, this plan too will fail, especially in plugging the grinding teeth; yet still it will, no doubt, often succeed. A practice which, I believe, was first proposed and practised by Mr. Harrington of this city, a respectable operating Dentist, is, to fill the cavity with some

*See Hunter on the teeth, pages, 148, 149. †Koecker, page 437.

powerfully astringent substance, as the soft inside of the nut-gall; this, by a gradual operation, hardens and obtunds the nerve until we are enabled to plug the tooth without exciting inflammation, which is the great danger in all cases of plugging teeth, having their nerves exposed. The gall should be carefully introduced, and a little wax put on its outside, so as to keep it in and exclude the external air: it is necessary sometimes to use the gall for some months before the irritability of the nerve is abated, so as to bear the plug without inflammation succeeding. By the two last mentioned methods we are most generally enabled to effectually cure the tooth, and preserve its vitality.

Destroying the nerve of the tooth is sometimes done by the use of caustics, strong acids, &c. but we at the same time destroy the vitality of the crown of the tooth, which causes it to lose its colour, and eventually to be lost or prove offensive to the mouth; and yet, in some rare cases, when great pain is present, and our only choice is to extract the tooth, or destroy the nerve, we may prefer the latter, and use the actual cautery (a hot iron) lunar caustic, nitric, muriatic, or sulphuric acids, caustic potash, or any caustic we choose, and after this, plug the tooth. But it is only as a dernier resort that I would ever think of destroying the nerve of the tooth; yet, in some cases, it seems to be more advisable than to extract the tooth. The peculiar circumstances which must determine either to the extraction of the tooth, or the destruction of its nerve, are very much influenced by the feelings of the patient, which may sometimes determine one way, and at other times the other. A tooth may be extremely useful in consequence of its being wanted to support artificial teeth, and we would rather destroy the nerve of the tooth than extract it.

The fourth stage of caries is after it has so long exposed

the nerve as, by frequent inflammation, acute and chronic, to cause its death. In this case, if the tooth retains its strength and stability to a considerable extent, and its root is sound, so as to be useful, as it may be in some cases, we may plug it, and it will often be useful for many years.

Deep-Seated Caries, or Caries proceeding from Internal Disease.

I am not aware that any author mentions any treatment for the cure of this disease, different from that of simple caries, nor do I know that any treatment is necessary, but after the bony abscess has burst out, as Mr. Koecker says it always will before it affects the membrane; but Mr. Fox says it affects in some cases the nerve before it appears outwardly. I leave the decision to others, for my part I do not think that deep-seated caries, occurs in more than one case of one thousand diseased teeth. The cure is the same as any caries, that of cleaning out the cavity, and if sufficiently deep, to plug it with gold.

To complete the subject of the treatment of carious teeth in general, I remark, that if the crowns of the grinding teeth, are so much decayed, as not to admit of a cure by the use of a plug, &c. they should be extracted; for if left, they usually exert a most baneful influence upon the remaining sound teeth, and upon the breath and health of the individual; and if the stumps of the front teeth are so far decayed as not to be useful, or if they affect the breath, health, &c. they should be extracted.

SECTION II.

OF EXOSTOSIS OF THE FANGS.*

One of the species of exostosis in bones is an enlargement arising from a deposit of bony matter, so compact in its structure, as very much to resemble ivory. This is that kind of enlargement to which the fangs of the teeth of some persons are liable.

The cause of this disease is obscure, and the slow increase in the size of the fang, is the reason why pain does not occur until a considerable augmentation of its bulk has taken place.

It is sometimes found to exist where the crowns of the teeth remain perfectly sound; in other cases, it appears to be the effect of indolent inflammation, arising from caries in the body of the tooth, and extending to the fang. This kind of disease does not produce suppuration; the gum continues quite healthy; but whenever pain occurs, as no permanent relief can be obtained without the extraction of the tooth, it becomes necessary, when the teeth are sound, to be very attentive to distinguish this disease from mere rheumatic affections of the jaw bones.

I extracted two teeth, the first molaris of each side of the lower jaw, from a lady, who had complained for a considerable length of time, of pain on both sides of the face, arising from each of these teeth. She described her symptoms to be a constant uneasiness, like the gnawing sensation of rheumatism, which continuing almost without intermission, exhausted her health and spirits. The

* Fox, Part II. pages 42 to 50.

teeth and gums were quite free from any diseased appearance, the pain, therefore, was considered as rheumatic; she had taken much medicine, and continued under the care of an eminent practitioner for a considerable length of time, without receiving any benefit. The gums were lanced, blisters were applied behind the ears, but all means were ineffectual; she at length determined to have both the teeth extracted. This was reluctantly performed, because they appeared perfectly free from disease.

When one tooth was removed, the cause of her complaint became evident, for the whole surface of the fangs was increased in size by the irregular addition of a quantity of bony matter. This induced me to comply with her wish of removing the other, which had precisely the same appearance. The cause of her pain now became certain; the increase in the size of the fangs, necessarily occasioned a distention of the alveolar cavity, and kept up a constant uneasiness. The lady was immediately relieved, and recovered her health and spirits, to the great joy of her family, who were nearly deprived of her society by reason of her excessive nervous irritability.

Where the disease has occured in teeth already carious, the persons have not been afflicted with extreme tooth-ache, but they have had occasional uneasiness, which at length has become more uninterrupted, and the tooth has projected to a certain degree from the socket, so that in closing the mouth, the tooth felt as if out of its natural situation, thus rendering mastication painful. When extracted, the fangs have been found enlarged.

Some persons will refer this appearance upon the fangs of the teeth to an original mal-formation; but so different is it in appearance from the smooth structure of any ill-formed, crooked, or diseased tooth; and when extracted, so much whiter than any other part of the fang; that it can only be referred to diseased action, occasioning a deposit of bony matter, as in other cases of exostosis.

Of this disease of the teeth, the most extraordinary case on record occurred to a young lady, scarcely twenty years of age. The following letter, from the surgeon who had attended the lady, and by whom she was introduced to me, presents a full narrative of the case.

Sir, Nov. 9th, 1809.

Miss ——, the young lady, who will deliver this to you, has been under my care for near twelve months with a very extraordinary complaint in her face, teeth, and gums. It commenced with a deep-seated pain in the face, confined principally to one side, returning most mornings at about eleven o'clock, and continuing several hours. This had gone on for near three months before she or her friends, thought it sufficiently serious to call in any medical assistance. When I first saw her, she had suffered great pain all that day, from the teeth, gums and face; on one side the gums were rather swollen and inflamed; and as one of the teeth was slightly decayed, I thought it most advisable to extract it, which gave relief till the next day, when the pain returned with still greater violence, so much so, that she was desirous of having the adjoining tooth taken out, which she fancied gave her more pain than the rest. This had the same effect as the other, only giving relief till the next day, when the pain returned with equal violence. I then tried scarifying the gums, cold lotions to the face, giving at the same time a brisk purgative and afterwards an opiate. This was continued for a short time without abating the pain, I then changed the plan for the more soothing one of fomentation and poultice, applying a fig to the gums, occasionally changing it for a crust of bread soaked in warm milk, taking at the same time a saline and opiate draught every four hours, but with just the same effect as the preceding remedies. In short, the pain in the teeth and face, the gums became partially ulcerated, and in the course of six months, I was under the necessity of extracting, at different times all the teeth in the lower jaw, excepting the four incisors, which very soon became affected in a similar way to the rest; these her friends would not allow to be drawn, nor was I anxious of performing the operation, as the removal of the others did not appear to give any permanent relief, excepting that the gums healed, and remained well where the teeth had been extracted. During this time, almost every remedy that could be thought of was tried, such as frequent scarifying of the gums, leeches, permanent blisters to the lower jaw and behind the ears, astringent lotions, as the infusion of roses with the tincture of myrrh, decoctions of bark, oak bark, infusion of galls, solutions of alum, argentum nitratum, salt and water, lemon-juice, oxymel æruginis, borax, charcoal and soda, tepid-bath, artificial sea-bath, and afterwards sea-bathing, seton in the neck, issue in the arm, &c. &c. with a great many other applications, which it would be useless to name. Internally she had taken strong purgatives, calomel combined with antimony, and afterwards continued alone in small doses to salivation, solutio mineral, solut. calc. muriat. bark, with nitrous acid, steel, lemon-juice in large quantity, tinc. opii. to the amount of qut. 60 at bed time, and repeated in small doses during the day at short intervals, cicuta, &c. &c. prescribed by an eminent physician in this place, without receiving little more than slight temporary relief from any one medicine prescribed. She has now all the teeth of the upper jaw, in a similar way to the lower; the palpebræ of one eye has been closed for near two months, and when opened, can discern objects but very imperfectly; the secretion of saliva has for some time been so copious as to flow from the mouth whenever opened. She is now come to London, purposely for advice, and I have recommended that she should call upon you.

I remain, Sir, your obedient servant,

T. S.

This letter not only fully describes the very afflicting case, but also shows that medicine under every form had altogether failed; of course no benefit could be expected from a repetition of any similar treatment.

At the time I saw the lady she was only able to take fluid nutriment; for the teeth of the upper jaw were so very tender, that the slightest touch caused extreme pain. As described by Mr. S. the flow of saliva was so considerable that, there was a continual necessity of discharging it. The lady herself said, she was assured she should never get well, unless all her teeth were extracted. I was however desired, if possible, to seek such relief as should prevent so painful an expedient, which should only be regarded as the last resort.

Dr. Babington and Mr. Cline were consulted, who prescribed a blister on the head, to be kept open by the application of the ceratum sabinæ. This was tried without success. The pain in the mouth, the soreness of the teeth, and the general irritation on the constitution, all combined to render the extraction of the most painful tooth advisable. This was the first molaris of the upper jaw, situated under that eye, the palpebræ of which had become closed.

The fangs of this tooth were much enlarged, and from the periosteum being greatly thickened, the fangs had the appearance of being cartilaginous. The removal of this tooth was attended with great benefit: as, in two days after the operation, the affected eyelids so much recovered as to open simultaneously with those of the other eye. This relief unhappily, was of short duration; and as the other teeth remained very sore, the lady determined to have them extracted one after another. She submitted to this operation every two or three days. The fangs of those teeth which had caused the most pain, were the most enlarged; but each partook of the disposition to exostosis.

The relief from pain which was experienced by the loss of the teeth was so great, that, with the utmost resolution, this afflicted lady persevered until every tooth was extracted.

After the loss of the teeth, from time to time, portions of the alveolar processes exfoliated, which rendered it necessary to scarify the gums: I am happy to say, that a material improvement has taken place in the general health, although not so perfectly as could be desired. One most important benefit resulted from the removal of the teeth, in arresting the progress of the other diseased actions; for the other eye had begun to be affected, and sometimes was so dim, as scarcely to enable the lady to guide herself about the house. In point of appearance, however, I had the satisfaction of completely restoring the lady; the teeth which had been extracted were replaced, as an artificial set, which with the greatest comfort, she has now used for more than twelve months.

SECTION III.

OF NECROSIS AFFECTING THE TEETH.*

When a bone, or part of a bone, has completely lost its living principle, it is precisely in the same state as soft parts when affected by gangrene; no restoration of the part can be effected; the surrounding parts become inflamed, and an action takes place which has for its object the separation of the dead from the living part. When the fang of a tooth has lost its life, the whole of the tooth becomes, in consequence, an extraneous body; and, as in bones, the cure of necrosis depends upon the exfoliation of the dead piece, so in the case of the tooth, the cure can alone be effected by its entire removal.

This disease usually affects teeth which are perfectly free from caries; and it is more particularly confined to the front teeth, the others being rarely affected in this way. When the fang of a tooth has lost its living principle, the socket becomes inflamed, the gum appears of a darkish red colour, loose in its texture, and matter begins to be discharged. In some, the discharge is from two or three orifices through the gums, opposite to the extremity, or the middle of the fang of the tooth; in other cases, the matter passes out at the neck of the tooth. In all there is an uneasy pain, and the discharge of the matter is very disagreeable.

During the progress of this disease, the alveolar processes are absorbed, and the teeth are loosened, from which great inconvenience arises.

---

* Natural History and Diseases of the Human Teeth, by J. Fox, pages 50 to 52, London, 1814.

In the early stage of this disease, considerable benefit attends the scarification of the gums; the loss of blood abates the inflammation; and, as it is very unpleasant to lose a front tooth, we may, by repeatedly lancing the gums, arrest the progress of the disease for a considerable time; but, when it has proceeded so far as to loosen the tooth, it is better to extract it, especially as the whole of the uneasiness arises from the tooth being an extraneous body; the discharge then ceases, and the gum becomes perfectly healed in a short time. After extraction, the fang of the tooth is always found to be very rough; in most cases, it is dark coloured, being of a deep green, brown, or black colour.

*Of the disease resembling Spina Ventosa.**

Spina Ventosa is the term usually given to that species of tumour in bone, which is originally an abscess forming in the centre: the ulcerative process removing the bone from the inside, whilst there is a corresponding increase on the outside.

This disease, according to my observation, is confined to the incisors and cuspidati of the upper jaw; as it produces upon the gum and socket similar effects to the disease last described. The seat of the malady is in the cavity of the tooth; the vessels ramifying on its membrane acquire a diseased action, by which the membrane becomes thickened, absorption of some of the internal parts of the tooth takes place, and the opening at the extremity of the fang also becomes enlarged. This disease of the membrane is attended

* Natural History and diseases of the human Teeth, by J. Fox. Pages 52 to 54. London, 1814.

with the formation of matter discharging itself at the point of the fang into the alveolar cavity, which, being rendered more porous by the process of absorption, affords an easy exit. During the progress of the disease, the gum covering the alveolar process becomes inflamed, and acquires a spongy texture; the matter passing from the socket makes its escape into the mouth by several openings through the gum, which is thus kept in a constant state of disease. The discharge, which is generally considerable, produces great fetor of the breath, the taste is constantly affected, and the socket is gradually absorbed until the tooth becomes quite loose.

When the tooth has been extracted, I have usually found the membrane sprouting at the end of the fang, the internal part of which is much enlarged, and the external part has a rough, scaly appearance; also, during the progress of this disease, the body of the tooth changes in appearance, and gradually acquires a dark colour.

The only treatment which can be observed here, is to scarify the gums occasionally, and to wash the mouth frequently with an astringent lotion; for this purpose, the infusion of roses with tincture of myrrh is very beneficial. As no cure of this complaint can be expected, the extraction of the tooth should be recommended as soon as the gums have acquired a truly diseased appearance; for, if the disease be allowed to take its natural course, the gums become so extensively affected as to induce absorption of the alveolar processes belonging to the neighbouring teeth, which is followed by their consequent loss.

SECTION IV.

*Of the removal of the enamel by the denuding process.**

This is a disease producing a change in the teeth, by which they acquire an appearance unlike that of caries, but attended with a loss of substance.

The tooth does not, as in caries, become softer, nor, like that disease, does it originate in inflammation, but it consists in a removal of the enamel from the bone of the tooth, as if by solution and gradual abrasion.

It affects the incisors much more frequently than any other teeth, and, in all the cases which I have seen, its operation is limited to the exterior surface of the teeth.

The first appearance is in the enamel of one or more of the incisors becoming thicker, and appearing as if a small portion had been scooped or filed out, occasioning a slight depression. This removal of the enamel continues until so much is taken away as to leave the bone exposed: as this denuding process, according to Mr. Hunter's term, advances, the tooth changes in its colour, gradually becoming yellower, as the bony part is more exposed. When the whole of the enamel is destroyed, part of the bone is also removed; the remainder acquires a brownish hue, is very highly polished, and will often remain in this state for a number of years.

I have seen a few cases in which the teeth have been so much wasted, as to have all the anterior part removed; but yet the natural cavity has not been exposed, for the bone has remained in a prominent line, as if it were defending that particular part, and thus preventing pain.

---

*Fox, pages 54 to 56.

Sometimes teeth thus affected become tender, very susceptible of cold, and are made uneasy by the use of acids.

I am not able to assign any cause for this loss of the enamel and part of the substance of the tooth, especially as it is confined to that portion of the teeth which could not be acted upon by the friction of one tooth against another. I have observed it both in healthy and delicate persons. As it appears to be connected with some cause which may produce a solution of the enamel, it is very possible that the saliva may have some influence, and that the friction of the lips may contribute to the removal of the enamel.

The only means to prevent a rapid progress of this disease, is to avoid whatever may contribute to it; therefore, as all acids act powerfully upon the teeth, their use as an article of diet should be forbidden; and, whenever there is any necessity for employing a medicine which contains an acid, persons should be extremely careful to rince the mouth, and wipe the teeth immediately afterwards with a cloth.

SECTION V.

OF THE WEARING OF THE TEETH BY MASTICATION.*

The mouths of some persons are so constructed, and the teeth so placed, that when the jaws are closed, the incisors not being so long as they usually are, meet each other at the cutting edges. Thus a variety is formed from the usual mode, which is, for the incisors of the upper jaw, when the mouth is closed, partially to overlap those of the under jaw.

---

* Natural History and Diseases of the Human Teeth, by J. Fox, pages 57, 58, London, 1814.

When the teeth meet in the manner above described, they all act upon each other, and the jaw has a much more extensive lateral motion. This occasions a greater friction in mastication, by which the teeth gradually wear away a part of each other. In some persons they become worn down equally, all round the mouth, whilst in others, who have acquired a habit of masticating their food on one side only, the teeth which have been in constant use are worn down, the others remaining quite perfect. This same circumstance also happens, if persons, by reason of caries, have lost several teeth in the early part of life, those which have remained have become very much worn away. I have seen a gentleman, whose teeth were so much worn down, as to have the whole of the crowns removed, leaving only the fangs in the jaws, even with the edges of the gums.

It is not unfrequent for teeth, in this state, to become tender; the application of cold or acids excites considerable pain, but this generally soon subsides; for during the time that the teeth are wearing away by their action on each other, a process goes on in the cavity, by which their sensibility is destroyed; the vessels take on a new action, and deposit ossific matter, until the whole cavity is completely obliterated. This circumstance also happens very frequently in the teeth of old people, which accounts for their not being so liable to the tooth-ache.

SECTION VI.

OF FRACTURES OF THE TEETH*

The teeth are liable to be fractured by blows, which may be inflicted either by accidents, or from malicious intentions.

* Natural History and Diseases of the Human Teeth, by J. Fox, pages 58 to 65, London, 1814.

The incisors of the upper jaw are the most exposed to these accidents. Boys, in their various amusements, occasionally receive blows in the mouth, which not unfrequently occasion fractures of the front teeth.

In falling upon the face, the teeth are sometimes struck against a stone; in throwing of stones at each other, one may be received against the teeth; in an incautious attempt to catch a cricket-ball, the force of which is not sufficiently spent, it may come with violence against the mouth: in these, and other similar ways, persons are subject to fractures of the teeth: also in the mastication of food, hard substances, such as a splinter of bone, or a small stone, or a shot in game, may unexpectedly be bitten upon, at which time the muscles of the lower jaw, being in very strong action, exert a force sufficiently powerful to fracture a perfectly sound tooth.

The treatment of these cases will depend much upon the extent of the injury. If a small piece be broken off from the point of a tooth, nothing more will be necessary than with a fine file to make the rough edge smooth.

A tooth rarely becomes carious in consequence of an accident of this kind; for, if there be no predisposition in a tooth to decay, the mere removal of a small portion of it will not cause caries.

A fracture of a tooth occasions inconvenience in proportion to the injury done to the cavity of the tooth. If it should extend nearly into the cavity, having left only a thin piece of bone to cover it, the person will be subject, for some time, to pain, on exposure to cold air; this, however, is generally cured by a deposit of bone taking place within the cavity, by which the nerve is defended, and the tooth may remain during life without exciting further trouble.

If the fracture should extend into the cavity, the membrane will be immediately exposed, and inflammation will follow. In this case, the treatment must be regulated by the age, and peculiar circumstances of the patient. If the accident should have happened to a youth under fifteen or sixteen years of age, it would be better to extract the tooth, because the teeth on each side, will gradually approach each other, so that when he is arrived at maturity the loss may never be observed.

It is to be understood, that I am speaking of accidents occurring to the permanent teeth; blows received by children under five or six years of age, can only injure the temporary teeth. Sometimes, by accidents, one or more of these are beaten out; this never fails to produce alarm in the minds of the parents; but, as in a short time a removal of these teeth must have been effected by nature, or performed by art, it cannot be considered as a permanent injury.

If the case be neglected for some time, the inflammation extends to the fang and socket, and produces a considerable gum-boil, which can only be cured by the extraction of the tooth.

When an accident of this kind occurs to a person more advanced in years, the loss is very considerable, as the appearance of the mouth, and also the speech becomes thereby much affected.

In Plate III, fig, 9, is a representation of two central incisors, which were broken by a fall. Fig. 10, is the posterior view of these teeth, the fracture of which will be seen extending into the cavity.

In an accident of this kind affecting either one or both teeth, if the person should apply for assistance, immediately after the accident, and before any inflammation has supervened, I should recommend that the tooth or teeth be extracted with great care, When this has been done, the cavity in the tooth should be cleared out as much as possible, and some gold-leaf be introduced, so as completely to fill it up.

After the cavity has been thus stopped, the teeth are to be restored to their sockets, and there to be confined by a ligature: they will soon fix, and in a few days be as secure as ever, and may afterwards remain, without inconvenience, for a great number of years.

If the fracture of a tooth should be so great as in fig. 11, the patient must submit to extraction; or if he should be desirous to preserve the appearance of his mouth, he may be recommended to have the remainder of the tooth filed away, so as to make the fang even with the gums; and, in the manner hereafter to be described, have a tooth fixed to the fang by means of a pivot.

When a blow has been received upon a tooth, so as to loosen it, if the person be young, it will become fast again; but it gradually looses the whiteness of its colour, and at length acquires a bluish tinge.

When the like accident occurs to a person rather advanced in life, a disease usually takes place about the fang, which eventually affects the socket, the tooth becomes very loose and must be extracted.

A young gentleman had the central incisors broken by a cricket-ball, as represented in fig. 9. The fracture did not extend into the cavity, In this case the teeth were filed, so as to remove the irregular portion, and bring them as nearly as possible, into a line with the other teeth.

Fig. 10, represents a posterior view of the central incisors of a young gentleman, who, falling on his face, struck his mouth against a stone. So much of the teeth were broken off as to uncover the membrane; the entrance into the cavity is described by the dark spots, *aa*. Immediately after the accident, the mere touch of the tongue passing over the exposed part of the membrane occasioned extreme pain; in a short time inflammation extended to the socket, the lip became very much swollen, and a considerable quantity of matter was formed. The parents being very desirous to preserve the teeth, made use of every means to abate the inflammation; but, as the gums remained thickened, and the discharge of matter continued, they were at length obliged to consent to the extraction of the teeth: on examining the fangs, they were found covered with a considerable quantity of lymph, which is a common consequence of a neglected accident of this description.

In fig. 11, is the representation of the teeth of a young gentleman who had the central incisors broken by the blow of a stick; being anxious to have the deformity removed in the best possible manner, he was willing to submit to any means that should be recommended. I stated to him the necessity of preserving the fangs, for the purpose of fixing other teeth in a permanent manner; but, perceiving that the sensibility of the exposed membrane was very great, I concluded that he would not be able to endure the pain attendant on the common mode of destroying the nerve; I therefore determined to extract the teeth partially, and return them back into the socket; after which I introduced an instrument, and passed it up to the extremities of the fangs, without occasioning the least painful sensation. Union of the fangs to the socket, took place in a few days, when the remainder of the crowns of the teeth was filed away, and other teeth fixed.

If a blow be inflicted with sufficient violence to remove a tooth from its socket, it may be returned again; and, if secured to the other teeth by a ligature, it will become fast in a few days. I have known a case in which a tooth had remained out of the socket for six hours, and yet, when returned, became again perfectly united. It will be necessary when a tooth has been out of the socket for some time to introduce a probe, and remove the coagulated blood; the fang may then be inserted with ease, and inflammation will be avoided. But when the teeth have been loosened or beaten out by a blow, and the alveolar processes have been injured, or fractured, the teeth will never become perfectly fast; inflammation arises, and nothing but extraction will effect the cure.

SECTION VII.

ODONTALGIA.

Tooth-Ache.

This is one of the most painful affections to which the human system is liable. Its proximate causes are inflammation of the membrane lining the affected tooth or teeth, and the transfer of nervous or rheumatic affections to the teeth. It is well known to all surgeons, that inflammation taking place in confined parts, as in those which are seated beneath fascia, as in whitlow within the bones, &c. are on this account rendered far more painful than when they occur in unconfined parts as in the cellular tissue near the surface of the skin, &c. Inflammation is a simple operation of nature, set up for the removal of obstructions, for the union of divided parts, or to restore the integrity of an organ, which has lost some of its substance, as in the formation of new bone when a portion has been lost by necrosis, or to expel some foreign body or matter from the system, and it may be excited to protect the surface of any organ from the contact of some injurious or irritating substance as cantharides, &c. &c. I will not enter into a detail of the various causes exciting inflammation, but content myself with remarking, that the difference in the phenomena of inflammation as to their different severity, &c. probably does not depend upon any specific difference in the action, but the various differences depend on the different parts affected, as to their irritability and distensibility, and the violence of exciting causes, &c. &c. Inflammation, as I before remarked, is an action, a simple operation of nature; this action is set up by the moving powers of the part where the irritating cause is located, and the object of it is to relieve the system of the irritating agent. These moving powers for the support of their own action depend on a principle derived from the arterial blood; and as their action is necessarily increased, so in order to support it, they must have an increased quantity of arterial blood, and as they command the capillary arteries, they stimulate these last to bring an increased quantity of the fluid they circulate; this of course distends all the capillary vessels of the part, which produces a morbid or unnatural sensation which we call pain, and the violence of the pain, will ever depend upon the degree of the action; and the distensibility of the part, or of its power of swelling the capillary arteries of the part becoming distended with blood, produces the redness and swelling. I have now said all that I need say, to explain, at least to myself, the reason why an inflammation of the lining membrane of a tooth, is so extremely acute, because so confined, that swelling cannot take place; but as I have spoken of inflammation in general, and in some measure explained my views of this subject, and attempted to explain the cause of the pain, swelling, and redness, which usually occur in inflammation, I will now presume to offer a word upon the heat of inflamed parts, and of animal heat in general, hoping that the candid reader will pardon the digression. I again repeat that the arterial blood, affords a principle which supports the *action* of the moving powers of the system in every part. This principle is received by the venous blood in the lungs, which converts the venous to arterial blood; the principle is oxygen, and with it caloric in a *latent state;* the blood thus made arterial passes to the heart, and thence to the capillary arteries in all parts of the system. From the arterial blood in the capillary arteries, the oxygen received at the lungs, is taken off by the moving powers, whose action it supports, whilst the caloric is set free, which produces animal heat, and this shows why inflamed parts have their heat so much above the other parts of the system, because their moving powers act on more blood than the other parts. When the oxygen is taken off at the capillaries from the arterial blood, then this last becomes venous blood, and traverses from the surface to the lungs, to again receive its wonted supply of oxygen and caloric, and possibly to exhale a quantity of carbonaceous matter. I think the human system has two sources of support. From the stomach and alimentary canal it receives that which supports the integrity of the organs, and from the lungs, a principle which supports their action. The first is supplied by our industry, the second is the widely extended gift of the Almighty. Wide is the field of facts and observations which prove and substantiate the foregoing positions; but this is not the place for their discussion, and therefore I only here advance these hints, in hopes that some investigating mind may take up the subject and prove or disprove it. The confined situation of the nerve, blood vessels and lining membrane of the teeth, is such that when any irritation is applied to them, a most violent action may, and often does commence, but as the power of distention is so exceedingly limited, that on this account the most excruciating pain is felt; in many cases a peculiar throbbing pain, which is synchronous with the beat of the arteries; sometimes the pain will be like a shock returning at intervals. I had a case but a short time since, in which the patient expressed the utmost anxiety to have the teeth (for two were affected) extracted instantly, and could hardly wait to have the instruments applied for their extraction.

Tooth-ache usually occurs in defective teeth, whose nerves by the progress of caries have become exposed, but is not generally considered, I believe, by any judicious dentists, to be occasioned by the progress of caries itself, but by the application of cold, or of some irritating agent—as by wounding or bruising the nerve mechanically, or what often is the cause of tooth-ache, dental operations performed upon the teeth whose nerves are exposed, plugs applied to irritable nerves without being prepared for the operation, &c. In the progress of scurvy, the chronic inflammation of the alveolar membrane often changes to acute, and extends to the nerve of the tooth, which compels the patient to have it extracted. I think cases may and often do occur where rhuematic affections extend to the jaws and teeth, and occasion great pain in the latter. Females, during pregnancy, I have often noticed to be very subject to this affection, more than at other periods, and probably because at this time a general plethora of their system is apt to take place.

Although tooth-ache is usually occasioned by the application of cold to nerves exposed by a decay of the bony part of the teeth; yet inflammation may take place in the membranes of teeth otherwise perfectly sound, and proceed to the formation of pus. Mr. Fox mentions a case of this kind and observes: "Some time ago, I was applied to by a gentleman, who complained of an acute pain arising from one of the molares of the under jaw: as I could discover no appearance of caries in it, I advised the loss of blood from the gums, with a view to remove the inflammation in the socket, or other parts connected with the tooth.

This treatment was by no means effectual, for the pain continued with scarcely any intermission: the gentleman therefore determined to have the tooth extracted. In attempting this operation, the tooth broke off at the neck, and completely exposed the internal cavity. Fortunately, this accident proved to be satisfactory, as it afforded an opportunity of ascertaining the cause of the pain. The membrane lining the cavity of the tooth had become so highly inflamed, that it had proceeded to suppuration, and the cavity of the tooth was filled with pus. Immediately after the operation, the gentleman was perfectly relieved, and had no return of pain. In a similar case, instead of extracting the tooth, I should recommend the drilling a hole at the neck of the tooth, into the cavity, in order to make an opening by which the matter might escape."*

Some persons have doubted whether matter could form in the internal part of a tooth, and at the same time the tooth, in all other respects, sound. That matter may be formed in the internal part of a tooth there cannot be a doubt. I was lately informed by a highly respectable physician, and now assistant surgeon in the U. S. Navy, that he had a case of the kind. A person called upon him to have a tooth extracted which was in extreme pain. He extracted the tooth and at once relieved his patient. The tooth was not in the

---

* Fox, Part II, page 12. Note.

least carious; from which circumstance he was induced to saw it apart in order to examine the state of the nerve, blood vessels, and lining membrane within; he found the latter in a high state of inflammation and the cavity filled with pus.

Several other cases have been mentioned to me by dentists. I give one from the work of Fauchard.

*Disposition to a fistula of the gums, by an abscess in the interior of a tooth.**

M. Desjardins, surgeon, called upon me to see conjointly with him, old Father Rose, Liquor Merchant at the Place de Grève. This patient experienced such violent pains along the whole extent of the chin, which prevented him entirely from sleeping at night, so that in the day he could not attend to his business. As no spoiled teeth could be seen, neither were any of the teeth susceptible to impressions of heat and cold, we thought this case might be regarded like the sequel of a flux, or some humour lodged in this part. The patient was treated accordingly, but without any success. At length the pains having become insupportable, I was called for. I then examined the lower incisor teeth; I perceived nothing at the time; neither was the sound to me of any advantage. The other teeth were not painful, they were sound. The lower part of the gums of the painful teeth appeared to us only slightly inflamed, but without real swelling or fluctuation. A small eruption of a purple red colour, situated on the gum of the right incisor tooth, was all that could be particularly seen; and which was not sufficient to decide upon the extraction of this tooth any more than the others. In

---

* Jourdain Tome 2. Pages. 317, 319.

this uncertainty, I asked for a lighted bougie and placed it against the two teeth. By the reflexion of the light we assured ourselves that the incisor nearest to the canine tooth was the cause of all this malady. In fact, the enamelled substance appeared to be wan and undulated. At length, and for more security, I pierced the eruption, and there came out bloody serum. The stillet traversed the maxillary substance, and came against the root of the tooth in question, which I extracted. We afterwards broke it; the canal of its root and its great cavity was filled with a very fetid black humour. The same day the operation was performed, the patient found himself really eased of pain, and with the assistance of some emollient gargles, the malady completely disappeared in a few days.

*Observation on a Canine Tooth, and on the pus that was formed in its cavity, which was evacuated by a perforating trepan.**

"The 12th of November, 1724, M. Tartanson, regular Surgeon of Paris, and ancient Prevost of the Society, was attacked with a cruel pain in the incisor and canine teeth of the lower jaw. He called upon me to know what so sharp a pain could proceed from, without the teeth being carious, being only a little worn at their extremities. After having examined, and touched them with my sound, I knew which one it was, and I assured him that he had but one canine tooth only on the right side of the same jaw, that was sensible, and which caused him this severe pain; which proceeded from

---

* Fauchard, pages 470, 471, 472, 473.

this tooth being more used than the others at its extremity, the nerve that was contained in its cavity having been more exposed to the air than those of the other teeth.

"I told him, that I was persuaded there was purulent matter contained in this cavity, and that he ought to have the tooth perforated for its evacuation; that by this means the pain would soon cease, and the tooth be preserved. After I had persuaded M. Tartanson of the utility of this operation, I took a graver that I used as a perforator; when I carried the point to the extremity of the tooth in the place where its cavity was, and turning it to the right and left, and left and right, I commenced opening this same cavity; at length I took a drilling instrument, which I made use of for turning in the same manner, to widen and deepen the opening which I had already commenced, and as soon as the cavity of this abscess in the tooth was opened, there came out of it considerable pus and blood; which I shewed this person by means of a mirror, in presence of Sire Larregee, his son, Surgeon. This appeared rather singular to M. Tartanson, although well versed in his art, and indeed it is not common to see this disease. If other authors have reported before me diseases nearly similar, I do not believe that they thought of before making use of proper means to cure it, of which the principal is to trepan the tooth, as I did on this occasion, to give exit to the matter shut up in its cavity.

"M. de Nain, of whom I have already spoken, had many teeth attacked with the same malady, which gave him much pain: I cured them all by the means I have just mentioned. Some months after I plugged his teeth, without their having since given him the least pain, and he can use them like the other teeth.

"Since then Madame, of the religious order of Saint Bennet, Convent of Chasse-Midi, being attacked by a severe pain caused by a similar malady of the first little molar tooth on the right side of the upper jaw, she had recourse to me: I made use of the same method as before with so much success, that the pain ceased almost immediately, and this religious woman preserved her tooth.

"It should never be neglected to trepan a tooth on a similar occasion; whether this operation is performed on the skull or other bones, to give exit to the matters which are diffused in the cavities of these bones, where they are formed contrary to the order of nature."

Cure.

As Odontalgia is usually caused by an irritated state of the nerve and lining membrane of the affected tooth or teeth, consequently our plan of cure must be, as far as is in our power, to remove or prevent the influence of the exciting causes, and, at the same time, make use of those curative measures which soothe the irritated nerves. But it is sometimes the case that no remedy which our patients will allow us to use will be of any service, and we are compelled to extract the tooth. In all cases when the molar teeth are affected and so far decayed as not to be of use if preserved, and plugged, &c. they ought to be extracted or excised. The canine and incisor teeth, if they are affected, ought not to be extracted; but if all our endeavours to quiet the inflamed nerves should fail, then the tooth should be cut off at the very edge of the gum, and the stump treated on the principles which will be laid down in the chapter on the preparation of the stumps of teeth for the reception of artificial ones. By these means we shall be able to preserve the stumps of the canine and incisor teeth, on which the crowns of natural teeth may be engrafted in the most perfect manner, so that, as far as the articulation and appearance are concerned, they will prove as useful as the first teeth. I think this direction is of the first consequence, that the incisor and canine teeth should never be extracted, but cut off, and their nerves treated as before referred to. In this way we shall prevent the falling in of the lips by preventing the absorption and removal of the alveolar processes, which will not be absorbed away if the stumps are left, and certainly will be if they are extracted. And, as we have before observed, the stump of the tooth is not deprived of its vitality when the nerve and lining membrane are destroyed, but continue to support their vitality by their connection with the alveolar membrane which lines the socket and covers the fang of the tooth. There is no method of fixing artificial teeth that is as good as upon sound stumps of teeth, and it should be an object of the greatest solicitude to preserve the stumps of these teeth instead of extracting them, and the pain of it is never as great as the pain occasioned by their extraction. Natural teeth may be fixed upon stumps of teeth so as to be worn for years and to elude detection, even from the most experienced eye. If no tooth is fixed upon the stump, this last may be preserved to be of great use to the patient for many years. I have thus far anticipated my subject, and will here remark, that the inflamed tooth should not be extracted or cut off, unless we are unable to alleviate the pain, or, in case of a tooth or a stump which could be of no use. In cases when the teeth would be of use if the inflammation was relieved, it ought to be our most solicitous endeavour to relieve it, which we may do in a great many cases by removing, as far as in our power, all the exciting causes, and then applying to the nerve and tooth some strong stimulant, or andoyne and astringent combined, or the astringent alone. In the pharmaceutical part of this work will be found a considerable many odontalgic formula. Some of these preparations are often of good effect; and if they are, we may continue to diminish the irritability of the affected nerve until we are enabled to complete a perfect cure by plugging the tooth. Different kinds of caustics are sometimes made use of to destroy the affected nerve: in general the practice is a bad one, and yet circumstances may arise when we shall choose to cauterise the nerve rather than to extract the tooth, when our other remedies fail, and after this to plug the tooth. Suitable caustics will be mentioned in the pharmaceutical part.

It has been proposed never to extract any tooth that has its nerve affected, but to excise it, cut it off, including the molar teeth and all. I will, in this place, insert a communication of this kind, and to this effect, from Mr. Fay, to the Society of Arts, in London. I give the gentleman's words, and leave the reader to do as he pleases. He says, "In the centre of every tooth is a little cavity, in which is expanded a nervous pulp, forming the principal seat of sensation in that organ, the nervous twigs pass through the roots of the teeth, by very minute passages into this cavity, when they are spread out. The base of this cavity is situated a little above the level of the neck of the tooth, and it struck me, that when caries had extended so far as to expose this nervous matter to the various agencies, from which, in the healthy state of the parts, it is protected, it would be easy to remove that part of the tooth containing the cavity, the seat of the pain, and thus allow the sound roots to remain in their sockets undisturbed, to support the adjoining teeth; as it is a notorious fact, that entire removal of one tooth, however easily performed, causes the adjoining ones to become prematurely loose, and ultimately to fall out, in consequence, principally, of the absorption of the alveolar process. Minutely to describe how this happens, would occupy too much space, and

I mention it merely as a well-known fact, to show the value of allowing the root or fangs of a tooth to remain. This operation I have called the operation of Excision, and I recommend it as a most valuable substitute for the extraction of the teeth, in the majority of cases of caries, but by no means to supersede it altogether, as there are, and must ever be, cases requiring the entire extraction of the teeth, when disease has proceeded beyond a certain point, as for example, beyond the common cavity, which I have cursorily described, or when the jaw itself is diseased.

"The instruments employed by me in this operation, are forceps, accurately fitted, like those for extraction, to the necks of the teeth, but having fine, well-tempered, cutting edges; these edges must be carefully applied on the necks of the teeth, as close to the gums as possible, taking care to keep the edges parallel to the edges of the gums, which are to be depressed a little with the inferior surface of the blades of the forceps, so as to bring the cutting edges fairly beneath the enamel, which in the adult, is the criterion of being below the common cavity of the tooth. Then, with a gradual application of pressure on the handles of the forceps, the tooth is in an instant snapped off at the neck, and the common cavity, the seat of the pain, is thus removed, leaving the patient a painless, bony surface for mastication, a firm prop for the support of the adjoining teeth, and a basis for an artificial tooth, if it should be required. I may mention here a fact *never before noticed*, namely, that the openings by which the minute canals terminate in the common cavity, become soon after plugged up with bony matter, which thus affords a permanent protection to the interior of the stump, and presents a continuous and firm surface for after life. In addition to these advantages, the operation is performed even on the largest teeth, in a moment, and consequently, at a great saving of suffering, which should be the grand object of all sound surgery."—*Trans. Society of Arts*, xliv. 70. *Taken from Littell's Museum of Foreign Literature and Science*, No. XX, *for August*, 1827, pp. 189, 190.

The foregoing communication of Mr. Fay was shown to me by a friend, since commencing this work, and the reader will notice, that what I have recommended for the front teeth, canine, and incisores, Mr. Fay has for all the teeth, namely, excision. How far his practice will be adopted, time will determine. He intimates, that if a tooth is extracted, it loosens the adjoining ones, and causes them to become prematurely loose, and ultimately to fall out. This, to a certain extent, is true, as regards to its loosening the adjoining teeth, which it does, in a very small degree, if some teeth are extracted; as for instance, the canine teeth, which will loosen the incisores, if they were before in a crowded state, but if otherwise, it has this effect very slightly. As to its making the other teeth fall out, I think, in a healthy state of the gums and the other remaining teeth, this effect never takes place; this depends on the number extracted: the teeth, to a certain extent, support each other. He likewise observes, that filling up of the end of the minute canal, in the stump through which the nerve passes, with bony matter, after excision, was never noticed, until his communication was given.

Mr. Hunter long ago remarked, that when the teeth become worn down so low as otherwise to expose its cavity, this became filled with bony matter. He has devoted two pages to this subject, and given plates of two teeth thus worn down and filled up with osseous matter.*

* See Hunter on the Teeth, Part I. pages 108, 109, and Plate XIV, figs. 24 and 25.

I will not say, but what the practice of excising the grinding teeth, whose nerves are inflamed, instead of extracting them, may, in a great many cases, be expedient; and I think the subject well worthy of consideration and experiment. When this affection arises from constitutional causes, as when rheumatic or nervous pains affect those teeth which are sound, we ought to endeavour, by warm application, anodynes, aperients, &c. &c. to relieve the affection without extracting the teeth. In some very rare instances, grubs, insects, &c. have been lodged in the antrum maxillare, and by preying upon its membrane have reached the membrane lining the fangs of some of the teeth, which at times are found to perforate the antra. I saw a case of this kind reported in the public papers, which was said to have occurred, I think, in Germany. The subject of it, a young lady, went to a respectable surgeon, almost frantic with the tooth-ache, and he extracted the affected tooth; and at different periods, I think, she lost nine teeth; when, upon the extraction of the last, a living grub passed out through the alveolus from the antrum. I am not able to find the paper, or assert the truth or not of the story, or whether other cases are recorded or not of this kind; but it is easy to conceive, that such a case might happen, for the ova of an insect might be deposited on a flower, and snuffed up the nose, and in this way be conveyed to the antrum, where it might be hatched, and produce these unpleasant and dangerous effects. I merely give the story as a hint which may lead to the detection of similar cases. We ought on no account to neglect this affection, but relieve it if possible, immediately, as pain is a sensation by which nature warns us of insidious and dangerous foes.

I had almost forgotten to mention that in some instances, it has been practised to extract pained teeth, and then replace them in their sockets, where they are allowed to remain and grow again as before. This is only done as a dernier resort, when every other has failed. It will then remain at the discretion of the judicious practitioner. Cauterising the nerve and sensible parts of the bony substance of the teeth has been done but with indifferent success. I conclude the subject with Mr. Delabarre's observations, who says, * painful teeth are cauterized to obtain two results. The first, to destroy the painful nerve ; the second, to put an end to and dry up the caries. The instrument that is used for this operation is various in its shape, on account of the caries to be operated upon. To fulfil the first indication, the instrument is made red hot, and it is quickly applied to the cavity where the nerve is to be destroyed. It succeeds sometimes very well in making the tooth insensible ; on other occasions it is preferred to put into the caries equal parts of caustic potash and acetate of lead ; the use of this means is less terrifying to the patient ; plunging rapidly a small silver sound, or a soft hog's bristle in the dental canal ; is also successful, by destroying the nerve, is such a manner as to render the tooth insensible and admit of its being plugged. This process is much less painful, and should often be prefered to cauterization.

But at length when a caries is dried up, or to stop the progress of erosion, or atrophy of the teeth in youth, in order to make them insensible to the action of the air and food, another method must be resorted to. This is by frequently repeating the operation with an instrument hot, but not red hot, that the desired success is obtained. This operation is a delicate one, and requires practice to judge the

* Odontologie Sur les Dents Humains, page 60, par C. Delabarre, Paris, 1815.

degree of heat that is proper to give the actual cautery. I operated upon teeth in this way, which were changed for the better, in a manner to be wondered at.

CHAPTER IV.

OF THE DISEASES OF THE GUMS, SOFT PARTS, &C.

I shall notice three diseases of the gums.

First, Scurvy, so called by Messrs. Hunter and Fox, and the Devastating Process by Mr. Koecker.

Secondly, Cancoris.

Thirdly, A preternatural growth of the gums, and of tumours from them.

First, Of Scurvy of the Gums.

This disease is one of very frequent occurrence, and often most deplorable in its consequences. It is one that as far as my knowledge extends, is very little understood by either surgeon-dentists, or by the physicians or surgeons of this country.

It is a local inflammation of that part of the gum which is situated around the bodies and fangs of the teeth, usually first affecting the gums covering the front incisors of the under jaw, next the grinding teeth, and lastly, the incisors of the upper jaw. It often affects persons whose teeth were otherwise perfectly sound. It affects all classes of persons, and all ages, from two years, (in whom it is often fatal,) to old age. It is this disease which usually occasions the loss of the teeth in old people, which but for this would have remained useful to the individual during their life time. This local inflammation often and generally goes on to suppuration, and matter is formed around the tooth, and is constantly discharged for years, and by mixing with the saliva, is not perceived except in its effects.

Scurvy is a disease which appears to be very common, or occurring to nearly all classes of persons in every nation.

* Mr. Koecker says it is a disease which seems to be confined to no particular climate, but is more or less prevalent in every part of the world. I have observed, says he, the inhabitants of most opposite countries, the Russians, the Germans, the French, the Italians, the Spaniards, the Portuguese, the English, the Africans, the East and West Indians, and the inhabitants of the United States, to be all more or less liable to it.

Similar causes, ceteris paribus, in general, produce similar effects, and as the organization of the human frame is the same every where, so if exposed to similar causes of disease similar diseases will follow, especially if those diseases have a specific character; and this explains to us the reason, why inhabitants of opposite countries have similar diseases, because exposed to similar causes of disease.

Symptoms.

This disease is usually very insidious in its first attack, and often, says Mr. Koecker,† it may continue for years, without being detected by the patient or his surgical attendant. As we have before had occasion to observe, the periosteum or membrane covering the fangs of the teeth, appears to be derived

---

* See Koecker, page 273.

† See Koecker upon the Teeth, Part II. page 276.

from the gums, and to receive its blood from the same source; and when the gums have been diseased, the lining of the socket and the covering of the fang become sooner or later affected; after the gums and the membrane lining the socket and covering the fang become affected, the teeth become loose, feel tender, matter is discharged around them from under the gums; pain begins to be felt more or less before this time, depending upon the peculiar irritability of the gums, which differs considerably in many persons. Upon examining them, we usually observe that they are red, swelled, and very tender, often covered with a dirty, yellowish matter, resembling the yellow fur upon the tongue in some states of fever. They bleed on the slightest touch, the use of a hard brush, eating any thing hard, or even sucking the teeth will produce bleeding; constitutional symptoms at times take place, and the health of the patients is often greatly affected. The gums sooner or later begin to retire from the teeth and are absorbed away, which exposes the fangs of the teeth. The alveoli also are absorbed away, until finally the teeth having become entirely loosened and pushed out of their sockets, which gradually fill up at the bottom, one after another drop out, until the patient loses all his teeth. Often his health greatly improves, and he is almost rejoiced that his teeth are gone. There is one circumstance which I do not know to have been noticed by any author, and it is this, that while the tooth is very loose, the gum and socket entirely absorbed away, so that the tooth merely is confined by the membrane at the end of the fang, and by the nerve, blood-vessels, &c.; yet it will be apparently alive, and its internal circulation will be vigorous and healthy. This shows the wisdom of the great Author of Nature, who has provided the teeth with two sources of support, so that if one fails, a measurable assistance is obtained from the other.

Very often as soon as the gum has retired from the body, and some part of its fang is exposed, caries will take place on its surface, and it will become very tender and extremely sensible to almost any impression. The slightest increase or decrease of temperature, will occasion more or less of uneasiness and pain in the affected teeth; peculiar pains will be felt passing along the dental nerves. Those teeth which become elongated, in consequence of the filling up of their sockets from the swelling of the periosteum covering their fangs, by this change in their position are constantly pressed upon by the opposing teeth, which presses them upon the tender and irritated periosteum, and causes a farther increase of pain, until the patient becomes quite wretched, and in some cases it becomes a pleasure to have the teeth extracted. In children this disease is often attended with very alarming and sometimes fatal consequences. In them the irritability of the gums and of the general system is far greater than in adults. Their gums become much swollen. The periosteum lining the alveoli and covering the fangs of the teeth, becomes inflamed, extending to the maxillary bones, which immediately loosens the teeth. Suppuration soon takes place about the bodies of the last, accompanied with a considerable discharge of matter. The teeth are covered with a dark, filthy sordes. The system becomes generally excited, accompanied with symptoms of high irritation. The periosteum covering both jaws becomes affected, and in many cases, the general excitement of the system is so great, that united with all the other distressing, local symptoms, proves the death of the patient.

The gums at first generally appear unusually red, and very sensible, but after the disease has continued for some time in a chronic state, they often appear very pale, and seem to have lost much of their usual healthy action. Small swellings, like granules, are at times noticed, which are very sensible and bleed readily; they will be often noticed in this state, whilst the surrounding gum appears pale and almost destitute of vitality.

Causes of Scurvy.

The causes of this affection are constitutional and probably local. This disease is always produced by local causes, which act on susceptible persons.

Constitutional Causes.—First, any thing which produces an increased irritability of the system on persons who are naturally irritable, or possess a considerable mobility of the system, as is most perfectly demonstrated in those cases where this disease attacks the gums of children, the mobility of whose systems render them extremely liable to be affected by it (children who live much on animal food)—the improper use of mercurial remedies, especially when taken so as to excite salivation; and if this is long continued, it is apt to bring on this disease in an aggravated form—frequent attacks of inflammatory fever—chronic inflammation of the stomach—a general plethoric state of the system, accompanied with a peculiar inflammatory diathesis—scorbutic and scrofulous taints of the general system, &c. &c.

The inordinate use of spirituous liquors, by producing an inflammatory state of the system, may predispose to this affection.

Mr. Koecker* notices the use of narcotic medicines; smoking and chewing tobacco, &c. With respect to this last cause, namely, chewing and smoking tobacco, I cannot say but it often causes this disease, or predisposes to it; but in

* Koecker on the Teeth, Part II, page 282.

my practice I have seen ten cases of it in persons who never used tobacco, either by chewing or smoking, where I have seen one case which has occurred in persons who use tobacco; and with respect to the injurious effects of narcotic medicines, I must say, that I have not seen any case which seemed to be excited by these medicines; nor can I explain to myself the manner in which they have this effect. Any cause that vitiates the saliva, whether constitutional or local, tends, more or less, to produce this disease.

Local Causes, &c.—These are probably always present, in a greater or less degree, in every case of this disease. They are, first, every kind of foreign matter lodged between the teeth and the edges of the gums, as for instance, tartar, which is generally deposited between the edges of the gums, on the bodies and fangs of the teeth, and is the most common cause of this disease, (Mr. Koecker says, that he never saw this disease unless tartar was present; also a greenish corrosive mucous is often present,)—a vitiated state of the saliva—diseased teeth and dead teeth, and dead loose stumps of teeth, &c. &c.*—improper operations upon the teeth, such as filing, when they are tender—scaling of the teeth improperly and imperfectly done—uncleanliness of the mouth and teeth, especially during sickness and the exhibition of medicines—the use of improper tooth-brushes and tooth-powders—(And among these Mr. Koecker mentions charcoal,† which he says increases the disease by its mechanical irritation, occasioned by its cutting quality. In this respect Mr. Koecker may be correct; but although I have seen it used in a great many cases, I never saw it produce this effect: nor have I ever seen but

---

* See Koecker, On the Teeth, pages 282, 283.

† See Koecker, On the Teeth, Part II, page 282.

once, a case of scurvy when charcoal was for a long time freely used. As to its cutting quality I think if rightly prepared, and finely and perfectly pulverized, it will not often have this quality)—irregularity in cleaning the teeth—cleaning them a few times, and then suffering them to remain for several days without any cleaning, I think, often greatly hastens the progress of this disease—irregularity of the teeth themselves may often predispose to it after this affection has advanced so far as to loosen some of the teeth, and the membrane covering the fangs has become tender and inflamed, which in nearly all cases it does, before the teeth are much loosened; then almost every thing that touches the loosened teeth seems to aggravate the disease. Mastication with them irritates the alveolar membrane, and soon becomes so painful, as to be avoided entirely. They are elongated and pressed upon by the other teeth, so that it causes pain, even to close the teeth upon each other. The general health is now apt to suffer, and an irritable state of the system takes place; this reacts upon the diseased gums, until Nature, if I may be allowed the expression, considering the teeth foreign bodies, sets up an active absorbing process, by which she removes the alveoli, and the gums covering the teeth, and the alveolar membrane, so that, at last, the teeth seem only to stand upon the ends of their roots, which rest on the jaw; they soon fall out. This is a gradual work, and often requires from five to fifteen years. Acute inflammation may, at times, take place.

Those teeth which are deepest and firmest in their sockets naturally seem to remain longest in the mouth, and vice versa. Even constitutional diseases sometimes arise from this disease, and in the chapter upon diseases produced by diseased teeth and gums will be noticed.

Treatment of the Scurvy of the Gums.

To effect a permanent cure of this disease it is necessary to obviate all its exciting causes. As it always depends more or less on local exciting causes, our attention should be directed to the state of the teeth and gums themselves. All the teeth that are diseased, if so much so as to be impossible to be cured by the means which have been and will be directed for the cure of diseased teeth, should be immediately extracted; likewise all dead and useless stumps of teeth. Mr. Koecker says,* a molar tooth, which has no antagonist, should be drawn, and all dead teeth. Those teeth which from their irregularity appear to influence the disease, if their irregularity cannot be obviated, should be drawn. The operation for extraction of the teeth should be performed at the same sitting, for the effect in checking the diseased action is greatly increased if all the teeth we purpose to extract, are extracted at the same time. I think this of great consequence, for we must bear in mind that a diseased action has been continued for a long time in the gums and alveolar membrane, and it is, sine qua non, an object of indispensable moment that we change this action and excite a new and healthy action in these parts, in order to a permanent cure of this disease. The bleeding from the sockets should be encouraged by directing the patient to rinse his mouth with lukewarm water of a temperature that is agreeable to him, until it spontaneously ceases, which it will generally do in a short time: subsequently, for several days, the patient should use some gently astringent wash. The following are those directed by Mr. Koecker,† which he says he has found to

* Page 287. † Pages 288—9.

be the most useful. "Take clarified honey, three ounces, vinegar one ounce; this, diluted in the proportion of three table-spoonfuls to a pint of warm sage tea or water, may be used frequently through the day.

"Take of clarified honey and of the tincture of bark two ounces each, mix and use as above.

"Take of honey and the tincture of rhattania two ounces each, mix and dilute as above.

"Take of honey and the tincture of catechu one ounce each, mix and dilute as above."

These are the different preparations which Mr. Koecker directs to be used during the day of extracting the teeth; some of these preparations, by way of experiment I have used, and have not been as well pleased with them as the following:

Take the inner bark of young green oak two pounds, to this add water six quarts, put all into some suitable vessel and boil it for several hours, and if necessary, add an additional quantity of water; after the water becomes fully impregnated with the qualities of the bark, this last may be taken out and the liquor boiled so as to have two quarts, which should be strained and put in a glass bottle. This liquor generally answers extremely well, and seems to heal the diseased gums and promote a healthy action in them better than any other remedy I have been able to procure, with the exception of the decoction of the nut-gall, which is still more powerful. I have found that fresh green oak bark was much better than the same bark when it had been kept dry for some time. This wash used freely for eight or ten days will generally prove of the greatest utility. However, some of the preparations recommended by Mr. Koecker, or some other gentle astringent may be used with great advantage. The one I have mentioned has always proved so effectual in my practice that I have rarely used any other except by way of experiment. Mr. Koecker intimates that now we had better wait ten or fourteen days before we again operate upon the teeth; but cases will often occur, especially in young persons, when we perhaps may not be obliged to extract a single tooth. That it is proper to wait some considerable time between the different operations, I believe in many cases to be expedient, yet in others, all may be done the same day, as in case 31st, mentioned by Mr. Koecker.* The expediency or not of doing much upon the teeth at once must be left to the judgment of the judicious practitioner, which will be directed by the circumstances of the case.

If there are any teeth which ought to be extracted, this, as I said before, should precede all other operations. After this the foreign matter should be removed, whether we wait a few days before we attempt the operation or not. The operation of scaling or cleaning the teeth, as an operation will be considered in a separate section upon that subject hereafter. We must now proceed to clean the teeth in the most perfect manner. The tartar will often be found collected under the gums, pressing upon the alveolar processes, also between the teeth, and adhering on the lateral parts of the teeth when their surfaces oppose each other. No pains should be spared to perform this operation in the most perfect manner, for much depends upon its being perfectly done, and the operator should be provided with suitable instruments for the purpose, and exert the utmost care and tenderness in operating; and very often, and most generally, it will have to be repeated once or twice, or more times, before the teeth will be perfectly clean. After this operation, and between the several

---

* Page 295.

operations, an astringent lotion may be used, as the one from the oak bark, until the gums become quite well. When we find a carious state of the fangs or bodies of the teeth, as sometimes will be the case, we must use the utmost care in cleaning them, as they are often very tender, and great pain is excited upon touching them. The carious teeth must be removed or treated upon those surgical principles which will be considered when we consider the several operations necessary for the cure of diseased teeth. Scarifying the gums, I have no doubt, in some cases, will be found of the utmost utility in the treatment of this complaint. The section on that subject will detail the manner of performing the operation of scarifying the gums.

In the intervals between the several operations we should direct the patient to use a soft brush until his gums will bear the impression of a hard one. A hard brush at first proves too irritating. From the well known and valuable property which the argentum nitratum (lunar caustic) has in allaying the irritability of abraded and ulcerated surfaces, I very early suggested to myself the propriety of using this remedy in cases of diseased and ulcerated gums, especially when the latter state is noticed around such teeth as we do not wish to extract; and after this, upon reading Mr. Fox's work, I had the pleasure of finding that I had fallen into the same views which had been entertained by that eminent dentist.* Mr. Fox says that if the gums hang loosely about the necks of the teeth, much good will be derived from the use of the argentum nitratum in solution. If only a particular tooth, or two or three are affected, we may use a pretty strong solution, applied with a camel's hair pencil to the edges of the

* See Fox on the teeth. Part II, page 81.

gums of those teeth which are affected. This remedy will usually communicate a new action to the diseased gum and greatly promote their cure. He also says that if a good deal of offensive matter is discharged from the gums about the necks of the teeth, &c. we may use a weak solution as a wash to the whole mouth. I have used this solution, and can most cheerfully recommend it as a valuable remedy in the cure of these diseases. In cases when the mouth is in a somewhat unhealthy state, and the breath is affected in consequence of it, this remedy is very valuable. However, in many cases, we can cure this disease by the means before mentioned, without having recourse to the use of the argentum nitratum.

After bad teeth have been extracted, and the remaining teeth have been perfectly cleaned, and the astringent wash with the brush, which has been recommended, and a dentrifice I shall hereafter mention, have been used for a few days, we generally notice a striking change in the appearance of the gums; and in many instances, a great change in the health and spirits of the patient. We soon notice a healthy appearance of the gums. In those cases where there was an unnatural redness, we notice a decrease of this colour; the swollen gums, which seemed to shrink from the teeth, now fall around and embrace them, and the abraded surface around the fang often perfectly unites to it. If we have before observed an unnatural paleness, we now notice a return of colour; and, in fact, every symptom and sensation of disease soon disappears. If any of the teeth which remain are diseased, we must treat them as has been before recommended in the chapter on that subject, only remembering that an unusual degree of care is required when operating upon them, so as not to excite fresh irritation by rude and unreasonable operations. It will not be a great while before we shall notice, that those which were previously loose, will become quite firm, and that the tenderness of the membrane lining their sockets, will be entirely removed. After the first operation for removing the tartar, and subsequently, for several weeks, or longer, if necessary, the patient should be directed to use a strong astringent dentrifice; for which see the chapter containing the several formularies for dentrifices. If there should be any constitutional causes which seem to continue the disease of the gums, and retard their cure, recourse should be had to those remedial means, which shall, if possible, remove the peculiar constitutional affection. Mercurial medicines should, if possible, be most sedulously avoided for a considerable time after we have restored a degree of health to the gums, for they will readily become diseased upon a repetition of those causes which first impaired their healthy action. We must likewise direct our patient to use those means which shall prevent a re-accumulation of the tartar. The teeth should be faithfully washed with a brush suited to the state of the teeth, remembering as a general rule, not to use our brushes so hard as to excite much irritation in the gums, or to those teeth which may be somewhat tender, and the dentrifices may be used at first with hardly any mechanical property in them, and gradually increased until the patient can use dentrifices of a mechanical nature, as great as is ever proper for the teeth. In the chapter upon dentrifices I shall give a great variety of formula, from which may be selected those which shall be proper and agreeable, remembering, as I before said with regard to tooth-brushes, that our rule and guide must be the effect of the dentrifice upon the teeth, the gums, and the feelings of the patient; for our measures should never greatly irritate the two first, nor occasion much pain to the patient. For the farther and complete illustration of this subject, I here subjoin the three following cases out of many that I have had the pleasure of curing, and would here observe, that I have ever been able to cure this disease, in every case, in which I have been allowed to follow the principles of practice which I have here developed.

Case I.—Mrs. —— F——, a lady, aged about 46 years, of the first respectability, residing in the District of Southwark, Philadelphia, applied to me in the month of July, 1827, with a very diseased state of the gums and teeth. She said, she entirely despaired of any person being able to restore her gums and teeth to a healthy condition; as, although she had applied to several of the first dentists in this city, she had never been able to procure any treatment or remedy which had been of any service to her; and, indeed, one or two dentists had told her, that her disease was incurable. I assured her she need not despair of being perfectly cured in a short time. Upon inquiring the length of time in which she had been affected with this disease of the gums, I found they had been diseased about fourteen years, and that at the time her teeth and gums were first affected, she enjoyed very good health, and was of a full flesby habit, which was to a certain degree peculiar to her family, and that four or five years after her teeth and gums became diseased, her general health began to suffer; she was troubled with various nervous affections; her digestive organs became considerably affected; she was constantly more or less afflicted with pain in her gums, teeth, and maxillary bones. Many of her teeth became loose, attended with great tenderness of the alveolar membrane, and pain in masticating her food, which prevented the course of healthy digestion; and from having been of a full and flesby habit, she had become, at the time I saw her, very thin and spare. Also that in the time she had had her teeth cleaned, and some of them, which had become carious, had been plugged; but it was evident, that these operations had been of little permanent advantage. In some instances, the caries had proceeded so far as to affect the lining membrane of some teeth, which caused so much pain as to oblige her to have them extracted. Upon examining her teeth, I found she had lost all of them upon her under jaw, except five, which were one right bicuspid, the canine, and one right lateral incisor, and the left dentes sapientia; and that of these five, three were very much diseased; two of which had lost their vitality, and were very loose, around whose fangs the gums had been very considerably absorbed away, and in a constant state of suppuration, discharging a considerable quantity of offensive matter. She had, I think, eleven teeth remaining on her upper jaw, to wit: the canine and incisor teeth, and one bicuspid, and four molares. All of these teeth were more or less diseased except one of the molares, and three front incisores. Her gums, as I before noticed, were in a state of suppuration around some of the teeth of the under jaw, and the gums covering the under jaw appeared very pale. On the upper jaw the gum was unnaturally pale, having several small swellings in different parts about as large as small peas, which were very sensible, red, and inflamed, and bled very readily upon being irritated.

As she would not consent to have any of her upper teeth extracted, I extracted the two on the under jaw that had lost their vitality, and around whose fangs the gums were in a state of suppuration. After this, I partially cleaned her teeth. As I was not, on account of the bleeding, able to clean them perfectly at one sitting, I also scarified the small inflamed swellings upon the gums of the upper jaw; I then gave her some of the oak-bark decoction, and also gave her a very soft brush, directing her to rinse her mouth freely three times a day for several days, with the decoction before mentioned, and at the same time to pass the brush gently over her teeth and gums, so as to excite a gentle action in the latter. In about ten days I plugged those teeth which required it, and carefully removed all the remaining tartar. I directed her to continue the use of the decoction and brush as at first, and directed her to use a suitable tooth-powder upon the principles before mentioned, for some time. Eight or ten days after this I again examined her mouth, and found a most remarkable amendment in all the symptoms; the tenderness of her gums and teeth had greatly abated; the gums had assumed a very healthy appearance; the unnatural paleness was exchanged for a mild, florid, and healthy appearance; pain and uneasiness had entirely left her jaws and teeth. I had occasion again to scarify one of the small granular swellings I had before mentioned, which completed the cure of her gums. In the course of five or six weeks, her remaining teeth, or many of them became quite firm, and have assumed a very healthy appearance. Subsequently I replaced her front under teeth, with an elegant set of natural teeth, mounted on a gold plate.

Case II.—Mrs. M——, residing in Catharine-street, called on me accompanied by her daughter, an amiable young lady aged 14 years, and requested me to examine her daughter's teeth and gums; and observed to me that they had been in a state of disease for about two years; that she had applied to two very respectable physicians, whose names were familiar to me, stating to them her daughter's case, and requesting their advice; and they examined the young lady's teeth and prescribed for her, but their prescriptions had been of no avail. She had also applied to one or two dentists without any benefit, and she expressed great pleasure upon my assuring her that in all probability a perfect cure could be effected in the course of a few weeks. The young lady was of a sanguine temperament. Her gums upon examination, appeared considerably swollen and inflamed, they had in some parts retired from the teeth, upon which there was a considerable deposit of tartar. There was but a slight appearance of decay upon any of her teeth, which were very regular and beautiful. In this case the disease appeared to depend upon an irritable state of the gums, increased into diseased action by the tartar deposited around the necks of the teeth, and in interstices between them. The indications of cure were, first, to allay the diseased action which had taken place in the gums around the teeth; and secondly, to restore a healthy action, and to cause the gums to heal around the necks of the teeth, as they are wont to do in health. This all I was enabled to accomplish in the most perfect manner, by at once removing all the tartar that was deposited around the teeth; which I was enabled to do at one sitting, and after this I directed her to use the oak-bark decoction, with a light brush for a few days, and then to use an astringent dentifrice at least twice a day for sometime, and to increase the hardness of her tooth-brushes, until she could without pain use a hard one. By this treatment in the course of three weeks, her gums were rendered perfectly healthy.

Case III.—I will mention but one more case of this affection, as I have already continued the discussion of this subject much farther than I at first expected; as I feel the utmost anxiety that whoever reads this chapter, may have a perfect and clear idea of this disease and of the causes which produce it, and of those means which, if properly used, will always render the cure easy and perfect.

W—— L——, Esq., a gentleman of about forty-five years of age, and of a remarkably good constitution, called on me in the month of September last, and requested me to examine his teeth and gums, which I did, and found a very peculiar irregularity of the incisor and canine teeth of the under jaw. The canine teeth had advanced forward so far, that they had protruded the right lateral incisor entirely out of the circle of the teeth, and within the mouth; and the right front incisor was turned around, so that it stood exactly edge-ways between the cuspidatus and the right lateral incisor like a wedge; its natural front and back sides being against the side of those teeth I have before mentioned, namely, the right cuspidati and the left front incisor. The left lateral incisor was also considerably diverted from its natural situation, so that the proximity of the canine teeth, and the very irregular crowded state of the incisores, presented the appearance upon looking down upon the edges of the teeth, of six teeth, as it were, all in a block. The gentleman could not recollect of any circumstance or accident by which these teeth could have been thus forced into such a singular mass, being shaped more like a square block, than like a circle of teeth as they naturally appear. The other teeth appeared to be quite healthy, and their gums likewise, and in a natural position, except that they all seemed to incline forward more than natural. From appearances, this mass of teeth had occasioned some considerable irritation, by the peculiar and great irregularity of their position. Some tartar was deposited around their necks; and an active process seemed to have been going on for a long time, in order to remove all these teeth. The right lateral incisor was pushed up, and its alveolus so completely absorbed away, that it had not even the appearance of a socket; it was supported mechanically by being pressed upon by the right cuspidati and the left front incisor; and the nerve and blood-vessels which entered its cavity appeared to be in a healthy state, and the tooth itself did not appear to have lost its vitality. There was no apparent suppuration about its fang. I have observed in those cases when suppuration does take place about the front under incisores, that the disease soon advances so as to destroy their vitality. In this case, I extracted three of the irregular teeth, and by cleaning the others, and using the wash as before directed, and an astringent dentifrice, the diseased gums were perfectly cured, and the gentleman's teeth and gums to this time remain perfectly healthy.

When the scurvy attacks the gums of children, as it readily inclines to do, we are are very often obliged, besides our other curative measures, to scarify those parts of the gums which are most affected. Its attacks in these cases are most frequently made during the first dentition, and after some of the teeth have passed through the gums and the others are passing, matter is lodged around the teeth already above the gum, which excites some irritation, and this united to the pain of the other teeth which are passing out, and the irritation all united, occasions in some cases a very alarming degree of constitutional excitement, and inflammation is apt to be very extensively spread through all the gums, lining of the alveoli, and to the maxillary bones. In these cases we must be governed by circumstances, and the urgency of the case. Leeches may be applied to the gums, extensive and pretty deep scarifications, and gentle aperient medicines ; the teeth should be cleaned with the greatest care, and afterwards the oak-bark decoction, or of the nut-gall, will be found almost invaluable, and a perseverance in all the measures before recommended must be enjoined. At the time of the second dentition, before all the first teeth are shed, and during the cutting of the second, great irritation at times arises, generally in children that eat a considerable animal food, and do not observe proper cleanliness of their teeth. The following case will illustrate all that I wish to say at present on this subject.

Mrs. M——, a respectable lady, living in Tenth-street, Philadelphia, sent her son, a child between five and six years old, to me, that I might cure a very unpleasant state of his gums and teeth. Upon examination, I found that the under front incisores of the infant teeth were shed, and had been succeeded by the permanent ones; that the deciduous upper incisor teeth were very loose, and the under lateral incisores also, and the gums around these loose teeth, were greatly inflamed and swollen, and were in the worst state of suppuration that I had ever seen in any case, and all the teeth and gums were in the most offensive state. I immediately extracted all the loose teeth, very carefully cleaned the remaining, and freely scarified the gums, and gave the person who came with him a bottle of the oak decoction, with directions to use a soft brush freely over his gums with the decoction, and to observe the most perfect cleanliness; and also that if any relapse of his disease appeared, to let me see him again, and as I have not heard from him, I conclude he is well.

In conclusion, I must say, that the most assiduous attention is necessary on the part of the patient, to the state of his teeth and gums. The former ought to be kept perfectly clean, and for this purpose he should have tooth brushes, so as to clean the teeth, both on the inside and out. He may use tooth-picks made of ivory or horn, or something of that kind; (one made from a common quill may answer very well—metalic tooth-picks should never be used;) and with these he may remove any matter between his teeth which the brush might chance to leave. All irritating dentifrices should be avoided, and those composed of some astringent and tonic, combining some mild ingredient which shall act mechanically, in conjunction with the other means to remove all foreign matter from the teeth. By these means he will be able to preserve his gums in a healthy state, and his teeth firm and beautiful. Definite rules cannot be given which shall perfectly suit every case, but it is believed that enough has been said to enable the judicious physician and surgeon-dentist to adapt these principles and remedies to the successful cure of every case, in all their varieties, provided their efforts and directions are seconded by the solicitous compliance of the patients.

SECTION II.

Cancrum Oris.

This is a term applied to a distressing and dangerous affection attacking the gums of children and often terminating fatally. It has prevailed to an alarming extent in the Children's Asylum, located in the south part of this city. In the third number of the North American Medical and Chirurgical Journal, for July 1826, we have a description of this disease, from the pen of Dr. H. B. Coates, at that time one of the attending physicians of the children's Asylum before mentioned.

In this ingenuous and well written paper we have condensed a great portion of what is now known of this disease. As I have seen but few cases of this disease in its malignant form, I shall presume to extract so much from Dr. Coates' paper as to give the reader an idea of its history and treatment. Passing over the introduction and reference to authors, among whom we notice the names of Pearson, Senmertus, Vander Wiel Muys, M. Berthe, Candeville, Van Swieten &c., who described or referred to a similar disease—noticing that the disease has been found mostly in marshy or low countries—that the Asylum is exposed to malaria, the water impure, the diet of the children meat once a day, molasses, indian mush, &c.—breakfasts and suppers, bread and milk, we come to his description of the disease.

*Description of the Disease.**

"The ulcer of which we speak, may begin in many parts of the mouth. In by far the greater number of cases, however, it commences immediately at the edges of the gums, in contact with the necks of the teeth, and, most generally, of the two lower incisors. A separation is found here, which exhibits a slight loss of substance at the extreme edge of the gums, and, as far as I have observed, a whitishness of the diseased surface. In some cases, though not very frequently, this is preceded by a slight swelling and redness. In this state the disease may continue for a long time; and I have reason to believe, that patients have remained thus affected, during the whole period of three months, for which I attended the Asylum. At one time when the disease was at its height, threatening several patients with destruction, I found upwards of seventy children, out of a population amounting to about 240, more or less affected with these ulcerations. No remarkable change is at this stage observable in the functions of the little sufferer, except a general air of languor and weakness. The appetite and the muscular activity continue, but are somewhat reduced, not sufficiently, however, to disable the child from attending school, taking the air, or

* North American Med. and Surg. Journal, vol. II, pages 11 to 17.

continuing his ordinary practices. In this state, no symptoms of irritation have been at all discovered. The skin is cool during the day, no pain is complained of, and no account has ever been given me of any nocturnal paroxysm of fever. It would appear to be purely a state of asthenia; we are, however, by no means certain, that there was no concealed irritation in the system. We were, of necessity, obliged to depend, in a great measure, upon the reports of nurses, and other females, and these were liable to overlook, or mistake for mere weakness, the signs of an obscure disease. In this manner, commencing cases were frequently not discovered, and nothing was done till the affection had made further progress; and this continued until the ascertained existence of the epidemic in the house, combined with the recollection of its former ravages, had excited an alarm which led to the inspection of the mouths of all the children in the institution.

The disease, in this form, must be within the curative powers of nature; as, if this were not the case, we should hear of more numerous unfavourable terminations. It has seldom, however, if at all, been within my power to witness this tendency; and when not controlled by a particular treatment, the cases have almost always remained stationary, or increased in severity. Its first progress is, most generally, by extending to the edges of the gums round other teeth; frequently affecting a large portion of the dental arches. A very early progress is, however, mostly effected down the length of the tooth, in the direction of the socket, and, in this way, the disease commits great and unsuspected ravages. When it reaches the edges of the bony socket, the tooth begins to be loose, and when drawn, exhibits portions of the fang, including parts which had been contained within the alveolus, entirely denuded of their periosteum. Indeed, from observation, I should say that the latter membrane was the part which was the most peculiarly liable to injury and death from this disease; and it is by no means clear, to my apprehension, that this is not frequently the commencement of the complaint. The injury generally proceeds with augmenting rapidity, especially when it has affected the deeper parts: and it is while in the act of rapidly spreading that it occasions gangrene.

In the production of gangrenous sloughs, it much resembles the descriptions usually given of sloughing ulcers. A portion of the parts immediately subjacent to the ulcer loses its life; this rapidly separates, and, before or after a complete removal, a fresh slough is formed in the same manner. They are generally black, with ash-coloured edges. I have not been able to discern a change of colour, the production of vesicles, or any material tumefaction, as antecedent to the gangrene. There is, generally, by this time, an increased heat in the parts, with the sensation termed "calor mordens." The discharge, now, for the first time, becomes acrimonious, giving pain when it comes in contact with cuts in the fingers, and excoriations are produced on all parts in contact with the sloughing ulcerations, as the lips, the cheeks, the tongue, and the adjoining surface of the part where the ulcer is situated.

As soon as the external gangrene has reached the level of the edge of the body socket, and frequently much sooner, the adjacent portion of the latter is found deprived of its life, forming a necrosis. The death of the periosteum in the socket, at least that of the fang of the tooth, precedes, by some interval of time, that of any portion of the bone itself.

When gangrene is formed, a fever of irritation is generally developed. In regard to the time at which this takes place, there is a great diversity in different constitutions. It has appeared to me to depend, principally, upon the inflammation of the mouth, which is secondary to the original disease, and, in most cases, to arise from the acrimony of the discharge. It is aggravated by loss of rest, want of nourishment, and, probably, by putrid matter finding its way into the stomach. To this latter cause I also refer a diarrhœa, which almost uniformly comes on towards the close.

There are accounts of a similar disease having begun on the inside of the cheeks. I have, however, never seen a well marked instance of this; the cases which were supposed to be such having, in every instance, been also found to exhibit ulcerations at the edges of the gums. That the disease spreads from the gums to the cheek, is a fact which I have often seen exemplified. It is, indeed, the most usual termination of bad cases. After producing gangrene and necrosis in the gums and alveoli, and after the discharge becomes, as above stated, acrimonious, a gangrenous spot is not unfrequently found about the opening of the Stenonian duct, on the inside of the upper or lower lip, opposite the incisors, in some other part of the inside of the lip, or cheek, or in more than one of these situations at the same time. Whether this be owing to excoriation from the discharge, or to some other cause, I cannot say; it has, however, in every instance which I have seen sufficiently early to witness its rise, been subsequent to the symptoms previously described.

When the gangrene reaches the cheek or lip, however, very active inflammatory symptoms are uniformly developed. In the cellular substance of these parts, they assume the well-known characters which have been attributed to the phlegmonous species. We have a great thickening forming in the cheek, a large, rounded, prominent tumour, with great heat and pain. Sometimes redness is perceived externally;

but, more frequently, the great distension of the skin of the cheek seems to empty the cutaneous vessels, giving to the part a smooth, polished, dense white appearance, very much resembling the effect of a violent salivation. I have no doubt that this is the tumour described by Poupart, and alluded to in an earlier part of this paper. Great thickness and hardness have always occurred in the other situations where this gangrene has approached the external cellular masses of the face; in the lip, however, they are less remarkable, perhaps, from the smaller amount of cellular texture. After reaching this stage, a black spot is frequently seen on the outer surface of the swelling. This spreads rapidly, and has always been, in my own experience, the immediate harbinger of death. It is proper to state, however, that I have heard it said that cases had recovered in this city, in which the gangrene had produced a hole through the cheek. Under what physician's care this occurred, I have never learned.

In two cases it commenced in the fauces, and was marked by the same unsuspected progress. In one of these, the little patient was remarked to be languid, but had no positive external marks of disease. The mouth was examined, and found healthy; but no suspicion of the real situation of the disease was entertained, till after three or four days more, when he complained of a slight sore throat. A large gangrene of the tonsils, half arches, and pharynx, was now found, and the event need hardly to be told.

The closing stage of this affection is marked by large gangrenous patches in the gums—deep fissures between these and the teeth—the latter loose, or falling out—large pieces of the alveolar processes, often containing the roots of several teeth in a state of entire necrosis—the whole lining membrane of the mouth suffering a violent excoriation—the whole adjacent external cellular substance hard and swelled—large gangrenous spots in the inside of the cheeks or lips, occasionally extending quite through to the outer surface—a total incapacity to sleep or to take the least food—fever—a swelled abdomen and diarrhoæa.

Dissection.—The inspection of the body after death had never thrown much light on this obscure affection.

Pathology.—The nature and production of this disease are certainly very obscure. We may, however, as in other branches of knowledge, attempt to record and develope what knowledge we possess respecting it, carefully separating truth and reason from conjecture. We have already said, that its access was very frequently preceded by no marks of visible disease, or at least, none that attracted attention. The little subjects were, apparently, in merely a drooping or enfeebled state. In other instances, the ulceration follows a common remittent or intermittent fever; insomuch that, at one time, whenever a child was brought to the nursery for fever, it was expected, as a matter of course, that his mouth would become sore. In other cases, as we have already had occasion to say, it is quite possible that a concealed "inward fever" may have existed; and this is rendered the more probable from the circumstance of their losing their appetites. In the instance where the body was opened, we have seen that the original disease was hepatization of the lungs, and yet it is quite probable, that this affection had caused, as it often does, that species of disease, which a rapidly spreading pathology refers to a slow inflammation of the stomach and intestines. With regard to marks of this last not having been detected by me, it is evident that I am in the same situation with a very numerous body of other observers.

The local appearances at the commencement, did not appear to be of an inflammatory nature, at least generally. If the gums were really the first part affected, it was not so; as these parts when inflamed, as they frequently are in affections of the teeth, exhibit decided soreness, pain, swelling, and an increase of redness. The ulcerated part was in about nine cases out of ten paler than natural; and then neither soreness nor increased heat was perceptible, except in a few cases, in which the mouth was generally hotter than natural, though it was not in a striking manner referrible to the gums. In a few cases, distinct redness, and a slight swelling, were perceptible round the ulcer. These patients generally did better than the others. If on the other hand, we suppose the original derangement to have taken place in the periosteum, we shall be enabled more easily to explain some of the phenomena. We then reason thus; the whole of the body had shrunk considerably from disease, and the circulation being deprived of a part of its usual vigour, the periosteum, apart possessed of little vitality, was unable to bear the additional extension which it underwent across the unyielding bone of the tooth. The blood ceased to circulate in it, and it died. Ulceration of the adjacent parts followed, as a matter of course; and these parts, especially the periosteum being possessed of but little sensibility, the sympathies of the other part of the system were but little interested, until an extensive portion of the mucous membrane of the mouth, or a mass of cellular substance became affected. We certainly see that in every case but two, the disease commenced in contact with the teeth. This doctrine will also explain the rapid and deep penetration of the ulcer along the roots of the teeth, and the destruction of the bone. We may recur to the statement, that a portion of the fang of every loose tooth, was always found deprived of its periosteum.

In the two cases excepted, we have seen it apparently begin in the mucous membrane of the fauces; and indeed the manner in which it generally spreads from the gums to the cheek and lips, seems to me unquestionably to indicate a greater liability than common, to gangrene in more than one part of the mouth.

The soreness and pain of the socket, which forms a part of most tooth-aches, might have been reasonably expected here; but neither was ever complained of, even when the teeth were loosening; and, as no fever existed at this time, the original irritation can hardly be considered as inflammatory; excepting perhaps the cases which exhibited redness, and slight swelling of gums.

*Prevention**.—Our precautionary measures should be directed to the predisposed or commencing state already described; to the prevention and cure of fevers, to the removal of "febricula," and other internal disorders, and to the general restoration of strength. Finally, its commencing state should be watched, and promptly met, and success I believe will always attend our endeavours.

† The remedy which beyond all comparison succeeded best, was sulphate of copper. The usefulness of this substance, though known at Salem, New Jersey, was discovered at the asylum, the mistake of a nurse. It had been previously used, in lotions of the strength of 11 grs. or 111 to the ounce of water, and with little advantage.

Observing that the empirical remedies said to have succeeded, were as I considered them, immoderately strong, I

---

* North American Med. and Surg. Journal, Vol. II. page 18.

† North American Med. and Surg. Journal, Vol. II. pages 20, 21.

urnished the nurse with a common solution of sulphate of copper, and with a vial containing 72 grains of the sulphate in an ounce of water, for the purpose of being progressively to the other at different periods. This stronger solution was applied, by mistake, instead of the diluted one; and it was the first remedy which had produced a rapid tendency to a cure. I finally settled down, after various trials, in the employment of the following:

℞ Sulph. Cupri, - - - - ʒij.
Pulv. Cinchonæ, - - ℥ss.
Aquæ, - - - - - ℥iv. m.

S. To be applied twice a day, very carefully, to the full extent of the ulcerations and excoriations.

The cinchona here is not absolutely necessary; but operates by retaining the sulphate longer in contact with the edges of the gums.

Simple ulcerations and small gangrenes, as well as the troublesome excoriation, when not in the last stage, yield promptly to this remedy; the good effect being generally visible from the first application.

Dr. Fox, my friend and fellow-labourer in the asylum, had already taught me that it was important early to extract the teeth. I was not, however, sensible of the full extent of this rule, till after examining the fangs of some of them which were drawn. The separation of a portion of the periosteum from the fang, within the socket, which was universally found whenever the tooth was loose, among two or three hundred specimens, proved the existence of the disease in a deep and narrow crevice, into which it was impossible, by any contrivance, to insinuate the lotion. This cavity was laid open by extracting the tooth, and when the remedy was applied, the sanatory effect was surprisingly prompt. From this period forwards, the universal rule was to extract all teeth the moment they were discovered to be in the slightest degree loose; and "the blue wash" above described became the standing remedy."

In reviewing this paper of Dr. Coates, there are two points upon which I wish to dwell for one moment, to wit: its pathology and treatment.

First, its Pathology. I do not wish to discuss the pathology advanced by Dr. Coates, but pass at once to what I conceive its true pathology. It commences a simple inflammation of the gums spreading in some cases to the neighboring parts, which, under some circumstances, and in some constitutions terminates in gangrene. This position I think will be readily granted when we consider for one moment its predisposing and exciting causes as directly and indirectly conceded by all those who have treated of this disease.

Predisposing Causes.

First, The disease in its malignant form attacks those children only who are of exceedingly debilitated habits, in whom the vital energies are greatly impaired—living under the influence of impure and unwholesome air which depresses the vital powers of all persons, but more especially of children—their light diet, impure water, and, most of all, the frequent attacks of febrile diseases, and suffering the operation of considerable medicine, all contribute to reduce the constitutions of these little sufferers to a state of organic weakness, as hardly to be able to resist the slightest injurious impression. In proof of this, I will mention a case I lately saw in the children's Asylum, of cancrum oris which terminated fatally. The mother of this child was a common drunkard. The child had never known good living or good treatment, and immediately after being admitted into the Asylum was attacked with measles. Although it survived the attack and course of measles, yet after this it was but the wreck of vitality: so exceedingly depressed were the powers of this child's system, that before the attack of the cancrum oris, a slight scratch upon the finger induced an inflammation which was not arrested until the finger was mortified and sloughed away to the second joint. Another fact in proof of our foregoing position is, that this disease is most apt to supervene soon after the conclusion of febrile diseases; so much so that when a child is recovering from fever, &c. the nurses are especially directed to notice its mouth. Another fact in corroboration of our principle is, that this disease forms, as says Dr. Coates, "the principal source of anxiety and trouble during the winter season." At this season the vital energies of children, and especially of those of the poor, are more depressed than at other seasons of the year. I forbear to mention any more particulars which might be noticed of the predisposing causes, except in the treatment of fever, the free use of mercurial medicines, which, if exhibited to any extent, always render the gums and lining membrane of the mouth, &c. more or less morbidly irritable. *See case of this kind in notice of disease of the maxilla by Koecker.*

Exciting Causes.

One uniform fact, with one or two rare exceptions, asserted by Dr. Coates, and admitted by all others who have spoken of this affection is, that it commences upon the gum, around the necks of some of the teeth, usually some of the incisores, thence passing along the tooth to the alveolus and neighboring parts. We have noticed the vitiated state of the constitution, and that even a slight scratch might be, and was productive of gangrene. We are now prepared to assert that the exciting cause of the inflammation in the gums, &c. is the same in these children as we find it to be in instances of almost every day's notice, among the children of the better sort of citizens, which, however, seldom becomes malignant, from the healthy constitutions, &c. of these children, to wit: acrimonious and foreign matter deposited under the gum and resting on the necks of the teeth, and passing, in some instances, to the alveolus. This foreign matter we have found uniformly to be the cause of inflammation in the gums as fully detailed in the chapter on scurvy, in this work, and by Mr. Koecker. In proof of this assertion, I will notice a few facts in the history and treatment of this disease.

Firstly, We have noticed that it always commences around the necks of the teeth.

Secondly, That the early extraction of the teeth, around which the gums were affected, was absolutely necessary in nearly all cases treated by Dr. Coates.

Thirdly, That cleaning the teeth with a tooth powder and brush, used as a prophylactic remedy has almost eradicated the disease from the house.

Fourthly, That the second dentition has completely arrested the disease and predisposition to it, by ejecting the deciduous teeth with the acrid matter on them, and the replacement of new and clean teeth, with a consequent healthy state of the gums, &c.

Dr. Coates suggests that the disease is not in its commencement of an inflammatory nature in all cases, although he admits it in many. The present medical attendants of the house all admit that in every case it does commence with inflammation. I believe at this time the idea of gangrene supervening without inflammation, except from mechanical obstruction of the circulation is nearly exploded.

In a few rare cases the disease commenced in the fauces, and on the inside of the cheek. This does not, for one moment, militate against our general principles, for foreign matter may, and does often adhere to the fauces, as the tartar of the teeth, and, we are disposed to believe, that diseases in the soft parts about the posterior part of the mouth are not unfrequently produced from this cause. On the inside of the cheek, and especially in the mouth of the stenonian duct, tartar is often deposited, proving a frequent source of irritation. In conclusion, it is believed that we may fairly assert that cancrum oris, in its causes, commencement, and first stages, is identical with the common scurvy of the gums, described by Hunter, Fox, Koecker and myself; but that under peculiar states of constitution, as before detailed, gangrene supervenes. One fact which positively demonstrates the assertion, is, that hundreds of children will be affected for a long time with what are called the first stages of this complaint, without ever passing to a malignant form, and when a malignant case does occur, it is seen in children whose organic powers are so debilitated as hardly to sustain life. In proof of what we have said, cases can be shown where, from a debilitated state of the system, gangrene has even taken place from operation about the mouth in adults. Jourdain relates of death in this way, from the extraction of a tooth.* I will now take a brief notice of the treatment, without detaining the reader with a lengthy disquisition of the subject.

Treatment.

I only wish to speak of the local treatment of this complaint, which should be prophylactic and remedial.

---

* Jourdain, Tome 1, page 489.

In the prevention of this disease our object should be to remove from the teeth all acrimonious and foreign matter, and to prevent a swollen and lax state of the gums. These two objects will be readily effected by the use of a tooth-brush, and appropriate dentifrice. The brush at first should be very soft, so as not greatly to irritate the gums, and should be changed for a harder one when the gums will bear it. The dentifrice should combine astringent and alkaline properties, so as to neutralize all acid and acrimonious matters in the mouth, and by its astringency to remove from the gums all tendency to an irritated and spongy state. Of these formulæ will be found in the pharmaceutical part of this work.*

The mouths of the children should be carefully noticed. and perfectly cleaned, at least once a day. When the disease has actually assumed an active and malignant form, it was the practice of Dr. Coates to rely chiefly upon the use of the sulphate of copper as a remedial agent, which he remarks was accidentally discovered to be useful, and "became the standing remedy."

The practice of the present physician in attendance at the children's asylum, in addition to prophylactic remedies, nearly as I have recommended, is, as soon as the disease assumes an active and malignant form, in addition to leeches, blisters, &c. externally to apply the undiluted nitrate of silver to the inflamed part. We have before remarked, and it is well known, that few remedies possess such almost specific virtues in allaying diseased action upon irritable surfaces, as the

---

* I will insert a very appropriate one in this place.

R. Pulvis Galla	. . .	℥i	
Cinchona	. . .	℥iii	
Sapo hispan.	. . .	ʒi	
Carb. Sodæ	. . .	ʒi	Mix.

lunar caustic, and especially when applied to inflamed and irritable gums; and in this disease it is found highly beneficial. The sulphate of copper is also used, but the medical attendants are now satisfied that this latter remedy, often from its acrimony, is itself a cause of inflammation. In looking over the records of some cases, I was struck with the fact. Another injurious property of this remedy, and one of serious moment to the enfeebled child, is, that a part of the wash is often swallowed, which uniformly produces violent vomiting, which in some cases, no doubt, by enfeebling the child, has hastened rather than retarded the fatal termination. I do not know as we are to expect any other benefit from the sulphate, than from its astringent properties. When I first began to treat diseases of the gums, I made use of the saline astringents, as the sulphate of zinc, sal saturni, &c. but I soon remarked their acrimonious qualities, and immediately exchanged them for the vegetable astringents, as quercitron bark, pulverized galls, &c. which last, without any acrimony, is as powerfully astringent as any remedy we desire.

SECTION III.

TUMOURS FROM THE GUMS, CARTILAGINOUS EXCRESCENSES, DISEASED GROWTH, &c. &c.

Independently of scurvy and cancrum oris, the gums are liable to other states of disease, such as tumours from their cartilaginous excrescenses, diseased growth, &c. These are almost uniformly produced by some irritation in or near the gums, occasioned by the influence of dead pieces of bone, diseased fangs of teeth, or of the teeth themselves, &c. &c.

Decayed teeth and stumps are sometimes the cause of a diseased action in the gums, in consequence of the irritation produced by them upon the gums. These last, at times, make an effort to grow over the stumps, but the irritation experienced from the latter often induces a preternatural growth of the former, which is a kind of fungous excrescence. I have seen a case of this kind, which had attained to a considerable magnitude. Tumours, perhaps, occasionally grow from the gums, not connected with diseased teeth, and which are much firmer than those produced from the irritation of dead teeth and stumps, and are often the subject of surgical operations. Mr. Fox removes them usually with a ligature, as they are apt to bleed profusely from excision.

I give the following remarks and case from Mr. Fox's book upon the subject of tumours, produced by stumps of teeth, as being applicable to perhaps every case of this kind. He says,* "Some time since, Mr. Cooper was applied to by a lady who had an enlargement of the gums of the lower jaw, which nearly filled up one side of the mouth: there were several decayed stumps of teeth remaining, around which this enlargement of the gums had taken place. Mr. Cooper sent her to me for the purpose of extracting the stumps, intending when these had been removed, to extirpate the tumour. The stumps being embedded in the gums, the operation was unavoidably attended with laceration of the excrescence, and consequently a considerable hæmorrhage. A few days after, the tumour became very flaccid and dark coloured; it then sloughed away in large pieces, so that a cure was effected without any other operation." This, I think, will be found to be the case with all these tumours produced by the irritation of stumps of teeth. Take away the cause and the ef-

* Part II, page 82.

fect ceases. As regards the hard and firm tumours which grow from the gums, and are not connected with diseased teeth or fangs, they should be removed by the use of a ligature drawn round their bases; and if this is broad, a needle may be passed through them, carrying two threads, and then each thread may be brought around on each side and tied, so as to firmly embrace the tumour, and it will soon slough away.

Excision in these cases has been practised in some instances, but the objection which has been raised to this, is the profuse hæmorrhage which occasionally follows, so as even to require the actual cautery to arrest it. In other cases, the hæmorrhage is slight, but the fungus is apt to be reproduced, so that probably the safest and most advantageous mode of removing these tumours, is by the use of the ligature.

I will introduce a case of this kind, remarking that in every case of tumours from the gums, a critical examination of the gums should be had, with a view of detecting any fangs of teeth which may possibly remain in the jaw, and produce the swelling.

*Case XXV.**—About the year 1815, a lady from the interior of Pennsylvania applied to Dr. Physick respecting a tumour of her gums over the left cuspidatus. It was of a spongy nature, and about the size of a walnut, greatly disfiguring the face, and preventing the patient from shutting her mouth.

The attending surgeon of the family had repeatedly operated upon it, and had removed the tumour twice with a knife, and I believe, on the second occasion made use of the actual cautery, but never to the effectual extirpation of the

* Koecker, pages 264, 265.

tumour. Dr. Physick objected to operate until he had obtained my opinion respecting the teeth. By a very careful examination of the gums, I found that a small part of the root of the left lateral incisor remained very deeply seated in the socket, and suspecting that to be the irritating cause, I proposed its removal, which was accordingly done immediately after Dr. Physick had extirpated the tumour. The lady left Philadelphia with the intention of returning, if a proper cure should not prove to have been effected; but as neither Dr. Physick nor myself ever heard any complaint from her before I left Philadelphia, there seems to be no doubt of her perfect recovery."

I could mention very similar cases, but I deem it unnecessary.

*Cartilaginous Excrescence of the gums.**

It is about thirty-six years ago that I was called with Allertius Baringue, surgeon, to see a woman that had a large tumour situated in the gum of the molar teeth. Her mouth was entirely drawn to the other side of the face, when she was seized with spasms. We advised her to not delay too long having this tumour removed: she would not consent to it; but seeing that this excrescence increased so fast in such a short time, and in such a manner, as to hinder her from taking food, she changed her sentiments. We embraced the tumour with a brass wire which we tightened every day. The excrescence receiving nothing to augment it, fell, and we saw it was altogether cartilaginous. We then applied such remedies to hasten the cure as appeared to us proper. On a

* Jourdain, Tome 2, pages, 334, 336.

similar occasion, the vessels not being varicose, I believed a two-edged instrument might be used with success; and in case of some arteries bleeding that were here given off, the hæmorrhage might be stopped by compression, or by the actual cautery. The remedies that are used after the operation ought to be taken from the class of dessicatives and spirits &c.: suppuratives would be useless.

Baldiunus, Epist. Med. 7, page 19, makes mention of a cartilaginous excrescence of the gums that a woman aged more than forty five years carried on the left jaw. They commenced with small glands like warts, and became as large as a pomegranate, hanging out of the mouth, in consequence of which this woman could take in nothing but drink, and sometimes thin aliments, but this was what she could not do without much trouble, it being necessary for her to use her little finger to push them into the mouth. This excrescence fell four times by means of a wire passed around it; and of course this woman got entirely well.

Ambrose Paré, Liv. VIII. Chap. IV. Page 188, speaks of having seen these excrescences so large that they came out at the mouth, and entirely deformed the visage; and that he had extirpated them while supple by inserting them with a double wire, and had also used hot iron; and that the flesh became sometimes cartilaginous, and even osseous in time. "I have amputated them," says this author, "that were so large that parts of them came out at the mouth; which rendered the patient most hideous to be seen, and there was no other surgeon that would undertake their cure on account of these excrescences being of a livid colour: and I did not fear this lividity which they had not in the least decided upon, but I had the boldness to cut, and even cauterize, the tumours, and the malady was entirely cured; not altogether at once, but at different times, on account of its reappearing as often as I cauterized it. The cause of it was, a small portion of the bone of the alveolus where the teeth are inserted, being altered; and to remedy it, we must cure these excrescences as soon as possible; for when they are small and rooted, they are easy to cure, and will be found only a slimy humour, which, by little and little, hardens and makes it very difficult to cure."

Blasius Obs. IX. Part VI. page 79, speaks of a cartilaginous excrescence of the gums he cut with the scissors.

*Daniel, Miscell. Curios. Dec. 1. ann. 2, Obs. LV. page 379; Scutter, Obs. LXXXII. page 301; Donatus, Lib. V. Hist. Miral. Med., speak also of similar excrescences cured by the ligatures.

"If, after it is cured," says Albucalis, Lib. II, Chap. XXXIII. this flesh begins to grow again, as it sometimes happens, it must be cut a second time, and burnt, and then it will grow no more." What is here said by Albucasis is in conformity to the principles of Ambrose Paré; but for burning, the actual cautery is preferable to all other means.

The ligature and the two-edged instrument may be used for extirpating these tumours; but circumstances ought to direct us in the choice of the different means employed; for these operations require the greatest consideration. Tacitus Luzitanus, Prax. admiral. Lib. 1, Obs. XCIII. page 22, "reports a woman of a melancholic temperament having a hard flesh on the gum of the lower jaw, which in the space of a year became so large that it equalled an egg in size. It gave her much pain, and exhaled a stinking smell, on account of a fetid sanies that came out of a little ulcer in the tumour. The most prompt remedy was to extirpate it; but after the operation the hœmorrhage was so great, which not having been able to stop, the patient was lost.

* Jourdain, Tome 2, pages, 336, 338.

There is every reason to suppose that in this malady the bone was carious; the ulcers fistulous, and the nature of the pus sufficiently indicative. In a similar case, I should have preferred the actual cautery to the two-edged instrument. I should have carried the first even as far as the bone, and after some similar examples which have fallen into my hands, to the extent of the exfoliated caries, the ferment being absorbed, the tumour would be destroyed insensibly of itself. It is judged necessary to repeat the actual cautery as often as the malady makes its appearance. I have had a poor woman under my care who had a tumour very nearly similar to that of which Lusitanus speaks of. It occupied the space of four incisor teeth of the upper jaw. The teeth were all carious. I extracted them. The tumour had two fistulous openings, which run in the direction of each tooth, and which furnished to each a fetid humour. With the actual cautery well heated in fire and double-edged, I made but one wound of the four fistulous openings: I touched the bone that was carious, which was repeated seventeen times in the space of three months. In proportion as the exfoliations were made, the tumour diminished. The patient was cured near the end of the fourth month. In fine, the Surgeon-Dentist, volume I, page 190, makes mention of two considerable excrescences of the gums. He speaks also of some of them which acquired in the order of time an enormous size, and degenerated into a bony or stony consistence, strongly adhesive, and almost making but one body only with the osseous parts to which it was intimately united.

These last excrescences, of which the author speaks, could not be removed with the ordinary scissors, nor with the bistoury, the scalpel or other instruments of this class, nor yet with the ligature. Then as they appear to resemble and enter the class of exostosis, recourse must be had to a kind of cutting pincers, sometimes to instruments that are used for extracting the teeth, or to flat scissors, straight or curved, to gouges, &c. all according to circumstances. In all these cases the principal cause of the malady should be removed at the time when it is possible to do so. Equal attention should be given to the positive state of the bone, and not to make a useless compromise, or expose it for want of attention to the action of the air or other impressions that might prove hurtful to it."

I will give the following which is mentioned by Mr. Koecker.

*Case.**

The following is a letter which was handed to me by Miss B——, Manchester street, London, in the beginning of the month of May 1825. The history it gives, is perhaps one of the most distressing cases of its kind, concerning a lady of great respectability and rank in Scotland, of about thirty-eight years of age. Its contents indeed are not less remarkable for the manner in which they display the uncommon fortitude of the unhappy sufferer, than for the striking confirmation which they give of the facts which I have detailed in the foregoing chapter, as well as of the description I have given respecting the present state of dental surgery.

Considering this evidence as most useful and important, I beg to submit to the reader, the whole of the fair sufferer's most interesting and affecting communication.

---

* Koecker, Part I. pages 111 to 117.

"My dear,—

"I have been so ill since I wrote you last, that I have not been able to answer your kind letter. As I can express myself easier to you than to a stranger, I shall endeavour to give you some idea of my present state, and you can give my letter to Mr. Koecker. Constant faint gnawing pains in my gums, membrane of the mouth, and cheeks, accompanied with considerable swelling of the latter, which are always blotched, inflamed and irritated, just in the way some people's faces are affected when suffering tooth-ache; my very nose is swelled and inflamed, and the muscles of the under part of my face so contracted and drawn upwards, that I cannot swallow any thing but liquids. My mouth is contracted with slimy saliva. In bed I have constant twitches in my gums, like what I could figure electricity; sometimes my face and gums burn like fire, and sometimes feel as if every nerve and blood-vessel were filled with ice, and the sheets near my mouth are wet with saliva; all these sensations often run down behind my ears, to my neck and arms, and at these times I have a great hurry and agitation of spirits, and aching across the breast and heart. To me, one of my greatest tortures, is the extraordinary inflation of gums, particularly towards the roof of the mouth; they feel as if they absolutely tore from the bone, hove up as it were with wind, and my jaws feel twice too large for my mouth, the pressure against my face is such. The same sensation often proceeds to my cheek bones, which increases the swelling of the muscles, and the dragging up of the under jaw. I must now go back in my history, that Mr. Koecker may know the progress of the last five years of my continual misery; but, unluckily, I fear it is impossible to make any one understand my sufferings, they are too various and complicated. You know I always blamed my teeth as the cause of all my sufferings; but I am now convinced that the disease is in my gums, and remains of the alveolar processes; and as I was told that was a part of his profession Mr. Koecker was supposed to be very skilful in, it makes me very anxious to have his opinion. You will remember how long (many months) the sockets of my molar teeth stood open, and even when they did heal up, the gums were full of morbid sensibility. When I last saw you, I had only about five front teeth remaining, and eight below; about 1818, they began to ache a little, and as usual to irritate and inflame my cheeks; the five upper ones began to spoil, but I fought on with them to the winter 1819, when the inflammation and the various sensations I have mentioned before as now suffering, increasing, and the teeth themselves aching, I had them pulled; the gums swelled and inflamed most dreadfully, the horrid sensations in the roof of my mouth increased, and my face was as bad as ever. In about a month the wounds healed, but the gums remained swelled, and became a hard white gristle. After suffering many months I had the gums opened, they were so hard and thick the dentist said they were like bone, the sockets were not the least absorbed, of course rough, and in some parts exfoliated. The gums were kept open near a month, and caustic applied to excite absorption. In the course of this process, the point of a tooth was discovered in one of the sockets and extracted; it was a full grown eye-tooth, which for want of room had never made its way down; I was easier as long as the gums were open; but just where I was when they healed up and resumed their state. Some months after, my under jaw became affected, the teeth there were not spoiled, but became so painful to the touch, that I could bear nothing in my mouth to touch them. My lips became very tremulous, and my hands trembled so, that I could neither feed nor dress myself; when warm in bed they ceased, but from the moment I rose and began to speak, or let the air into my mouth, I never ceased trembling, and the dry retchings (which you remember how tortured I use to be with) increased so as to bring on vomiting. I suffered in this way for eleven weeks, when in despair I had all my remaing teeth pulled; the tremblings and retchings quickly abated, and in a few weeks completely left me, and I have never had them since; my under gums even before the teeth were pulled, were a hard gristle, and almost as white as the teeth. My gums have been often opened to give me relief, but as nothing will induce them to suppurate, I get no advantage, the wounding only increases the hardness: these gums seem to me to act as levers pressing on the nerves and blood-vessels, and keeping up a constant inflammation and irritation in my mouth and face. Under an idea that my complaint proceeded from neuralgia, I was advised to have the mental nerves divided at the chin, which did no good, and has created such hard tumours on these places, that I think their pressure on the side of the jaw is the cause of the twitching pain of my under lip, and the contraction of the muscles. I would take it as a great favour if Mr. Koecker would say, whether he thinks he could be of any use to me here, until I am able (which, alas! I fear I am not) to come to London, or if he could give me any advice which I might desire to be done here, and if he will be so very good as to mention what are the different kinds of diseases he has ever met with in the gums or alveolar process, and his mode of treatment. There seems to be an idea here, that if the sockets are not carious, there can be no disease there, but I think Mr. Fox mentions otherwise. My upper gums had not been touched for four years, till a week ago, when a part was opened that was very troublesome and much swelled;

the bone was full of points and inequalities, and rough, sounding gritty like sand; there was a great deal of thick slime like white of an egg, mixed with blood; some nitrous acid was put upon the wound to try and keep it open a little, but in vain: it is covered already with a new gum, and the old thick parts gaping open; I am sure if these old swelled gums could be got away, I should suffer less. I should think there is about the eighth of an inch of the socket remaining; the ridge of the under jaw is as sharp as a knife, and so painful to the touch when I press it, that it makes my face, ears and neck burn; my lips are painful and drawn in. I was advised to try false teeth, but they increased my sufferings ten-fold, which is very hard, as the clinching of my jaws adds much to my sufferings; my eyes are beginning to be much affected, which must plead an apology to Mr. Koecker for this sad scrawl, which I think you will need to help him to decypher. There are various opinions respecting my complaint: one says it is a nervous complaint at the origin of the nerves, affecting the extremities of these nerves; others say it is a nervous affection of the dental nerves and their ramifications on the face; and others are of opinion it is an affection of the covering of the bone. I am satisfied it is in some diseases of the antrum. Could it injure me to have the antrum opened to ease my mind? There is one place where I think there is a part of a fang of a tooth, which I am certain was broken, as the dentist burnt the tooth without letting me see it; perhaps that may torment me."

CHAPTER V.

DISEASES OF THE MAXILLA.

It is not my intention to discuss this subject at much length, but as the surgeon-dentist often witnesses them, and as they may have a connexion with diseased teeth, or the irritation of dead ones, I presume to say something upon it, and introduce a few cases which conclusively have, in some instances, their connexion with diseased teeth, &c.

The maxillary bones are subject to inflammation, mortification, and likewise to bony growths or deposits around them, of which I shall hardly take a cursory notice.

In the upper jaw the antrum maxillare is occasionally subject to inflammation, formation of pus, mortification, to cancerous growths, and in some cases, accumulation of mucus. I subjoin a history of these affections from the pen of Messrs. Fox, Koecker, &c. referring the reader to a case which came under my own observation, and described in the section upon Phthisis, as caused by bad teeth, &c. I will commence with diseases of the antrum.

* Inflammation in the antrum is often occasioned by diseases of the teeth, but it also occurs when the teeth are quite sound. Sometimes in examining the prepared bones of the head, one or more fangs of the large molares may be found passing into the cavity. In such a case, inflammation, excited by a diseased tooth, would speedily communicate to the membrane lining the cavity and cause suppuration.

I think mischief usually follows the neglect of an abscess of the antrum. The natural opening from the cavity is usu-

---

* Fox, Part II, pages 125 to 131.

ally rendered impervious; hence the matter is obliged to make its exit by an ulceration through one of its sides, which most frequently is that situated under the cheek. It is common to membranes under inflammation to become thickened, and as the opening into the nose is through a membranous part, it is probable that when inflammation takes place, it is in consequence of the thickening of this membrane that the opening of the antrum into the nose becomes closed.

During inflammation in the antrum, the patient at first conceives the pain to proceed from the tooth-ache, but if the tooth should not be diseased, a more accurate observation is made upon the peculiar sensations excited. The pain usually extends towards the forehead, in the direction of the frontal sinus, and a sensation of tightness and weight, with throbbing, is felt on the side of the face. In a short time the cheek becomes red, and appears as if swollen; it feels very hard, and on raising the lip a considerable fulness above the fangs of the teeth may be observed.

If the disease be not attended to in this stage, as the matter rarely passes out at that side leading into the nose, an absorption of the bone above the molares takes place, and the matter discharges itself through the gums; but this does not cure the abscess; the formation of matter still continues, and the ulcerative process goes on, until so great a destruction of the bone is caused as to render the disease incurable.

This case requires the same kind of treatment as abscesses in general, viz. an outlet to be made for the matter; the best mode of effecting this is by extracting one of the molares, and making a perforation into the antrum, through the socket of the fangs. If it should happen, that either the first or second molaris be carious, it will be proper to extract it; but when the teeth are perfectly sound, the second molaris is to be preferred, as the antrum descends the most at that part, and it is desirable to have the opening in the most depending situation.

When the matter has been discharged, the object must be to restore the parts to their former condition; with this view a solution of the tincture of myrrh is to be frequently injected, with a syringe, through the opening. As the inflammation subsides, the natural opening usually becomes pervious, and the injection will pass into the nose; and when this opening is restored, the discharge gradually diminishes; the gum may then be suffered to heal over the artificial opening, and a cure is effected. As there is always a disposition in the gum to close over the part from whence a tooth has been extracted, it may be kept open where the socket has been perforated, by introducing a piece of bougie, which, sticking at the upper part of the socket, and hanging just low enough to be taken hold of, may be withdrawn at the time of syringing, and then be again returned.

If the natural opening into the nose has become perfectly obliterated, it will be requisite to preserve an artificial one; this may be accomplished by wearing a silver tube in the perforated part, through which the mucus will constantly pass into the mouth, and future accumulations be prevented.

I have met with several cases of disease in the antrum, occasioned by carious stumps, in which a considerable enlargement, with absorption of some of the anterior part of the bone, had taken place. The extraction of these stumps has been followed by a great discharge of glareous fluid from the socket; the discharge continues for some time, but it gradually diminishes, until the part acquires a healthy state.

The antrum is sometimes the seat of formidable diseases, but these cases are not common. That which most frequently occurs, is the formation of a polypus, or fungous tumour, within the cavity. The usual progress of this malady is, that the tumour, having acquired a certain size, an absorption of the bone is induced by the pressure; this absorption commences in the internal part of the cavity, which is gradually rendered thin, until the whole is completely removed. The alveolar processes, and even part of the fangs of the teeth, are absorbed, when the remainder of the teeth becoming loose, irritate the gum, and must be extracted. The tumour continuing to increase, the cheek becomes much enlarged, and instead of bone or fungous substance, occupies the whole side of the face; at length ulceration takes place in some part, which, as it increases, is attended with so considerable a discharge of matter, that the strength of the patient is gradually diminished, and at length the disease terminates fatally.

The antrum is sometimes most dreadfully affected with cancerous disease. Happily, these cases are very rare; the only specimens that I have seen are in the possession of Mr. Heaviside and Mr. Taunton. The histories of these cases are very similar; the patients were both elderly women; at first they complained of pain in the side of the face, extending up to the forehead, and the eye, and back to the ear; these symptoms continued for about four months, when a tumour formed near the ear, from which, shortly afterwards, there was a discharge of very fetid, dark-coloured fluid. Ulceration then began in the cheek, over the maxillary bone, by which, after great ravages had been committed, their strength was gradually exhausted until death terminated their sufferings. These cases were about fourteen months in their progress.

In the patient under Mr. Taunton's care, the disease which was on the right side, occasioned the absorption of the os-maxillare superius, the os-palati, the os-malæ, the os-unguis, and the condyloid, and coronoid processes of the os-maxillare inferius; also there was an opening of communication from the orbit to the dura mater, by an absorption of part of the os-sphenoides and of the os-frontis; but the dura mater was not injured.

In Mr. Heaviside's museum is the skull of a woman, who had a disease of the antrum, attended with a very great enlargement: in the course of the disease an ossification in the substance of the tumour took place. Mr. Heaviside, who very kindly favoured me with drawings, is not in possession of any accurate history of the case. It occupied, in its progress, about five years. When it had existed about four years, matter began to form under the skin of the face, which ulcerating, was attended with a great discharge, under which the patient finally sunk.

A few years since, I had the opportunity of observing the progress of an antrum case in a respectable gentleman, Mr. W. The disease first exhibited itself as a tumour above the molares, occasioning a slight prominence of the cheek. By the direction of Mr. Cline, about once a fortnight I made an incision with a lancet into the tumour, which being attended with a considerable hæmorrhage, greatly diminished the tension which arose from the fulness of the vessels.

As the tumour increased, an absorption of the maxillary bone took place, together with the fangs of the teeth, which, becoming loose, were extracted. At length the tumour became so enlarged as nearly to fill the mouth, and by its projecting of the cheek, greatly deformed the countenance. By adhering to the occasional use of the lancet, the disease was retarded in its progress for about five years, when ulceration commenced, by the distressing effects of which the life of the sufferer was terminated in a few months.

Mr. Cooper is in possession of a remarkable case of ossification from both antra; a tumour projected from each antrum, which, by their gradual enlargement, effected such a change in the structure of the orbits, that the eyes considerably projected; at length the ossification proceeded upwards, and produced so much pressure upon the brain as to cause the death of the patient.

Mr. Koecker mentions having seen one case of diseased antrum. Mucus occasionally from obstruction of the canal leading from the antrum to the nose is accumulated in the antrum, of which I will insert an interesting case.

* The most interesting example of the effects of this lodgement of mucus in the antrum, is that recorded by Dubois: a boy, between seven and eight years of age, was observed to have, at the base of the ascending process of the upper jaw bone, on the left side, a small, very hard tumour of the size of a nut. As it gave no pain and did not appear to increase, his parents gave themselves no concern about it; when he was about sixteen, it increased in size, and began to be somewhat painful. Before he was eighteen, its augmentation was so considerable, that the floor of the orbit was raised up by it; the eye thrust upwards, the palpebræ very much closed, the arch of the palate pushed down in the form of a tumour, and the nostril almost effaced. Below the orbit, the cheek made a considerable prominence, while the nose was thrown towards the opposite side of the face, and the skin at the upper part of the tumour below the lower eyelid, was of a purple-red colour, and threatened to burst. The upper lip was drawn upwards, and behind it all the gums on the left side were observed to project much further than those on

* Waite, Surgeon-Dentists' Manual, page 81.

the opposite side of the face, and at this point alone, the thinness of the bony parieties of the antrum was perceptible.

The patient spoke and breathed with great difficulty; he slept uneasily, and his mastication was painful, the case was at first supposed by Dubois, Sabatier, Palletan and Boyer, to be a fungus of the antrum, and an operation was considered advisable.

In proceeding to this measure the first thing that attracted the notice of Dubois, was a sort of fluctuation in the situation of the gum, behind the upper lip; a circumstance which led him to give up the idea of the case being a fungus, though he expected that on making an opening, merely a small quantity of ichorous matter would escape, affording no kind of information. In this place however, he determined on making an incison, along the alveolary process, whereby a large quantity of a glutinous substance, like lymph, or what is found in cases of ranula was discharged. A probe was now introduced, with which Dubois could feel a cavity equal in extent to the forepart of the tumour; and in moving the instrument about, with a view of learning whether any fungus was present, it struck against a hard substance, which felt like one of the incisor teeth, near the opening that had been made. Five days after this operation, Dubois extracted two incisors and one grinder, and then removed the corresponding part of the alveolary process. As the hæmorrhage was profuse, the wound was now filled with dressings, which in two days came away, and enabled Dubois to see with facility all the interior of the cavity. At its upper part he perceived a white speck, which he suppo-ed was pus, but on touching it with a probe, it turned out to be a tooth, which was then extracted, in doing which, some force was requisite.

The rest of the treatment merely consisted in injecting lotions into the cavity, and applying common dressings. In about six weeks all the hollow disappeared, but the swelling of the cheek and palate, and the displacement of the nose still continued. In the course of another year and a half every vestige of deformity was entirely removed. (*Dubois, Bulletin de la Faculté de Med. an* 13, *No.* 8.

I will close this subject by two anomalous cases from the pen of Mr. Koecker, given in his late work on diseases of the maxilla, and one I have seen, and two from Fauchard not connected with the antrum. I will mention the one I have myself seen, which although I did not at that time understand its pathology, I am now fully satisfied was occasioned by the irritation of inflamed gums and teeth. The case occurred about seven years ago in the town of Georgia, state of Vermont. The subject of it was a boy of about seven years old, the tumour appeared to take its rise from the first permanent grinding tooth of the under jaw, which at this time was first passing the gum. The tumour soon after its commencement increased very rapidly, involving all that side of the face, pushing the tongue out of its place, and likewise extending back so as to press upon the esophagus, and upper part of the larynx of that side. The mouth was kept permanently open, and the cheek of the same side greatly protruded, so as finally to show one enormous mass of diseased growth. The child sunk under the progress of the disease, I think in about seven weeks. A great number of physicians residing in that neighbourhood saw the case, and I believe generally pronounced it cancerous, but I could not learn that any one of them was able to give any satisfactory conjecture of its cause.

I will give two cases from Fauchard of bony deposit on the lower jaw, merely with a view to hint to the surgeon the propriety of ascertaining the situation of the teeth in these cases.

Cases.

* "We have an instance," says Fauchard, "in the person of M. Holland, keeper of the Château de Moudon, who had carious molar teeth on the left side of the lower jaw; their caries was communicated to the alveolus; the alveolar processes spread it to the body of the bone; where considerable deposits were formed, which placed it in a short time in a very pitiful state. The king came to reside for some time at the Château de Moudon: M. de la Peyronie was requested to visit this patient. He found him in such a situation as obliged him to have recourse to a capital operation in order to save his life, and the repeated application of the potential cautery."

"M. Lambert performed on M. de Barca's son, about twenty years ago a similar cure; he had recourse nearly to the same means; he was actually obliged to bring away a part of the maxillary bone. This patient was radically cured, and the cicatrice was but very little seen."

"These two cases are of notorious publicity; they made much noise at court, and they were communicated to me by Mr. Anel, who had seen the two patients."

I will close this chapter with the cases from Mr. Koecker's late work, and one case of a fatal fungoid swelling of the gums given by Mr. Hill in the Edinburgh Medical and Surgical Journal, No. LXI. as follows:

† It succeeded to the extraction of a tooth in an atheletic man, aged 52, who had some uneasiness in the socket and adjoining parts for several weeks after the operation, but

* Fauchard, pages 248 and 249.

† The Study of Medicine, Vol. I. page 48. By J. M. Good, Boston. 1823.

which gradually disppeared. At the distance of about two months, a puffiness was discovered in the cavity formed by the loss of the tooth, preceded by a sense of soreness in the roof of the mouth. The excrescence soon assumed the character of a bleeding fungus, spread very extensively towards the roof, and so much affected the patient's speech, that it was difficult to understand him; at the same time the sublingual glands began to sympathize in the morbid action, to inflame and tumefy. At this period, "the mouth presented a spongy, bleeding fungus swelling, protruding the upper lip, and extending backwards to the centre of the ossa palati. The teeth on each side of the tumour were loose and divergent, appearing as though stuck in a thick jelly. The slightest handling of these parts produced a discharge of venous blood. I removed the loosened teeth, each of which brought away with it a large piece of fungus with the scalpel. I also removed the whole of this substance as clear as I could." This however, was not sufficient. Though the bones did not at this time, on examination appear diseased, both the maxilla, and os-palati so soon afterwards, and portions of them were separated by Mr. Hey's circular saw. Still the disease held its ground; it was scotched but not killed. Fresh and more extensive excrescences were protruded, and bid equal defiance to the knife and to various caustics. It does not appear, however, that the actual cautery was tried. "Feeling at length too feeble to labour, he suddenly adopted the resolution of retiring to his native place, as he said, to die." And truly enough he said. He retired into the country, and about three months afterwards, being less than a twelve-month from the attack, fell a sacrifice to pain, debility, and distress; at which time the tumour extended from the angle of the jaw to the top of the shoulder, surrounded by various others, one on each side of the nose, all moveable and elastic; the fungus on the gum filling the cavity of the mouth, rendering the speech inarticulate, and the poor sufferer's swallowing extremely difficult.

*Case III.**—Captain M——, of the East India Company, from Calcutta, laboured under a most distressing and complicated affection of the mouth, the effect of an unparallelled abuse of mercury, which had been exhibited only eleven months previously.

He came to England, accompanied by a medical gentleman, on leave of absence from his regiment, to seek for surgical advice, and visited Mr. Lawrence June 11th, 1826, soon after his arrival in London, who requested him to consult me immediately.

The patient was a tall, well-formed, handsome young man, about twenty-one years of age. According to his own statement, his health was originally excellent, and his constitution strong, and only one year previously he was in the possession of a complete set of teeth; they, as well as all their contiguous parts, being perfectly sound, regular, and beautiful; this was still evident from the appearance of the remaining parts, which in the morbid and dead state, evinced the most striking evidence of their previous perfection.

All the teeth, although entirely free from caries, or any disease of their bony structure, were now perfectly dead, and only mechanically held in their sockets. The periosteum was also totally destroyed, either by absorption or corrosion. The alveoli were not only dead, but in a state of putrefaction; their upper edges all round the semicircle of the mouth, being from an eighth to a quarter of an inch exposed, and exhibiting from their cadaverous appearance, a

---

* An Essay on the Diseases of the Jaws, &c. &c.—By Leonard Koecker, London, 1828, pages 63 to 69.

very frightful aspect. The gums were partially destroyed, and the remaining portion of them either gangrenous and sloughing, or in a state of inflammation and suppuration. The disease had already extended to the maxillary bones, and their osseous structure as well as the periosteum of their cavities, was more or less under the influence of inflammation, suppuration, and mortification; but more especially the left side of the upper jaw, which was already much increased in size, accompanied with a correspondent swelling of the cheeks. The face was flushed, and the skin had a bloated erysipelatous appearance, and the patient suffered excessive pain of the whole mouth, the jaw-bones, and other parts of the head, as well as of other more remote parts of the system.

There was a constant flow of viscid, ropy discharge from the mouth, like that of great salivation, mixed with greenish matter, and accompanied by a fetid, cadaverous odour, emanating from this fluid, and the dead and morbid parts, and so exceedingly offensive as to be almost insupportable to the bystander.

The malady was also particularly complicated, as well as highly aggravated by a great many adhesions of the muscles of the jaws to each other, which had taken place during the excessive salivation previously mentioned, in consequence of which, the unhappy patient had lost almost all power of moving the under-jaw. From these causes, the teeth were mechanically pressed into their dead sockets, and by this unnatural and permanent pressure, the absorption and exfoliation of the sockets were greatly retarded, and the immense irritation already produced by the dead teeth and sockets upon the gums and other soft parts, highly augmented; not to mention that these adhesions particularly impaired the enunciation of the patient.

In addition to these evils, this almost complete closure of the mouth and teeth had, for a long time, prevented the patient from taking solid food, and indeed hardly admitted a sufficient quantity of fluids to preserve his deplorable existence, especially during a long and tedious sea voyage; an evil which would have been nearly destructive to the patient, had it not been in some degree lessened by the removal of one of his incisors. He laboured under excessive debility and nervous irritability, accompanied by fever and general emaciation; in short, his general health had suffered to such a degree that his life might be regarded to be in a most precarious state.

Treatment.

The principle indication of treatment in this interesting case was evidently to relieve the inflammation of the surviving osseous and soft structures, by promoting the exfoliation of the carious sockets and other bones, and more especially, by removing all the dead teeth. These operations, however, were rendered particularly difficult and painful by the fixed state of the under jaw; to this the great debility of the patient added another very considerable obstacle, notwithstanding his surprising fortitude. The following treatment, however, was adopted:

June 12th, 1826.—Seven dead teeth were removed, and the patient directed to wash his mouth frequently with a mixture of the tincture of myrrh, honey, and sage tea.

June 16th.—Two dead teeth were extracted, and the use of the mixture continued. The patient's health and strength were already improving, and by the extraction of his front teeth, he was enabled to take some nourishment.

June 19th.—Four teeth more were removed, the health of the patient still continuing to improve. Some parts of the sockets had come away by exfoliation. The patient complained of pain in the jaws.

July 7th.—I found our patient almost recovered, and in excellent spirits. Mr. Lawrence, who had seen him a few days previously, had taken away the greater part of the remaining teeth and sockets, which had become so loose as to be removed without much difficulty.

August 11th.—Captain M. visited me, to state that all the remaining dead teeth and sockets had been removed some time previously, by Mr. Lawrence. His health had much improved, and his mouth was healing very rapidly. His speech, however, remained very defective; a misfortune principally owing to the almost total loss of motion of his under jaw. He intended in a few days to depart for Ireland, to visit his relations and friends, and to return after some time to submit to the necessary operations to cure the adhesions of his mouth, agreeably to the advice of Mr. Lawrence, and then to supply the deficiency of his teeth by a double set of an artificial masticating apparatus.

*Case IV.** Mr. S——, from ——, a gentleman of about fifty five years of age, of a very robust and plethoric constitution, and constantly active habits of life, gave the following statement of his case.

His health had been generally good, but during the last six years he had sometimes suffered from swellings of the face, accompanied by an erysipelatous appearance, and heat of the skin, as well as an abtuse pain particularly situated in the nose, and its surrounding parts.

* An Essay on the diseases of the Jaws, &c. &c. by Leonard Koecker, London, 1828, pages 79 to 84.

About eighteen months previously to his coming to town, he discovered a small excrescence in his nose, followed by a considerable discharge of fetid greenish matter. His surgical attendant removed the tumour with the forceps, assisted by the application of lunar caustic, but without effecting a permanent cure. The disease continued after a variety of surgical treatment, and its repeated extirpation was uniformly followed by returns of the excrescence. The general health of the patient becoming evidently affected, he was urgently advised by his physician and surgeon to visit London, in order to avail himself of the professional talents of Mr. Lawrence. On an examination of the case, this gentleman instantly detected the actual disease as well as the particular exciting cause. Viewing it as a case of osteo-sarcoma of the nose, and suspecting the state of the teeth to be the cause of the disease, he directed the patient to take my opinion with respect to the condition of his mouth.

By a careful inspection I found the whole of the gums and sockets more or less suffering from that disease, of which I have more particularly treated in the 2nd part of my Dental Surgery, chapter III, p. 270, under the title "Of the Devastation or Absorption of the Gums, and Sockets of the Teeth." These parts were in a state of great inflammation and suppuration, his teeth were much encrusted with green tartar, and many of them so far deprived of their gums and sockets as to have become very loose, and their preservation was not only impossible, but their retention appeared to be a powerful exciting cause of the disease of the mouth, notwithstanding they were entirely free from caries. The upper and under cuspid teeth were much out of their natural line; and from the permanent irregular action of one jaw upon the other, the lateral incisor, cuspidatus, and first bicuspis of the left side of the upper jaw had been deprived of their vitality, the fangs of which, by their irritation, had produced the exostosis.

The tumour adhered to the mucous membrane of the left nostril, and was about two-thirds of an inch in length, and a quarter of an inch in diameter; and I gave it as my opinion that a permanent removal of the exostosis, and a complete cure of the disease, could not be obtained without the extraction of every tooth, which, from the loss of its vitality, or deprivation of a considerable part of its sockets, and irregularity of its situation, acted as a powerful permanent exciting cause of the disease; and the truth of this assertion will be particularly proved by the sequel of the case.

The Treatment.

It was in the beginning of March, 1827, when the excrescence was removed by Mr. Lawrence, and soon after the operation, the patient called on me, and stated that it was the request of this surgeon, that I would do every thing the case might require.

March 9th.—Five teeth were extracted, and the patient directed to wash his gums with an astringent lotion eight or ten times a day.

March 13th.—Two teeth were removed, and the use of the lotion requested to be continued.

March 16th.—Four teeth were extracted and the removal of three teeth more was particularly urged, but the patient would not submit to the operation.

March 21st.—The teeth were scaled, and the use of a proper powder and brush directed.

March 27th.—The scaling of the teeth was repeated, and every direction given to preserve a perfect cleanliness of the mouth; I again very particularly explained the necessity for the removal of the remaining injurious three teeth, which were the lateral incisor and cuspidatus of the left side of the upper, and cuspidatus of the right side of the lower jaw, but nothing would induce the patient to submit to the supposed disadvantageous loss of them. Having already so much recovered his general health from the removal of the stated eleven teeth, and the local disease seeming to him also to be very rapidly improving, he hoped that the extraction of these three teeth might prove ultimately unnecessary, and he insisted, at all events, upon giving them a sufficient trial, before submitting to their removal.

After returning home to the country, the local disease continued to improve, but did not perfectly subside; some inflammation remained, and a return of the tumour was apprehended; in consequence of which the gentleman visited London again, and on consulting Mr. Lawrence, that gentleman now positively insisted on the extraction of the three teeth I had pointed out as the cause of the irritation kept up in the affected parts.

May 10th.—These three teeth in question were extracted.

May 15th.—The teeth were again scaled and all the tartar perfectly removed.

After this complete removal of the local exciting causes, the inflammation and pain in the nose almost immediately subsided, and healthy inflammation and absorption of the diseased gums and sockets followed, as well as a complete cure of the local affection.

The patient was now rapidly restored to vigorous health, which he has ever since continued to enjoy.

*"Dr. Regnoli, of Forli, relates a case, in which a fungoid affection of the maxilla and gums, was successfully treated

---

*An Essay on the Diseases of the jaws, and their treatment, &c. &c. by Leonard Koecker, London, 1828, pages 20 to 23.

by the removal of the alveolar process of both jaws. The patient, a woman of thirty five years of age, had had carious teeth from her infancy, and was almost constantly tormented with severe tooth-ache. She was, besides, subject to frequent erysipelas of the head and neck.

"Towards the close of 1824, she discovered a small tumour, behind the last molar tooth of the lower jaw on the right side. It soon ulcerated, and rapidly spread to the gums and alveoli of both jaws. These parts were much swollen, and considerably contracted the cavity of the mouth. The fungoid excrescences poured out blood on the slightest touch, and continually produced a thin and fetid discharge. The deformity was considerable, and the voice was altered. The limits of the disease were well defined, and the lymphatic system did not appear to be affected, but the patient experienced much pain; her countenance was dull and cachetic; she lost flesh, and had febrile exacerbations in the evening. In this state of things the patient was admitted into the Hospital at Pesaro, where, after having first performed the operation on the dead subject, Dr. Regnoli" [no doubt, after having divided both cheeks to a considerable extent at both angles of the mouth,] "removed the teeth and alveolar processes of both jaws, with the exception of the last molar tooth on the left side of the lower jaw, the socket of which appeared to be sound. From the situation of the parts, the saw could hardly be employed; hence, it was merely used to form a shallow groove in the most prominent parts of the bone, the separation of which was effected by means of a chisel and mallet. Actual cautery was applied to the bleeding vessels, and to such suspicious parts as were not accessible to the knife. The lips of the external wound were brought together by three gold needles, and the twisted suture.

"The first day after the operation, the patient referred her pain to the throat, rather than to the parts which had been operated upon. She had severe head-ach, which was attributed in part to the shock given to the head by the strokes of the mallet, and to the division of the dental nerves. The needles were removed on the fifth day. On the fifteenth, seventeenth and eighteenth, some portions of exfoliated bone were detached. On the nineteenth, the lips could be closed for the first time. By the twenty-third all tumefaction had subsided, the voice was improved, the catamenia which had been long absent, had reappeared, and the other functions were in a natural state. On the thirtieth the sole remaining tooth was removed, as it interfered with mastication. Five days later, she left the hospital in good health. The lips fell in a little, especially the lower, but the deformity was very slight. The voice, which had not quite recovered itself, was daily improving.

"Dr. Regnoli concludes that though the disease should return, the operation was still proper and necessary. Without it, he considers that death would have been inevitable, and he urges in its favour, that it incurred but little danger; that the practice of Dupuytren and Vacca support it—and that the disease does not always return.

From the description of the above case, I have no hesitation in positively asserting, that the mere extraction of all dead roots and such teeth as were loose, or suffering from complicated caries, would have been better calculated to affect an expeditious and radical cure than the above extremely painful and destructive treatment."

DENTITION.

This is a term applied to a beautiful process of Nature, by which the teeth are passed from the jaw through the sof parts and gain situations above the gums. In a majority of cases this process is effected with little pain, and without exciting any symptoms of constitutional sympathy; in others, great constitutional irritation is produced. In chap. 2nd, section 4th, was shewn the manner in which dentition is affected: in this section I only wish to notice constitutional and local affections, which are the result of difficult dentition.

In this process, the teeth, by their developement are pressed against the gum, which, by a process of ulceration, is removed. Such is the beautiful harmony of nature, that in a majority of cases, these two operations will proceed without, in the least, affecting the health of the individual, and he will be reminded of the approach and complete developement of the teeth only by a slight tenderness of the gums. In adults whose systems possess slight mobility, dentition is rarely productive of constitutional irritation, and seldom, indeed, does the cutting of any of the second teeth produce any bad effects, save in some rare cases with the cutting of the dens sapientiæ. In general, it is only in the premier dentition that the aid of the surgeon is required. Delicate children, possessed of considerable irritability and mobility of constitution, and inclined to costiveness, are most apt to be affected by the first dentition. In this process, if the gum is not absorbed away as fast as the young tooth grows, then it becomes distended, swells, and great irritation usually follows, indicated by fever, restlessness, fretfulness, crying, &c. The child often puts its fingers in its mouth, and is often quieted if this is done by its nurse: sometimes it will refuse the nipple, or if it attempts to nurse, starts back, as if hurt in the attempt.

Various constitutional affections are apt to arise, and nature appears to make, in many cases, a sanative effort to relieve the infant system. Among many, I will mention those which are the most common: Diarrhœa is apt to take place in some cases; in others, critical eruptions appear upon the skin, inflamed blotches, soreness behind the ears, and discharge of matter. In some cases an eruption somewhat resembling small pox will appear; at other times, a rash will come out on the breast, face, &c., called the red gum. If the irritation is not soon relieved, convulsions are apt to ensue, and often endanger the child's life. Upon looking into the mouth the gums appear swollen over the new tooth, and often extending some distance on each side of it. A great many anomalous symptoms are sometimes noticed, so that the physician or surgeon ought to be perfectly acquainted with the time when each tooth is expected to appear, so that if any singular symptoms of disease present themselves in the child, he may be able to detect the cause of them.

The surgeon or physician should likewise bear in mind, that all the diseases of infants do not arise from cutting teeth, and for this reason he ought to be perfectly acquainted with the symptoms which denote the appearance of new teeth, and the precise time when they are expected to appear, and also what teeth are expected; for if he does not understand these circumstances, he will often be led into erroneous practices, at once derogatory to himself, and most deplorably injurious to the child.

The treatment of children during dentition, must be regulated by the state of the system. No critical evacuation should ever be checked, if it is not excessive, or so long-continued as to greatly impair the strength of the child. If a gentle diarrhœa comes on, it may be encouraged by giving the child a few grains of rhubarb or magnesia, and if excessive, opiates may be given.

Blisters behind the ears are often useful, or upon the nape of the neck.

Leeches may be applied behind the jaw, or at the chin, or upon the temples, or on the cheeks.

The child may be allowed some soft substance, as a piece of bread, &c. to put in the mouth and its fingers, but hard gum-sticks it should not be allowed.

Washing the gums with a little laudanum and rose-water will be often found useful.

A copious flow of saliva at times relieves the child.

The child should be dressed warm, and kept as quiet as possible. If convulsions ensue, opiates, the warm bath, &c. are of essential service, and should never be omitted.

If there is great heat about the jaws, ether and laudanum, about equal parts, may be rubbed over them externally with great advantage.

But the remedy upon which we are principally to rely is the dividing the gums over the new tooth, so as to allow it to pass out.

This operation is often unsuccessful from not being effectually performed; but if properly done, it seldom fails to relieve the child. The lancet should be carried deep upon the tooth, so as to completely divide the gum over it, and if it is a double tooth, two incisions should be made in the form of a cross, so as to allow the large tooth to pass out, or entirely remove a piece of the gum. The bleeding which follows cutting the gums is of great service in relieving the irritation occasioned by the young tooth.

If properly performed this operation is perfectly safe, but if the surgeon does not ascertain the identical tooth which affects the gums, and does not then perfectly cut through them, the operation will be of little or not any benefit to the child, but on the contrary will occasion increased pain and distress; and hence I may again repeat, that unless the surgeon is perfectly acquainted with the manner of the growth, and the period of the developement of the teeth, he cannot treat the diseases of dentition with any just precision and correctness.

The common round-edged gum-lancet is a very suitable instrument for cutting the gums.

The second dentition is seldom attended with any considerable pain: rarely is any thing but slight scarifications required.

The cutting of the wisdom-teeth is at times attended with considerable pain, but may be usually relieved by cutting the gum, or blisters behind the ears, &c.

The gums after being divided, sometimes heal before the tooth passes out, but the first cutting, if well done, so destroys the firmness of the gums as seldom to require a second division, which, however, is sometimes necessary.

I do not wish to expatiate upon the great utility of incising the gums in cases of difficult dentition, but will merely present the reader with a case in which its great utility is fully demonstrated. It is given by Mr. Baumes in his Premier Dentition, from a work of M. Robert.

Case XXXIX.—An infant, after having suffered much from its teeth, died, and it was in the evening. M. Lemonnier having business there, was told unexpectedly, the infant had lost its life. After having accomplished his object, he was curious to know the state of the alveolus in a case where the eruption of the teeth had not made its appearance; he made a great incision on the gums. But at the moment when he was preparing to follow up his examination, he saw the child open its eyes, and show signs of life; M. Lemonnier called for assistance; the infant was freed from its winding-sheet; care was taken of it; the teeth came out; and the infant recovered its health.

M. Robert has deposited this case in the 2d volume of his Treatise on the Principal Objects of Medicine, page 311.

OF GUM-BOILS AND ABSCESSES.*

Carious teeth frequently become inflamed at the root, and suppuration takes place in the socket, attended with swelling and soreness of the gums. In these cases the same laws are observed for the exit of matter as in abscesses in general, viz. ulceration takes place in some part of its surface, so as to make an outlet for the matter in the best possible situation. When matter forms at the root of a tooth, the periosteum which covers its fang thickens, and in some cases becomes detached from it; the matter is accumulated as in a bag, by the extension of which, considerable pressure is made against the sides of the socket, the consequence of which is, that that part of the alveolar process, situated on the outside, becomes absorbed, rather than that within the mouth.

The ulcerative process continues until the gum bursts nearly opposite to the place where the point of the fang is situated, and thus the matter escapes from this natural opening; the edges of the opening are generally raised, having the appearance of a small, red fungus; sometimes, after the discharge of the matter, the inflammation will subside; but

* Natural History, and Diseases of the Human Teeth. By J. Fox, London, 1814.

the gum-boil rarely disappears, and a small fistulous opening remains, at which matter continues to be discharged; or, upon taking cold, persons are liable to a recurrence of inflammation, occasioning a re-accumulation of matter, but which is seldom attended with much pain. These gum-boils, being occasioned by diseased teeth, are seldom cured without their removal; but, as the operation of extraction cannot always be submitted to, means must be employed to render them as little injurious as possible.

At the first appearance of a gum-boil, that is, as soon as gums by swollen condition and soft feeling, together with the sensation of throbbing pain, indicate that matter is already formed, a puncture should be made with a lancet, in order to suffer it to escape; this will relieve the pain, and prevent any extensive effusion. Sometimes the tooth becomes very sore and rather loose, in which case it will never be serviceable, it would be far better to extract it, which will prove a cure to the gum-boil.

When the inflammation occasioned by a carious tooth is very great, we should be particularly careful to guard against its effects. The formation of matter is often so considerable, as to produce an abscess of no small extent. In some cases the matter is contained within a cavity, extending through the length of one side of the jaw. The teeth which produce the most distressing symptoms, are the dentes sapientiæ of the under jaw; when inflammation extends from either of those teeth to the contiguous parts, the swelling is speedily diffused over all the cheek, so as to close the eye, and cause a considerable hardness at the upper part of the neck, near to the angle of the jaw.

The muscles of the jaw are also affected by the adhesive inflammation, and they become so rigid that it is with great difficulty the mouth can be opened.

These cases require the utmost attention, for a large abscess is usually formed, which if left to itself, generally points externally; the ulceration extends through the substance of the cheek, there producing a most troublesome sore, which when healed leaves a deforming scar. To prevent these sad consequences, when the matter is formed, a free opening should be made on the inside of the cheek, into the softest part of the tumour.

A common notion exists, that it is dangerous to extract a tooth at the time the gum is inflamed; but this is erroneous. Certainly, at this time, the operation is attended with rather more pain than at another; but as the carious tooth is the cause of all the disease, the removal of it is the most certain, and always the most speedy mode of cure. In those cases where the mouth is closed, as this practice cannot be adopted, we must wait until the inflammation be sufficiently subsided for the mouth to be opened.

When inflammation and swelling of the gums and face arise from a carious tooth, they seldom subside without going into the suppurative stage. I have frequently attempted by leeches, cold applications, &c. to prevent suppuration, but have rarely succeeded; the progress of inflammation having been by these means only retarded, not prevented; for, after a certain time, it has come on with redoubled violence, and has gone through its progress; on this account whenever there is any considerable swelling, and the patient too timid to submit to the extraction of the tooth, or if the mouth be so much contracted that the instrument cannot be conveyed into it, I think it advisable to hasten the suppurative process by fomentations, &c. and as soon as a soft place can be felt on the inside of the cheek, to introduce a lancet, and discharge the matter. People very often continue poulticing a swelling of this kind, in order, as they term it, to bring it to a head: in so doing, they cause ulceration to take place through the substance of the cheek. If the tooth producing the abscess be situated in the upper jaw, it will discharge in the middle of the cheek; if in the lower jaw, the opening will be at the lower part of the jaw, either near the angle, or at the edge of its base.

These abscesses are rarely healed, the painful symptoms may subside, but the opening remains fistulous, attended with a consequent discharge of matter.

I have known persons persist in their attempts to heal these kind of abscesses for some months. One lady continued the application of dressings and lotions to a sore of this kind for two years, but with no benefit.

In all these cases the fangs of the teeth become very much diseased, and are the cause of the perpetual discharge; therefore no cure of these abscesses can be expected without the extraction of the tooth.

In these cases, at the opening where the matter was discharged, the skin rises and acquires a sort of fungous appearance, being very red, and of a loose, spongy texture: when the tooth has been extracted, the discharge gradually diminishes, and the external opening closes; but, as the inner part of the integuments have been destroyed by the ulcerative process, in healing the skin becomes contracted, and a deep scar or pit remains. From the situation and appearance of these scars, they are liable to be attributed by superficial observers to the effects of scrofula, which to a female, or a person of nice feelings, is always a source of uneasiness.

When teeth which have caused abscesses of this kind, are extracted, the fangs are found covered with a fleshy substance, which are granulations extending to the bottom of the socket; this being only an effort of nature to effect the healing process, and to fill up the cavity occasioned by that absorption of substance which always attends the formation of matter.

When unfortunately the patient is so much under the influence of fear, that neither acute pain nor protracted suffering is sufficient to induce submission to the extraction of the tooth, the inflammation of the jaw-bone is often so great as to terminate in the mortification of a large portion of its substance.

The process of exfoliation is necessarily a tedious one, the patient is in a continual state of uneasiness, and the mouth is constantly filled with an offensive discharge. As the process of separating the dead portion of the jaw from the living advances, the gums gradually recede from the alveolar processes; at length the dead bone begins to separate, it gradually becomes loose, and when it is completely separated from the bony attachment, it may be taken away.

In plate 1, are two specimens of the mortification of portions of the jaw-bone, in consequence of carious teeth.

Fig. 8 represents a portion of the superior maxillary bone, containing a central and lateral incisor, and the cuspidatus of the left side; this case occurred to a gentleman whose lateral incisor was decayed, he had pain for a day or two, when his gums and lip became swollen; in this state, instead of taking proper advice, he poulticed and fomented his face for several days in succession; a considerable quantity of matter formed and discharged itself under the lip; in this state it continued for some time; when he applied to me, I found that not only the diseased tooth was loose, but also the one on each side. I extracted the carious tooth, but found the socket quite rough, arising from the destruction of the periosteum. I told him I expected that the socket of this tooth would exfoliate: a short time afterwards I saw him again, when, on touching the other teeth, I perceived a motion under the gums, through the extent of the three teeth. Some weeks after, the whole became so loose, that a slight force brought it away. The parts then healed but not without leaving an immense cavity.

Fig. 9 exhibits a similar case, which occurred to a young lady, a patient of Mr. Williams in the Borough of Southwark.

This lady was tormented with the tooth-ache for a long period; her face swelled, and matter formed, but all the entreaties of Mr. Williams, and the dreadful consequences which he taught her to expect, could not raise in her mind sufficient courage to permit the tooth to be extracted. The consequence was, that a large piece of the jaw mortified, the bicuspides, in consequence of their attachment to the bone being destroyed by the ulcerative process, became loose, and being single fanged teeth, were easily taken away; at length the piece of bone was so completely detached, as to allow of its removal, bringing away with it the diseased tooth; at this time, the second molaris, having lost almost the whole of its support, was found to be so loose as to render it necessary to be extracted. Here is an instance where a person lost four teeth, and a large portion of the jaw, through an obstinate determination of not submitting to the extraction of the originally diseased tooth.

I saw also a woman in Bartholomew's Hospital, who from a similar cause, lost all the teeth with the alveolar processes of the anterior part of the lower jaw.

When abscesses form in the mouths of children, from diseases of the temporary teeth, the greatest care should be taken, as by an exfoliation of part of the jaw-bone, the teeth may be destroyed.*

* Vide Natural History of the Teeth, Part II. page 71.

A knowledge of the evils which may result from a carious tooth, ought to influence all persons who may be affected with this malady, to take such early steps for their prevention as prudence shall dictate.

Sometimes an indolent kind of inflammation will exist at the bottom of the socket of a carious tooth, occasioning a hard lump, or small tumour, of the size of half a nutmeg. In this state it will continue for months, with no other alteration than being rather sore, when, in consequence of a cold, a little active inflammation may arise.

These hard swellings should always be regarded as very dangerous, because, as during their indolent existence they have caused a certain degree of absorption of the inner part of the integuments of the face, if any active inflammation occur, it very speedily runs on to suppuration; and, as the skin has already become thin, ulceration to the external part takes place so rapidly, that I have known an opening formed through the cheek in a very few days. On these accounts I always endeavour to persuade patients to have any tooth extracted, which may be accompanied with any hardness, or swelling. It is also much better to submit to the extraction of any carious tooth which has produced an abscess; for it will be always a source of trouble, as well as occasion an offensive state of the breath.

I will, after what has already been adduced, introduce a few more cases and their treatment, which will sufficiently illustrate these affections, with one from the work of R. Wooffendale, who observes:

* "A lady, about twenty-one years of age, applied to me about four years ago, who had an open sore in the side of

* Practical Observations on the Human Teeth, by R. Wooffendale, London, 1783.

her face, nearly opposite the roots of the first large double teeth of the lower jaw on the left side, from whence there was a continual discharge of matter, over which she wore a piece of black silk to conceal it. About two years before, she had been under the care of an eminent surgeon, who had taken out part of a tooth, leaving the other part in: the discharge of matter was not, however, decreased by it, nor by any other methods used. She was attended by him three months without any advantage; at the end of which time she went home, she living at a distance from him. I examined the teeth, and found one root of the first large double tooth of the left side in the under jaw, which I suspect to be the cause of the complaint; the other root had been drawn by the surgeon as mentioned above. I recommended the remaining tooth to be taken out, which was consented to, and the operation performed immediately. The day following, the discharge from the wound was much lessened; she went home the next day, and I have since heard that she got well in a very short time, without any farther assistance."

The following case is mentioned by Mr. Koecker.

***Case* XX*IV*. Mrs. K. of Philadelphia, a lady about twenty eight years of age, had been suffering for some time from an abscess under the chin, on the left side. Being ignorant of the nature of the disease, she sought no surgical aid, under a hope that it would get well of itself; but it grew worse, and was attended with a constant discharge of fetid pus, with great pain in the whole jaw and mouth, extending as far as the ear. These symptoms at last became so violent as to produce general disorder and fever. At this time Dr. Physick was consulted, who, having discovered the malady to be a fistulous abscess passing through the under maxillary

* Koecker, pages, 262, 263.

cavity and bone, immediately suspected that the teeth were the cause of it; and desired that I should be consulted. On examination I found that three large grinders on the side affected, had been so completely carried away by decay, that the parts of the roots remaining were entirely covered by the gums, which were greatly inflamed.

1819. October 8th.—These roots, six in number, were extracted; and so effectual was the relief obtained from this operation, that in a very short time the patient perfectly recovered.

**Case* XXVI. Mr. L. of Pittsburg, consulted me on the 17th of May 1818, on account of an abscess which he had suffered for several years, in his left cheek, produced by the dead fangs of the left first upper large grinder.

He was about thirty years of age; had an excellent constitution, and enjoyed good general health. He had never suffered from any illness whatever. All his gums and teeth I found, to my great surprise, perfectly sound, although the dead roots above mentioned had excited considerable suppuration in the alveoli at their upper extremity and the maxillary cavity, and had forced an opening through the muscles of the cheek to the external surface. The discharge was so great that, during the time that the patient explained his case, two table-spoonsful at least of purulent matter ran out over the cheek. On examination, I found that nature had been so actively engaged in endeavouring to rid herself of the cause of this disagreeable malady, that the roots were quite loose and hanging on the outside of their respective sockets, merely attached to the gums. The removal of these roots, and the usual surgical treatment of the fistulous opening in the

---

* Koecker, pages, 265, 266.

cheek, effected a perfect cure of the disease in a short time. A considerable depression and scar, however, remained in consequence of the long neglect of proper treatment.

THE EFFECTS OF MERCURY UPON THE TEETH, &c.*

When mercury has been introduced into the system, certain circumstances occur which are usually regarded as criteria of its specific and constitutional action. The most evident of these are, an increased discharge from the salivary glands, soreness of the mouth, and fetor of the breath. The gums become tumid and spongy, are very tender, and liable to bleed; the teeth also become loose, and cannot bear the pressure necessary for the mastication of hard substances; this loosened state of the teeth arises from the thickening of the periosteum which covers the fangs, and by which the teeth are held in the sockets; the soreness of the gums is probably occasioned by that fulness of the vessels which the peculiar action of the mercury induces. These affections of the teeth and gums generally subside soon after the use of mercury is discontinued; the teeth again become fast, and the gums acquire their natural firmness.

A common consequence of the use of mercury is, an increased action of the absorbent vessels; and there is no part on which this action is more evident than the alveolar processes. On examining these parts in persons who have died during the use of mercury, they will be found much less dense, and of a more porous texture than the bone ought to be in its sound and natural state. The use of mercury is

---

* Fox, Natural History of the Teeth, pages 115 to 120.

therefore no uncommon cause of premature loss of the teeth, by inducing absorption of the alveolar processes: this injurious consequence, arising from the use of this remedy, is now greatly obviated by the improvment adopted in its exhibition, namely, by keeping up a longer but slighter action of it upon the system, rather than that violent one which accompanied the old practice of salivation.

Where the use of mercury is carried very far, the teeth, even during its exhibition, often become so loose as to drop out: in other constitutions, still greater mischief is experienced; there is a considerable inflammation of all the parts of the mouth, attended with great swelling and ulceration. This sometimes extends even to mortification of parts of the jaw-bones. It would not be difficult to collect cases of extensive mischief following an injudicious use of this valuable medicine; several striking examples of which have been presented to me by various surgeons of my acquaintance. In Plate V, fig. 2, is the representation of a large piece of the anterior part of the under jaw, containing the incisors and cuspidati, which exfoliated in consequence of a long-continued salivation.

Fig. 3, represents nearly the whole of the under jaw, which mortified and exfoliated; this person also lost almost every tooth of the upper jaw, which became loose and dropped out.

A very similar case occurred to a patient in Guy's Hospital, who applied for advice on account of great disease in his mouth, as the consequence of a late salivation. He had an exfoliation nearly similar to the last case, and it was surprising to observe how small a deformity attended the loss of so great a part of the jaw. During the progress of the exfoliation, so large a deposit of new bone took place around the dead portion, that it became, as it were, enclosed in a case; and after it came away, the new bone was rounded, and the gums healed over very perfectly.

Last year I saw a most dreadful instance of the injurious consequences of an improper use of mercury, in a lady, a patient of Mr. Norris, who had just arrived from the East Indies, where she had been salivated on account of a liver complaint. She had been advised to employ so much mercury, that she was literally poisoned; her mouth became completely ulcerated, and the whole constitution was so much affected, that she lay for some time in a state of insensibility. As she recovered, the soreness of the mouth rendered the opening of it painful and difficult; and as the ulcers healed, so much adhesion and contraction took place at the posterior part of the mouth, that it could scarcely be opened even to admit a tea-spoon; at length the contraction increased to that degree that she completely lost the power of opening it. Ou this account, she was under the necessity of receiving nutriment in the form of thick milk, soups, &c. introduced into the mouth by a large syringe, the pipe of which being curved, was passed into the mouth through an opening formed by the loss of one of the molares. In addition to these calamities, the great inflammation which had been excited, caused the mortification of nearly the whole of the alveolar processes of both jaws. On separating the lips, a most dreadful appearance presented itself; the gums had retired from the teeth, leaving the alveolar processes uncovered and quite black. I removed several teeth which had become loose, and in two or three places exfoliation was beginning to take place.

The constant discharge of matter made a very frequent syringing of the mouth with tincture of myrrh and water absolutely necessary, and had she not possessed a most exemplary patience and composure of mind, she must have been completely miserable.

Some time since a man became a patient in Guy's Hospital, who had been so injudiciously treated in a course of mercury as to cause a complete ulceration of the gums and the inner surface of the cheeks and lips. The consequence of which was, that, as the process of healing advanced, so much adhesion of those parts took place that the mouth could scarcely be opened. The man could only be relieved from this distressing situation by the dissection of the lips and part of the cheeks from the gums, which was performed by Mr. Cooper; the parts were then preserved from re-uniting by the interposition of lint, until they had perfectly healed.

During the use of mercury, when the mouth becomes affected, it should be frequently washed with a mild astringent lotion: for this purpose I have usually recommended the infusion of roses with a small quantity of alum; and, if the soreness of the mouth be very considerable, some tincture of myrrh may be added. During the exhibition of mercury, there is, usually, a considerable deposition of tartar about the teeth; to obviate the ill effects of which, it should always be removed as soon as the medicine is discontinued; the gums will then soon recover their healthy state, and material injury to the teeth be prevented.

In farther confirmation of this subject see case mentioned by Mr. Koecker, in the section on diseases of the maxilla, and another, which came under my own observation, upon cleanliness of the teeth necessary during sickness, &c. &c.

I have mentioned the foregoing effects of mercury, not under an impression that they often happen in the practice of our enlightened physicians, but that they have, and may happen, if mercury is exhibited to excess and care is not taken to obviate its dangerous effects upon the mouth, teeth, their appendages, &c. &c.

TOBACCO.

This article, as well as mercury, perhaps, is used or taken by as many different individuals as any other active or medical substance whatever. That under some states of the constitution it exerts an injurious influence upon the stomach and digestive organs, there cannot be a doubt. But whether it directly injures the teeth or not, has been disputed. I will give the opinions of a few authors upon this subject. Fauchard remarks:

*"The smoking of tobacco is also very hurtful to the teeth; it makes them black and ugly, and besides, if the precaution is not taken to cover the end of the pipe, the rubbing which it makes against the teeth never fails, in the using of it, by slow degrees to uncover their sensible parts. Experience proves this fact, and to which their has not been paid ordinary attention. This smoking produces bad effects; it heats the mouth, and a stream of cold air coming immediately in contact with the teeth, these two extremes might give occasion to the fixation of some humour in the tooth also, in the gums, or in some one of their neighbouring parts; which might occasion very inconvenient pains and defluxions, and caries also, which is the most mischievous of all accidents."

It is not my intention to prohibit the use of tobacco entirely. I know that the teeth are blackened by smoking, if great care be not taken to keep them clean, and to rinse the mouth often; but I know also that the smoking of tobacco may contribute to the preservation of the teeth, by procuring the evacuation of superabundant humours, which might by

---

* Fauchard, pages, 68, 69, 70.

acting upon, destroy them. My intention is only to remark, that immediately after having smoked, they should not be exposed in the mouth to any sudden impressions of cold.

"A dentist of this city, and a great enemy to tobacco, was not willing that it should be used by the nose, pretending it was pernicious to the teeth. It were to be wished that it might be moderately used; but even used to excess, I do not believe it has the power to do any hurt to the teeth. The use of it might be useful to persons subject to defluxions. Tobacco determines the humours to run off by the nose, and diverts, and prevents them from falling on the teeth, which is no small advantage.".

*"Smoking tobacco is also wrong, and is what makes them black and ugly, for they being heated by it in the mouth, and a cold air coming immediately in contact with the teeth, these two extremes might give occasion to some humour, either to the tooth or gums, which might cause pains, considerable fluxions, which are very inconvenient, and caries also, which, of all accidents, is the most mischievous, and for which the fewest remedies are to be found"

Longbothom, in his treatise or Dentistry, remarks: †

"The smoking or chewing of this herb is frequently introduced from the vehement pain of the tooth-ache, and with most constitutions paves the way to a far more dangerous disease than it is intended to remove, by its acrid and internally violent qualities, in the act of fumigation being inhaled; and the chemical oil which it leaves within the hollow of the teeth, disposes them to blackness and premature decay; which, though less obnoxious for the present, proves a lasting enemy to the mouth and stomach."

---

* Le Dentiste Observateur, par Courtois, pages 50 and 51, Paris, 1775.

† Longbothom's Treatise on Dentistry page 30.

I have had occasion before to remark that I have noticed persons having good teeth who had used tobacco, both smoking and chewing it, for a great number of years. On the other hand, I have seen persons with very bad teeth who used tobacco. In some constitutions tobacco removes its irritability; in others, it increases the irritability of the system. And when we look over the causes of caries, diseased gums, &c. we shall find that the fact respecting the operation of tobacco, which we have noticed, explains its good and bad effects on different individuals. There is an acrimony or impurity about some tobacco, which causes it to injure the teeth; but my observations, as to the effect of good tobacco, are, that by some individuals it may be chewed with impunity, and that smoking tobacco may be allowed; and, probably, used as an errhine it never injures the teeth; but as it is a dirty, and in many instances pernicious substance, perhaps its use might, with advantage, be entirely dispensed with.

CHAPTER VI.

SECTION I.

DISEASES PRODUCED BY DISEASED TEETH, &C.

I need not, in the commencement of this chapter, for one moment detain the reader in proving the well-known fact, that disease in one part of the living system may be productive of disease in another and remote part; or endeavour to explain the rationale of that mysterious sympathy by which this effect is produced. A vast many pathological facts are yet to be explained, whilst the few that have been are every day assailed by new and more plausible theories. At present the truly intelligent physician is satisfied with clearly understanding causes and effects of diseases; considers disputes respecting the modus operandi of the causes of disease to be, to say the least, unprofitable. In the subsequent chapter it will be my object to lay before the reader a few plain and undeniable facts which unequivocally establish the important principle, that the diseases of the teeth, the gums, and maxillar organs, exert a powerful and extensive sympathy with the rest of the system.

The diseases which I shall mention as produced by diseased teeth, gums, maxillar organs, &c. are the following:

Phthisis Pulmonalis.

Perhaps many persons may start at seeing this set down as ever being caused by diseased teeth, and consider its having a place here, as arising from the caprice or fancy of the writer, but which cannot be placed here either by facts or sound reasoning. Phthisis pulmonalis, the scourge of the human family, the destroyer of our race, the baneful siroc, whose course is marked by its destructive energies, that spares neither age nor sex, enumerates in the number of its causes, a diseased state of the teeth. If this is so, why are not these diseases known by the practitioners of medicine, and made an object of their especial attention? I answer, because in this country they form no part of the education of the student of medicine preparatory to his entering upon the practice of his profession; and after that period, either from the multiplicity of their engagements, or from a want of industry or enterprize, few of them ever enter upon those untrodden fields of disease, or their causes which had never been hinted to them, either by their preceptors or the authors they read.

The diseases of the teeth, or their destructive effects upon the system in general, are at present very little known to the medical practitioners of this country, although they have occupied the pen of a Hunter to detail them; and the name of Rush, has borne testimony to their injurious and dangerous consequences. Need I ask for greater names, or higher authority to give evidence or consequence to this subject? No, for none greater are wanted, or can be found. Their illustrious names are identified with the science of disease, and have descended to posterity as stars of the first magnitude in the horizon of their day, and shine as beacons for the guidance of distant generations. One of the first effects of diseased teeth, is to contaminate the air that passes over them; this they do, more or less, proportionate to the extent and state of their disease: in some cases very slightly, in others, the affected tooth or teeth are in a complete state of putrefaction, and the air which passes to the lungs, through the mouth and back, is greatly contaminated and rendered exceedingly offensive to every person near the individual, and oftentimes to the sufferer himself. It is to the writer of this, at times, a subject of astonishment to reflect upon the quantity of offensive matter thrown off from one or more diseased teeth; although the air which passes over them is changed every instant, still it is constantly affected, and rendered offensive, and the air of a close room is soon contaminated by the breath of such a person. We respire about 20,000 times in twenty-four hours, and yet for months and years, this vast quantity of air is rendered poisonous by one or more diseased teeth. How little does it avail an individual, if by every possible means the purity of the air is preserved, if no impurities are suffered to remain in the streets, his tenements kept clean, his apartments ventillated, or that he make distant journeys, at a great expense of time and money, for the benefit of pure air, and at the same time that he carry the very cloaca of filth in his own mouth? If this state of the breath, caused by bad teeth, so affects the olfactory nerves of a person near an individual having bad teeth, what must be its effects upon the delicate and sensible tissues of the lungs of the person himself? Nature has formed the lungs most delicate and sensible, and susceptible to the slightest injurious impression; she has also finely tempered the atmosphere for its safe and healthy reception in these delicate organs; but an accident or disease may render it impure, unfit for respiration, and cause it, instead of harmonizing with the lungs in the most perfect manner, and give to them and the whole system health and strength, to be a baneful influence, armed with pestilence, and scattering the seeds of disease over the lungs, and pouring the streams of deadly poison through every vein of the system. The matter thrown off from the teeth in a state of disease and putrefaction, and also some states of diseased gums, is very acrid in its nature, as is demonstrated by its vitiating the saliva so much as to cause it to dissolve and oxidate metals, even silver, and to tarnish gold: and we have noticed its effect upon the respired air, that it is present in a great degree in it, and consequently its acrid qualities are blended with it, and must render it extremely pernicious to the lungs. We know that many of our organs have the power of resisting, for a length of time, in a wonderful manner, the effects of injurious impressions; but with the lungs I am disposed to believe, that even slightly injurious impressions, if continued, will sooner or later prove to them a cause of disease and disorganization.

The records of medicine are somewhat barren upon this subject, but there is not a doubt but the reason of this is, because a vast majority of physicians and surgeons have never made themselves acquainted with the diseases of the teeth; consequently they have imputed phthisis to other causes, have seldom attended to the state of the teeth and gums, or the effects of their diseases upon the lungs, and yet conclusions drawn from well authenticated facts and the most logical reasoning, justify the assertion, that diseased teeth and gums do produce phthisis, and a few well authenticated cases positively demonstrate the alarming fact. We have only thus far considered the effects of diseased teeth on the respired air, and through this medium on the lungs, but we should also remember that the records of medicine, are full of cases when disease in one part, is produced by some irritation in another; for instance, a wound upon the head has been known to produce an abscess in the liver, and worms in the bowels, are known to produce dropsy in the brain, hydrocephalus; and a wound in the foot, to produce lock-jaw; and a small tumour beneath the skin of the leg, to produce epilepsy. If these apparently slight causes have produced such alarming affections of the system, is it unfair or unreasonable to suppose, that a diseased state of the teeth, or their being in a state of putrefaction and constant irritation and inflammation, should not, at times, produce the most fatal diseases in the general system and in the lungs, as well as any other organ. I will conclude these observations in the language of Dr. Rush. He says,* "When we consider how often the teeth, when decayed, are exposed to irritation from hot and cold drinks and aliments, from pressure by mortification, and from the cold air, and how intricate the connection of the mouth is with the whole system, I am disposed to believe they are often unsuspected causes of general and particularly of nervous dis-

* Medical Inquiries, Vol. I. pages 349 to 353.

eases. When we add to the list of these diseases, the morbid effects of the acrid and putrid matters which are sometimes discharged from carious teeth, or from ulcers in the gums created by them, also the influence which both have in preventing perfect mastication and the connexion of that animal function with good health, I cannot help thinking that our success in the treatment of all chronic diseases would be very much promoted by directing our inquiries into the state of the teeth in sick people, and by advising their extraction in every case in which they are decayed. It is not necessary that they should be attended with pain in order to produce diseases, for splinters, tumours and other irritants before mentioned, often bring on diseases and death, when they give no pain, and are unsuspected as causes of them. This transition of sensation and motion to parts remote from the place where impressions are made, appears in many instances, and seems to depend upon an original law of the animal economy."

There are so many causes of phthisis, that we are often unable to determine, in each case, what is the precise one; and the only positive proof is, the cure of the disease upon the removal of the supposed cause; and if we suspect a diseased state of the teeth to be the cause, and, upon having them extracted or cured of disease, the phthisical affection is cured, it is then often demonstrated that the teeth were the exciting cause. Dr. Rush quotes from a French writer, a case of phthisis cured by the extraction of some diseased teeth; this is positive proof. We must also remember that phthisis, excited by whatever cause, is cured by the removal of that cause only in its early stage, for after the disease has proceeded so far as to disorganize the lungs, it is probably never cured; the removal of its early cause then will have no effect. The following case occurred in my practice, which to me seemed conclusive, that the diseases of the teeth do at times excite pulmonary affections.

Mrs. S——, a married lady, aged about thirty-five years, residing in this city, with whom I had been acquainted for some months, sometime in May or April 1827, suffered me to examine her teeth. She was at the time troubled with a hacking cough, which she had had for several months, and said; "that she was afraid that she should have the consumption or had got it:" upon examining her teeth, I found that several of them were in the worst state of disease, and rendered her breath exceedingly offensive. I indeed wondered that the lungs of any person could bear the ingress and egress of such offensive matter. Upon assuring her that I thought her cough would be relieved by having her teeth extracted and cured, she consented to have it done. I accordingly extracted eight diseased teeth and stumps, and by a suitable application of remedies succeeded in rendering her mouth, teeth, and gums, perfectly healthy, and soon after this without the farther aid of medicine her cough left her, and her general health became perfectly good, and continues so to this time. I also am acquainted with a lady who has been affected with a cough for several years, and, as far as I can learn of her, it commenced soon after a diseased state of the teeth had taken place: at this time her teeth are in the worst state of disease, and the pulmonary affection is gradually undermining the powers of the system. I have urged her to have her diseased teeth extracted or rendered healthy by dental operations, but from an alleged fear of the pain attending it, she declines having any thing done for their cure.

The following case of phthisis, has confirmed me in the fullest degree, that consumption is occasionally produced by disease in the teeth, jaws, &c. June 10th of the present year, Dr. George M'Clellan of this city sent to me a patient of his, Mr. F—— P——, a gentleman resident in the south part of this city, aged about forty-five years, with a request that I would perform such operations upon his teeth and gums, as, if possible, to restore them to health; and likewise informed me that the antrum of the right side was extensively diseased. When this gentleman called, it was with difficulty that he could walk from the carriage into my house. The following was the state of his general health; extreme debility, great emaciation, pale countenance, slight hectic fever, fréquent cough, attended with a copious expectoration, tongue covered with a light flocculent fur, loss of appetite, dejection of spirits, &c. &c.

The following was the situation of his mouth, &c. The right antrum was extensively diseased, all that part of the jaw-bone of the right side situated anterior to the last molar tooth, and below the antrum, as far as the anterior symphysis of the superior maxilla, had mortified and been ulcerated away, so that all the upper teeth of that side, with the exception of two, which had been extracted, and the last molar tooth, were destitute of alveoli and hung loosely in the gum. The whole interior of the antrum was exposed by a very large opening, made by the loss of the two anterior grinders. A copious discharge of pus from the antrum, had been continued for a long time. On the left side of the upper jaw were several fangs of decayed teeth, and the soft parts around them ulcerated to the very bottom of their sockets, which were almost totally absorbed away. Upon a slight examination, I suspected that the left antrum was in a state of disease, but after removing the loose and dead fangs, and cleansing the cavity of the pus, I had the pleasure to ascertain, that the disease had not reached the antrum of that side. After considerable inquiry, I found that the diseased state of the antrum before mentioned, and the teeth of the same side, was of three years' standing; that the general health of the patient had been uniformly good, until a few months after the disease of the antrum was noticed, when his lungs became affected, attended with cough, pain in the breast, and expectoration. The gentleman informed me that since that period he had never been free from cough, although he had experienced temporary relief from change of air and travelling. With regard to the disease of the antrum, he paid so little attention to it, and kept it so private, that it was not known even to his own family or physician, until quite recently, when it became so aggravated as to force itself upon the attention of the patient, his friends and physician, who, greatly alarmed, immediately sought the assistance and advice of that eminent surgeon Dr. M'Clellan. Upon inquiring whether phthisis was hereditary in the family of this gentleman, he assured me it was not; that none of his relations or family had ever had it, that his father died an old man, of a fever, and that his mother was still living, and in the enjoyment of good health. It was the unqualified opinion of the gentlemen, of his family, and of his physician, that pulmonary affection proceeded from his teeth and diseased antrum, and what might appear rather singular, that for a year before the disease of the antrum was detected, the physician had imputed the exciting origin of the affection of his lungs, to use his own words, "to be somewhere in his head." The gentleman was a man of excellent habits, remarkable for his temperance and correct christian deportment. I immediately extracted all those teeth whose alveoli had been affected by the disease of the antrum, and the fangs and decayed teeth on the opposite side of the same jaw. I then partially cleaned his teeth, gave him an astringent wash for his mouth, and dismissed him with a request to see him at the expiration of one week; in the interval of which time, constitutional and local remedies were prescribed by Dr. M'Clellan. At the expiration of five or six days I again received a visit from him, when a few slight operations were performed, and in a very short time his mouth became perfectly healthy, with the exception of the diseased antrum, which continued rapidly improving. Under this treatment the health of the patient improved. For a short time nature seemed willing to rally the almost exhausted powers of life, but the excessively warm weather, joined to the previously extreme debility, and the harassing symptoms of his malady, urged the disease to a fatal crisis, and he died in July after I saw him.

It was the confirmed belief of the patient, that by an early attention to the disease of his antrum and teeth, the accession of phthisis, would have been prevented; and from this opinion I think few can reasonably dissent.

I think we may safely infer, although diseased teeth do not in every instance excite general diseases of the system and of the lungs, still like an insidious enemy, they are ever ready to unite with or exasperate other causes, so as to finally undermine the powers of the system. I have dwelt at considerable length upon this subject, and would earnestly solicit the attention of the Medical Faculty in general, to a critical inquiry into the state of the teeth in all cases of pulmonary affections, and there is hardly a doubt but what their enquiries would eventuate in the general conclusion; that a diseased state of the teeth and gums do very frequently excite pulmonary affections, especially in persons predisposed to them, and always aggravate these complaints, let them be excited by whatever cause they may.

SECTION II.

DYSPEPSIA PRODUCED BY A DISEASED STATE OF THE TEETH AND GUMS.

There are three ways in which diseased teeth, and gums, &c. may cause this distressing complaint.

Firstly,—By preventing a proper mastication of the food.

Secondly,—By the putrid and ulcerated matter which passes from the teeth and gums along with the aliment of the stomach.

And, Thirdly,—The irritation of a diseased tooth being often so great as to disturb the healthy functions of the system, and of the stomach in particular.

Firstly,—By preventing a proper mastication of the food. Mastication is one of the first steps in that series of processes by which the food is rendered subservient to the purposes of nourishing and supporting the animal system. It seems to be an indispensable requisite that in order to the accomplishment of healthy and speedy digestion that the food should be reduced to very small pieces. It is an old proverb that food well masticated is half digested.* This, with few exceptions, is an universal law of the animal economy The digestive powers of the stomach act with much more facility upon the food if finely comminuted, than if swallowed in large pieces; and, indeed, the practice of swallowing the food in large pieces, in almost all cases, sooner or later produces dyspepsia and greatly weakens the powers of the stomach. I need not enlarge upon this subject, for it is a fact known to every scientific practitioner of medicine, that the food must be perfectly masticated in order to be digested in a healthy manner; and one of the first and indispensa-

---

* Fauchard, Vol. I, page 64.

ble injunctions of the judicious physician to his dyspeptic patient is, to masticate his food with the utmost care, and never to swallow solid food, that is, not perfectly masticated. This becomes a *sine qua non*, for, without it, there is hardly a hope of ever curing the dyspeptic. The influence, in this case, is direct and positive; for if the teeth and gums are in such a state of disease as to prevent proper mastication of the food, dyspepsia must and will be occasioned and continued, from the causes I have before mentioned, and all the evils resulting from this cause, follow as certainly; and are shown as clearly, as any possible demonstration. I will not detain the reader by any more observations upon the influence of proper mastication upon digestion, but will refer him to almost every judicious writer upon dyspepsia.

Secondly,—Dyspepsia may be occasioned by the putrid and ulcerated matter from diseased teeth and gums mixing with the aliment and passing to the stomach. Upon this head of the subject I need hardly make a remark, as it must be self-evident to every reflecting mind, for no person can doubt that matter received into the stomach, which is the result of mortification and diseased animal secretion, must impair the tone of that organ, and vitiate, more or less, all the fluids of the system. The carious matter from decayed teeth is in a state of putrefaction, and the matter from ulcerated gums is the result of diseased animal secretion. I could mention many cases of this kind, but will mention but one.

Case.

P. S.—A gentleman residing in Front-street, called on me in April 1827, with a diseased state of his teeth and gums, at the same time mentioning to me that he had but little hope of having his teeth and gums restored to health, as he had been for some time under the care of one of the most respectable surgeons in this city, with whom I had the pleasure of a personal acquaintance, for the cure of his gums; that, although he had fulfilled his prescriptions, still they were of no use to him, and that he had had his teeth examined and operated upon by a dentist without any service. Upon examining his teeth, I found many of them were in a state of decay, and that his gums, in consequence of the tartar deposited around the teeth, and pressing upon and irritating the gums, were in a state of suppuration, and that the alveolar processes were much absorbed away—the front under incisors were completely dead; their sockets were nearly removed by absorption, and the gums surrounding them were in a complete state of suppuration, attended with a constant discharge of matter. He naturally seemed to possess a good constitution, but his general health was, at this time, much impaired, attended with obstinately dyspeptic symptoms. I think he had imputed all his dyspeptic complaints to the disease of his gums. I succeeded by cleaning his teeth and the use of the oak bark decoction to arrest the disease for some time, but as he refused to have the dead teeth and stumps of teeth extracted, as they always should be, I did not succeed in making a perfect cure of the disease. I mention this case to show how greatly dead teeth, and stumps, and suppurating gums, do affect the healthy action of the stomach, and also again to remind the reader that dead teeth and stumps must be extracted, in order to cure a suppurating state of the gums, and to remove consequent effects. For another case of dyspepsia produced by diseased teeth and gums, in consequence of not masticating the food in a proper manner, and in consequence of decayed and ulcerative matter passing into the stomach, see the case of Mrs. F—, narrated in the chapter upon Scurvy of the Gums. (*See Koecker, page* 110.)

And, Thirdly,—Dyspepsia may be occasioned by the irrita-tion of a diseased tooth being so great as to disturb the heal-thy functions of the system, and of the stomach in particular. It is a well known fact in the pathology of disease that ex-cessive pain occurring in any part of the system will derange all its healthy functions, and no organ is sooner affected than the stomach, as it is the centre of sympathetic action in the animal system. We have often noticed the deadly sickness produced by a slight injury upon delicate parts. The appli-cation of caustic to a wound will sometimes, in some individ-uals, have this effect; and hence, we can easily understand that an acute inflammation of a tooth will disturb the action of the stomach, as I have often witnessed. I will give one case of this kind from Dr. Rush's paper on this subject. He says, " soon after this I was consulted by Mrs. R——, who had been affected for several weeks with dyspepsia and tooth-ache. Her tooth, though no mark of decay appeared in it, was drawn by my advice. The next day she was relieved from her distressing stomach complaints, and has continued ever since to enjoy good health. From the soundness of the external part of the tooth and the adjoining gums there was no reason to suspect a discharge of matter from it, although it had produced the disease in her stomach. It is not my de-sire to protract the consideration of this subject any farther than will be necessary for a correct understanding of it. I have endeavoured to seize and display its principal points to the physician. We have seen that three distinct effects of diseased teeth and gums will, alone, and singly, produce dys-pepsia, and how certainly will they do it when all these ef-fects act upon the stomach in conjunction; and I cannot forbear remarking, in conclusion, that every practitioner of medicine, when prescribing for dyspeptic patients, ought to attend to the state of their teeth and gums, and if they are not in a state of health to have them made so by judicious dental operations.

Another remark we might make, and which was obligingly suggested to me by Dr. Chapman, the highly intelligent professor of the theory and practice of medicine, in the University of Philadelphia, which clearly proves the influence of disease in the mouth upon the stomach is, that dentition in infants, in a great majority of cases, excites diseased action in the stomach and bowels, manifested by the loss of appetite, nausea, and diarrhœa; and it is a fact notorious to the medical faculty, that the occurrence of dentition is apt to aggravate all other complaints which may be present, and especially those of the stomach and bowels of children so prevalent in the summer months, and so certain and well assured are they of this, that even the probability of dentition occurring during the prevalence of summer complaints, is ever productive of alarm, as they know that they will be aggravated, and the lives of their little patients placed in the greatest jeopardy.

The following case of dyspepsia, produced by a diseased state of the teeth and gums, is taken from the public lectures of the present professor of the theory and practice of medicine in the University of Pennsylvania, Nathaniel Chapman. M. D.

Some years since a lady came from a distant part of the country to this city in pursuit of medical aid, and placed herself under the care of Dr. Chapman. He found her labouring under every symptom of obstinate dyspepsia, by which her health and strength were greatly impaired. His correct and well-known acumen in the pathology of disease immediately led him into an inquiry into the state of her teeth and gums. He found that her gums were in a high state of inflammation, and that many of her teeth were loose and diseased. By the direction of Dr. Chapman, she applied to one of our most respectable dentists, and had her mouth and teeth placed in a healthy condition; and with the return of health in her teeth, gums, &c. every dyspeptic symptom left her, and she became quite well. After some time, and the lady's health seemed confirmed, she had a few artificial teeth placed in her mouth to supply some which she had lost, which either from not being well adapted and properly inserted in her mouth, or from some peculiarity in the lady's constitution, proved a source of irritation, and again brought on a return of the distressing dyspeptic symptoms, which compelled her to entirely dispense with the artificial teeth, when her health was again completely restored.

I will mention two cases of dyspepsia, caused by diseased teeth, which came under the notice of Mr. Koecker.

*Cases.**

Mr. F., a literary gentleman, in the neighbourhood of London, had been for some years under the medical care of Mr. J. Derbyshire, of Greek-street, Soho, on account of a constant state of derangement of his digestion.

Much sedentary occupation, and some excessive grief, had of late greatly augmented the distressing symptoms generally accompanying this cruel disorder. His disease had assumed the character of hypochondriasis. His spirits were so dejected, and the state of his bodily health was so low,

* Koecker, Part I, pages 110, 111.

that he was no longer capable of attending to his ordinary business.

Having had some conversation with Mr. Derbyshire on the influence of disease of the teeth upon the general health, that gentleman was induced, at his next visit, to inquire into the state of his patient's teeth, and learning that they were in a very deplorable condition, he proposed a consultation with me on the subject.

After a particular examination, I found every tooth in the patient's mouth more or less carious or dead, and all the gums and sockets in a very diseased state.

On the 27th of May, 1824, twenty-one teeth and roots were extracted, all of which were, more or less, in a state of putrefaction, three large grinders only excepted, which were either suffering from complicated caries, or producing morbid irritation upon the other parts from some other causes.

Four upper and two under incisors, two upper and two under cuspidati, and two under bicuspides; fourteen front teeth in all, were left remaining. These and all the other parts of the mouth were restored to perfect health in the course of about six weeks.

During the progress of this treatment of the diseases of the mouth, the general health improved very surprisingly; and after the restoration of perfect health to all the remaining teeth and their relative parts, the patient enjoyed uninterruptedly good health, and returned to his ordinary professional avocations.

*Mrs. P——, a lady of great respectability, under the medical care of Dr. Jule Rucco, of Leicester-square, had, some years since, continually suffered from dyspepsia, as well as from various kinds of nervous attacks of a very an-

* Koecker, pages 108 to 110.

noying and alarming nature. This judicious physician had for a long time suspected the cause, and frequently proposed to consult me. By the wish of the lady, however, the dentist of the family was at last sent for, and three or four teeth and roots were removed, which, according to the assertion of the dental attendant, were all that could be extracted. The disease, however, was only aggravated by this interference, and the sufferings of the patient increased more and more.

About six months after, the doctor again urged a meeting with me on the subject, and at last I was sent for. I found the lady labouring under a complete salivation, from an extraordinary sympathy of all the glands, in any way connected with the teeth. On the previous night, and indeed, for many nights preceding, she had been suffering such violent fits of convulsion, as to alarm the whole family. The face was affected with an acute erysipelatous inflammation, accompanied with head-ache, as also with considerable derangement of the digestive functions, such as sickness, vomiting, loss of appetite, &c. By examining the mouth, I found that the previous dental treatment had been but very partial, and I proposed the removal of every tooth and root which produced irritation.

The lady consented immediately to my proposal, and the necessary operations were performed on the 8th of October, 1824, when nine decayed teeth, some of them mere roots, were extracted. The patient was directed to rinse her mouth frequently with a diluted astringent lotion. By this simple local treatment, and by the further medical care of Dr. Rucco, she was perfectly cured in about a week after the operation.

Baglivi, one of the best medical writers of a former period, observes in his Canones de Medicinæ:—

* "Persons whose teeth are in an unclean and viscid state, though daily washed, have universally a weak stomach, bad indigestion, and offensive breath, head-ach after meals, generally bad health and low spirits; if engaged in business or study, they are irritable and impatient, and are often seized with dizziness. From weakness of stomach they are naturally somnolent, scarcely wakeful in the morning, and never satisfied with sleep."

I will mention one case more out of many I have witnessed in my own practice, where the stomach was affected by the state of the teeth.

July 2d of the present year, Mrs. S——, aged about 38 years, residing in Frankfort, was sent to me by one of our most eminent physicians, with a request that I would examine her teeth, and perform such operations upon them as I judged proper, to render them and the gums healthy. The state of this lady's health was miserable; she was harrassed with the most distressing symptoms of dyspepsia. Her digestion was very imperfect, the stomach irritated, loss of appetite, and a most melancholly depression of spirits. When she first called, it was necessary for her to repose herself for some time, before she could have her mouth examined. Upon examining her teeth and gums, I found nearly

---

* "Qui quotidiè sordidos, viscidosque dentes habent, licet eos quotidie abstergeant, ii ut plurimum sunt stomacho debiles, malè digerunt, ore fœtent, post prandium capite dolent, mæsti sunt, atque debiles: et si studiis, atque negotiis eo tempore dent operam, irascuntur, impatientes fiunt, capiplenio cum dolore corripiuntur; ad venerem minus proclives sunt: generaliter enim stomacho debiles, venerei non sunt, imò potius frigidi et impotentes. Debiles quoque stomacho, naturæ sunt somnolenti; mane vix evigilant, imò nunquam somno satiarentur."

Georgii Baglivi, Opera Omnia Medico. Practica et Anatomica, Lugduni, 1710.

all the former in a state of disease, and the latter were in a state of suppuration, much inflamed and swollen. A considerable deposit of tartar was formed around the necks of the teeth; in several instances their fangs were denuded of the gum by the deposit of tartar, and in fine her mouth was in a general state of disease. I need not detail the several operations by which her mouth and teeth were rendered healthy, as the principles of treatment are elsewhere in this work fully detailed. Suffice to say, that in about four weeks her mouth was perfectly well. The amendment of the general health after the first operations were performed on her teeth, was almost surprising, and would have been entirely so, to any person not acquainted with the immense sympathy between the mouth, gums, &c. and the stomach. Within five weeks after I first saw her, every vestige of disease in her digestive organs left her, and she was apparently in perfect health.

SECTION III.

PAIN IN THE EAR, AND FORMATION OF MATTER IN THAT ORGAN.

It often happens that painful teeth and those affected with complicated caries, are the cause of great pain in the ear, and occasionally affect the functions of that organ; and so great is the nervous sympathy between the nerves of the teeth and the ear, that remedies applied to the latter, will relieve pain in the former. Laudanum dropped upon a lock of cotton, and introduced into the ear, will often relieve the tooth-ache. This is quite a popular remedy. Upon the same principle or a knowledge of the same facts that the actual cautery has been applied to the antihelix of the ear to relieve pained teeth.

It is often the case, that persons suffering pain in their teeth, from cold, &c. find great and occasionally complete relief by simply filling the ear with cotton.

I will give a case of this kind from the work of the celebrated Jourdain.

*" A lady experienced for a long time, very severe pains in the ear on the right side. All the means were tried but in vain, to remove this painful affection. Eventually, those who were most discerning, asked her if she had not some carious teeth. She assured them that her teeth were very good, performed their functions well, and had never given her any pain. Nevertheless, she was advised to have her mouth examined. She addressed herself to me, and after the account she gave me of her case, what had been done, and the suspicions entertained, I examined all her teeth with the most scrupulous attention. Their first aspect was very imposing. At length proceeding farther in the examination, and removing the cheeks upon the wisdom molar teeth of the lower jaw, I perceived the one on the right side was carious very deeply externally, and that the internal part of the cheek was lodged in this caries. As the pains of the ear extended to the posterior angle of the jaw, and also a little along it's base, I beseeched the patient to have the true cause of her malady removed. This tooth having been extracted, the pains entirely ceased on the third day, and the malady never returned."

Mr. Koecker has given a case of disease in the ear from diseased teeth. He remarks,† " Miss G. of Philadelphia, about

* Jourdain, Tome. 1, page 486. † Koecker, pages 156 to 159.

16 years of age, was troubled with a complaint in her ears, attended with severe pain and discharge of yellowish matter from them, difficulty of hearing, much general debility, and great depression of spirits. No means had been omitted to obtain the best medical and surgical advice ; but it had been utterly unavailing. Her father and the greater part of her brothers and sisters were also hard of hearing, and some of them were sometimes troubled with a like discharge from the ears, although not to such an extent, nor accompanied with such severe pain. The case was consequently regarded as incurable, and supposed to be owing to some natural defect in the organization of the parts.

Nov. 23, 1818. She consulted me with a view of obtaining relief from the tooth-ache, by the advice of her brother, one of the few members of the family possessed of a perfect hearing. He had been some years previously under my care, and was greatly impressed with the belief, that the health of his teeth was one of the principal causes of the preservation of this sense, and for this reason he was induced to believe that the sufferings of his sister originated from the diseases of her teeth.

I found her exceedingly agitated, and so full of apprehension that she actually wept ; and I had the greatest difficulty in persuading her to let me look at her teeth. Having been previously apprised of the nature of her malady, I had already bugun to suspect it was owing to diseases of her teeth, particularly as she had been under the care of the most eminent surgeons and physicians, who, I had every reason to believe, would have been successful, if the disease had not been symptomatic. This opinion seemed confirmed by observing that there was no visible defect in the organization of the ears, and by the reflection, that if any defect did really exist, it was not likely to produce symptoms so violent, as those present, however it might affect the sense of hearing.

After a little consideration, I gave my opinion, that there was great reason to hope for a complete recovery, if she would allow me to investigate the case more minutely. The effect of hope was wonderful. She readily permitted me to examine every tooth, and every part of her mouth very particularly.

Her teeth were, generally, under the influence of caries, and the disease had penetrated to the cavity in some of them. They were all more or less encrusted with tartar, her gums and the sockets of her teeth were in an inflamed state, and bled at the slightest touch. The left under second large grinder was carious and painful, and the opposite one was also carious, and the crowns of the two upper second bicuspidati were nearly destroyed. There was but little room for the dentes sapientiæ, and knowing that in the warm and changeable climate of America, their formation is frequently hastened at a premature age, particularly in delicate and irritable constitutions, I readily suspected that their precocious formation, and the want of room for them to pass through the gums in combination with the diseases of the teeth, were the causes of the inflammation, and the pain in the ears."

Mr. Koecker obtained consent, and performed such operations upon her teeth and mouth, as to render them perfectly healthy, and in conclusion remarks,* "These measures were followed by great improvement of the general health, cessation of pain in the ears, as well as of the discharge from them. The hearing was good, but not quite so acute

---

* Koecker, page 161.

in the left as in the right ear. The gums and teeth were perfectly sound and beautiful. Care had been taken to preserve their natural shape and appearance, and particularly to prevent the stopping being visible on the exterior surface of such front teeth as had been filed.

"Before I left Philadelphia in 1822, I saw the patient frequently. Her health and spirits were good, and her hearing, if not perfect, was as good as that of any other member of her family."

SECTION IV.

INFLAMMATION AND PAINFUL AFFECTIONS OF THE EYES FROM DEFECTIVE TEETH, &C.

In some instances a remarkable sympathy is found to exist between the eyes and their integuments, and inflamed teeth.

A few weeks since a lady, residing in the northern part of this city, called on me with a request that I would examine her teeth, and extract those which were so far defective as to be incurable from dental operations. She at the same time showed me the fang of the first bicuspis of the upper jaw on the right side. The crown of the tooth was nearly all decayed away, and the fang was subject to frequent inflammation. It was remarkable that whenever the fang of the tooth was inflamed, the lining membrane of the lachrymal duct became inflamed so much as to entirely close the duct, and prevent the passage of the tears to the nose, in consequence of which they would be constantly trickling down over the cheek. For a considerable length of time the duct remained closed; at which period she called upon one of our oldest and most eminent surgeons, mentioning to him the state of her teeth, and showed him the diseased eye, duct, &c. and asked his advice. He at once said that there was no connexion between the disease of the lachrymal duct and the defective tooth—that the extraction of the tooth was not necessary, and that, in a few days, he would pass a silver canula down the canal of the duct, which would form a passage for the tears to the nose. The chronic inflamma- of the tooth, by the use of an antiphlogistic regimen for a short time, was reduced and relieved. With the subsidence of pain and inflammation in the affected tooth the inflammation of the membrane of the lachrymal duct was entirely relieved, and the tears passed by it to the nose. Some time after this, upon taking cold, an inflammation was again excited in the tooth before affected, and almost simultaneously with this, the lining membrane of the lachrymal duct, before mentioned, became inflamed so as to obstruct the passage of the tears. The eye itself was likewise much affected. She now called upon me to ask my advice. I proposed the immediate extraction of the tooth, to which she consented. The extremity of the fang was in a state of ulceration. The inflammation of the integuments of the eye and lachrymal duct immediately ceased, and the lady has remained in the enjoyment of good health ever since.

I present the reader with two cases of this kind from Jourdain.

*Opthalmia and loss of an eye by a defluxion on the teeth.**

A lady of Cologne was tormented for a long time with a defluxion on the last molar tooth of the left side of the jaw,

---

* Jourdain; Tome I, pages, 484, 485.

where there was erosion and caries. She was purged frequently by the advice of a physician, and cupping glasses were applied to the shoulders. But as she would not consent to the extraction of her tooth, the continual pain not ceasing, the irritation and attrition of the defluxion on the gums gave birth to an Opthalmia of the same side. Cataract and the loss of sight followed this opthalmia; because a part of the humours were dissipated, while the use of cold medicaments had condensed another part of the humours.

Singular Opthalmia.

A young lady from sixteen to eighteen years, had the second great molar tooth of the upper jaw of the right side extremely carious, without being painful, only in drinking or eating any thing too hot or cold. This reason was sufficient to oppose the intention I had to extract it; she consented to have it plugged, which I did with the greatest precaution. The following month, and about the time of her courses, the eye on this side became irritated and inflamed: the tooth became apparently loose. The time for her courses having passed, the opthalmia disappeared, and the tooth became solid. On another return of her courses, the same opthalmia returned, but more severe than the first, which also disappeared at the end of her courses. The accident re-appeared a third time: I removed the plug from the tooth—on the following day there was no more of the opthalmia, and the courses regular. After this third time I cauterized the tooth with red hot iron, and plugged it. New term of the courses, new opthalmia. I removed the plug from the tooth; the opthalmia disappeared. I put cotton in the tooth, and every day that I took it out I found it charged with a sanguineous and purulent humour of a very fetid smell. These accidents made the patient more reasonable, and solicited by her parents, she was determined to have this tooth extracted. After what has been said, it ought not to be wondered at that these opthalmias were repeated, and followed by like consequences. There was a discharge from this tooth when it was not plugged, but the plug prevented it; the refluxion fell upon the neighbouring parts, where the fluids themselves put it in motion during the term of the courses, and contributed to the swelling and irritation of the eye.

The reader is likewise requested to note how greatly the eyes were affected in the case of exostosis given by Fox, and inserted in our article on that subject. He will likewise remark the same effect in the dreadful case of cartilaginous growth of the gums communicated to him by letter from a lady in Scotland, and inserted in the section of this work under the head Cartilaginous Excrescences from the gums.

I will close this subject with one case from Mr. Koecker's Book.

*Case.**

"Alexander Stuart, aged sixty-four, had lost all his teeth from this destructive disease, except two upper, and one of the under cuspidati, which had been for some time very loose and painful. His sight had been declining for above fifteen years, and one of his eyes had been affected with incipient cataract for about five years. In January 1824, he requested my assistance for some acute inflammation of his mouth. One of the above canine teeth, the principal cause of the inflammation, was immediately extracted, and at the same time I gave my opinion, that by the removal of the other two, not only his mouth would be restored to perfect and perma-

* Koecker, pages, 278, 279.

nent health, but, most probably also, very salutary effects might be produced with regard to his sight: in consideration of this, he consented to their immediate extraction.

My anticipation proved just, for by this treatment the disease of the mouth was perfectly cured in one or two days, and since that period, not only has the general health of the patient been much benefitted, but the pain and weakness of his eyes have greatly diminished, and their sight has gradually much improved.

SECTION V.

NERVOUS AFFECTIONS.

Epylepsia and Hysteria.

The teeth being supplied with nerves from the fifth pair, exert, in many instances, a remarkable sympathy over distant parts of the system. The nervous affections which are occasionally excited by diseased teeth, are epilepsy, hysteria, hypochondriasis, rheumatic affections, tic douloureux, sympathetic head-ach, hemicrania, palsy, &c.

It is not my intention to discuss this subject at large, but to merely mention a few cases in reference to it, with a view only of pointing out the injurious effects of diseased teeth, as seen in their producing these diseases.

Dr. Rush mentions the following case of epilepsy, produced by diseased teeth. The doctor says, "Some time in the year 1801, I was consulted by the father of a young gentleman in Baltimore, who had been affected with epilepsy. I inquired into the state of his teeth, and was informed that several of them in his upper jaw were much decayed. I directed them to be extracted, and advised him afterwards to lose a few ounces of blood any time when he felt the premonitory symptoms of a recurrence of his fits. He followed my advice, in consequence of which, I had lately the pleasure of hearing from his brother, that he was perfectly cured." The following case of an hysterical affection I lately witnessed in my own practice: about the last of October, 1827, I was requested to call and see a lady, living in a small alley below Christian-street. I found she had been afflicted with a most distressing tooth-ache for about three weeks, and to that degree had the pain in her tooth affected her nerves, that any thing which was unusual, as any kind of mental emotion, &c. threw her into fits of hysteria; as for instance, when she sat in a chair to have her pained tooth extracted, she fell into a violent paroxysm of hysterical convulsions, and her mother informed me that when her tooth was in pain, without any other apparently exciting cause, she would have the hysteric paroxysms. As I found she could not be in any way composed so as to allow of extracting her tooth, I gave her a preparation of nitrous ether and pulverized alum, directing to apply it upon a piece of cotton to the diseased tooth, and directed them, as soon as her health and spirits would allow, to have her tooth extracted. I have never heard from her since.

SECTION VI.

HYPOCHONDRIASIS.

Hypochondriasis is usually an attendant upon a disordered state of the gastric functions; and all the cases of dyspepsia

I have seen, which were occasioned by diseased teeth and gums, have been more or less complicated with hypochondriasis.

SECTION VII.

RHEUMATIC AFFECTIONS.

Dr. Rush mentions the following case of a rheumatic affection of the hip-joint, occasioned by a diseased tooth. He says, "Some time in the month of October, 1801, I attended Miss O. C. with a rheumatism in her hip-joint, which yielded for a while to the several remedies for that disease. In the month of November, it returned with great violence, accompanied with a severe tooth-ache. Suspecting the rheumatic affection to be excited by the pain in her tooth, I directed it to be extracted. The rheumatism left her hip immediately, and she recovered in a few days. She has continued ever since to be free from it."*

I will give another case of a rheumatic affection, which was communicated to me by Dr. Dewees, of this city, and fell under the notice of Dr. Rush, by whom it was mentioned in his public lectures; and the subject of it afterwards came under the care of Dr. Dewees.

Case.

A lady, resident in this city, was attended by Dr. Rush, one entire winter, for an obstinate rheumatic affection, but during the cold weather his prescriptions were unavailing:

* Koecker, page 118.

her health recovered in some measure during the warm weather of the succeeding spring and summer, but her rheumatic complaints returned on the accession of cold weather, and she was confined to her room all that winter. Warm weather again relieved her from her rheumatism. At the commencement of the third winter, she was again attacked with rheumatism, as in the two preceding winters, when the doctor examined her teeth, and found that some of them were in a state of disease; these he ordered extracted, which done, she immediately recovered from every symptom of rheumatic complaint, and was free from them ever after.

SECTION VIII.

TIC DOULOUREUX.

This affection is now so generally known to be excited at times by diseased teeth, that very few intelligent surgeons, in cases of this kind, omit to notice the state of the teeth, and if they find any of them diseased, they, in all cases, direct their extraction. The following case of this kind was mentioned to me, some years ago, by the present professor of surgery in Yale College, Dr. Nathan D. Smith: as I relate from memory, I have entirely forgotten the date of the occurrence of this case. A young man, somewhere in the state of Vermont or New Hampshire was troubled with most acute and severe nervous pains and twitchings in his face, chiefly along the infra-orbitar nerves: this affection baffled the efforts of several respectable physicians for several months, I think four, when it was perfectly cured by the extraction of a diseased tooth of the under jaw. This case is remarkable for the sympathy be-

---

* Koecker, pages 279 to 281.

tween the nerves of the under teeth and those of the upper part of the face. I will continue a few cases of this kind from Mr. Koecker's book, and Mr. Bew's work on Tic Douloureux.

Mr. Koecker observes,* "Mr. J——, a gentleman of great respectability, a native of this country, but for many years a resident of Smyrna, aged about thirty-nine years, had suffered upward of ten years, from this distressing malady, attended by all its torturing symptoms, in a most unparallelled manner. His whole constitution, but particularly the glandular system, was so much affected as to produce swellings and indurations in the most distant parts, accompanied with great pain and inconvenience; but its effects on his head were frequently agonizing; indeed, he assured me, that so great were his sufferings, that he had been so far driven to despair, as to implore Heaven to relieve him by putting an end to his miserable existence. He repeatedly applied for the best medical and surgical advice that the country could afford; but the real causes of his sufferings were not detected; and such was the character of his disorder, that it baffled every exertion and all the remedies which were applied for many years. At length the effects of a sea-voyage, and a visit to his native country were proposed, and at the same time a trial of such remedial measures as he might be able to command in England.

Immediately after his arrival in London, this patient consulted Mr. Lawrence. This sagacious and disinterested surgeon soon suspected his teeth to be the chief cause of his malady, and recommended him to have my advice without delay, and to submit to any treatment I should deem necessary and proper.

---

* Koecker, pages 279 to 281.

On examining the gentleman's mouth, I found his gums and all his alveolar processes more or less diseased. His double-teeth, however, had most especially suffered; and so considerable a part of their sockets was destroyed, that their preservation was rendered altogether impossible. I therefore proposed their immediate removal; and although the gentleman was exceedingly nervous, he acceded to my proposed plan of cure without the least hesitation.

February 14th, 1826. Thirteen roots and teeth were extracted, and the mouth was subsequently cleansed with a gentle stimulant lotion, every hour or two in the course of the day.

February 21st. The remaining front teeth of the upper and under jaws were carefully scaled as far as the diseased state of their gums would allow of; and the patient provided with the means of preventing the re-accumulation of tartar. He was requested to continue the use of the lotion.

February 28th. The above operation was repeated, and cleanliness particularly recommended.

March 7th. The same operation was completed, and a perfect removal of the tartar was accomplished: the patient was also directed to proceed as before."

Thus, by the judicious management of the case, by Mr. Lawrence, and the above treatment, the patient was now, in less than one month, restored to perfect constitutional health. His mouth was rapidly recovering from a disease, probably of more than fifteen years standing; and the most important of his teeth were saved from total destruction, and permanently preserved.

Mr. Charles Bew says,* "A Miss E——, whose interesting

* Opinions of the Causes and Effects of the Disease denominated Tic Douloreaux; deduced from Practical Observations of its Supposed Origin, &c. &c. By Charles Bew, London, 1824.

appearance, pleasing manners, and elegant accomplishments, (though scarcely eighteen,) have been thus early, as an instructress, highly beneficial, having been medically recommended sea-air and recreation on the coast of Sussex, in the autumn of 1823, was attacked with what appeared, and was denominated rheumatic pains in the face, ear, and head, subsequently followed by deprivation of rest and appetite. The painful sensation being so unsteady as to position, and so fluctuative, as to effect, as never to have awakened even the slightest suspicion, even in herself, or medical attendant, as to the precise sphere from whence her suffering might have arisen; except, indeed, that in the height of some of her paroxysms, with her hand frequently placed on the parietal bones of the head, above the left temple, she would exclaim, "O my dear mother, I shall lose my senses! my face burns like fire, and something seems forcing up into my brain!" The distressing sensation thus depicted, and doubtlessly described to the physician, (who, as I hear, most kindly acted on the well-known liberality of principle in the faculty, "that sons and daughters of Apollo should help each other gratuitously, gave his attendance,) probably determined from the diagnostics delivered to him, that being similar in effect, it could be no other than a general bilious derangement of stomach, manifested to the head, through the immediate or recurrent channel of the sympathetic nerve.

Upon this supposition, the fair patient was treated with presumed hope of success, till after the usual routine of depletionary and repletionary exhibitions "in such cases recommended and provided," had proved abortive, with much time and attention lost, and little advantage gained, except from intermediate variety of suffering, and occasional imagination of amendment, as the supposed disease, (almost generated into reality) appeared to advance or recede, to or from convalescence.*

About this time, change of situation was suggested, and in conclusion, consigned the case to my inspection, in February, 1824.

I soon discovered, by the mode herein recommended, the immediate seat of my little interesting patient's complaint to be in the second bicuspis, or small grinding-tooth, in the left side of the upper jaw, a very small portion of which alone was visible. The disease generated by pressure of the neighbouring teeth, having devastated the tooth itself, in proportion as the accompanying paroxysms and the remedies proposed, had, to a certain extent, been active in the discomposure of her health and comfort.

The aborigine diminutive tooth, still more diminished by disease, having been declared neither useful nor ornamental, was quietly and gently (as well with regard to the sufferings of the patient, as to prevent the possibility of fracture) rendered incapable of causing further calamity to the fair owner, by removal. On examination, after extraction, the periosteum, or vascular membrane investing the root, appeared at the extremity swollen to the size of a small pea, which, on being punctured, sent forth on the lancet a quantity of fluid of the colour and consistency of cream, occasioning at once the confirmatory conclusion, that could the pain attendant on the inflammatory action, which had never ceased, and was then going on in this small, but largely excitable substance of

---

* All which may be easily conceived, when it is recollected, that the great sympathetic nerve forms a plexus, or combination with the fifth and sixth pairs, and is thus, through connecting consequence with the trigemenus, not only in complete association with the head, heart, and stomach, but also with the teeth, eyes, and ears.

bone and membrane, been continued to the fullest extent, the cessation of sensibility would have ended in exostosis; in other words, have produced a bulbous addition of bone, which the alveolar process would have promptly enlarged to the proportion of, rendering all attempts at removal by instruments, as difficult and abortive as it were to displace a screw from its position, having a nut unassailably attached to the opposite side.

* An elderly man of moderate independence, residing at New-Haven, in the county of Sussex, in the summer of 1820, who had been long unknowingly subjected to Tic Douloureux, designated by his medical attendant, "rheumatic affection of the face," at the anxious instigation of a friend, desired my assistance. Having announced the day and hour I would attend, I was introduced almost at the door of the person's house, to his medical practitioner, who, on hearing my name, announced himself as such, adding, that he had taken the opportunity of not being immediately wanted at home, to give me the meeting, his friend not yet having made his appearance, to state to me the hopelessness of his case, which he described as being decidedly rheumatic intermittent, which had remained immovable to every effort; concluding his observation by conceiving a mercurial course, the only remedy yet untried and most likely to be successful. Before he had quite concluded his observation he was called away, and his absence from the room succeeded by the immediate object of my visit, who came out of an adjoining chamber, wrapt about the head with linen cloths, like another resurrectioned Lazarus, meagre in form, pale in face, and feeble from debility.

---

* By Charles Bew. London, 1824.

From himself I learned that he had long been afflicted with this disease, which had not only made inroads on his health, but also on his imagination, having been subject to torment during the day, and interrupted repose during the night, as he in his own words described in a most unaccountable way, frequently starting from sleep, with the sensation of loud smacks on his face, as if from sharp irons, sometimes feeling as if they were cold, and sometimes hot; always appearing to have been inflicted by some one who had vanished on his waking. With difficulty repressing the smile, which already agitated my lip, at the tale of terror so gravely told by the truly grotesquely attired invalid, I begged him to be seated, and after unloading his head of its encumbering coverings, I soon saw the stump of the second bicuspis, pressing on the exterior periosteum or covering membrane of the first molaris, or large grinding-tooth, which, having excited inflammation, had become loosened in its tri-fanged socket, so as to occasion its descent to an insolated state of contact with teeth of the the lower jaw, in the grinding mechanism of mastication. The irritating pressure of the stump on the membrane of the molaris, (or perhaps when in full proportion before its fracture, which he said had been done by one of his kind friends, anxious to relieve him from pain,) had commenced the calamity which, with its attendant excruciations and the then state of excitement, admitted no hope of cure short of extraction. The tooth though formidable from size, was easily and safely removed, just as the medical attendant again entered the room, and relief of course afforded to a certain extent; but not completed till the expulsion of the stump some few days after, when every disagreeable sensation subsiding, health was established in the usual course, along with the conviction that two teeth, with much intermediate misery, owing to original bad management had been lost, which might otherwise long have remained members of his masticating system.

* A gentleman of spare habit and nervous temperament, holding a situation of trust and consequence in his present Majesty's Carlton House establishment, was long a victim to the distressing Tic Douloureux, originating in the pressure of the first and second bicuspides of the upper jaw; or what are called the two small grinding-teeth, during their uninterrupted process of pressure on each other's sides, which ultimately consigned them to destruction. He told me his misery was most extreme, and that one evening when worn down with the pain on one hand, and the various remedies recommended for his relief on the other, he had sought in repose temporary oblivion from the oppression of the complaint, he was on a sudden so attacked as to induce him to believe his life had been assailed by the stroke of an assassin. From the respite procured by repose, whether of short or long duration, he was however, soon disturbed, and his family alarmed by his piercing shriek, and demand for light. On his wife arriving at his bed-side with a candle, he eagerly inquired, who went down stairs? and then exclaimed, "some one has struck me on the face with an axe;" at the same time fearfully, and instinctively carrying his hand to the supposed cut, and then to the candle, as seeking confirmation of what in the first moments of his waking agitation, he had verily believed to have happened. The period of these paroxysms was previous to my appointment as dentist to his majesty's household; but subsequent acquaintance with him having enabled me to trace the course, and the consequence of the severe complaint to which he had been subjected; I could only comment on the peculiar position from whence

* By Charles Bew. London, 1824.

he had been assailed with pain, upon the philosophic principles of volcanic calculation, the force and data of whose destructive fires, are only to be ascertained by the situation and extent of its extinguished craters; as by the portions of the teeth remaining in the immediate vicinity of the maxillary sinus, I was soon enabled to account for, and explain the extent of the malady, which had so long militated against his health and happiness.

I will give a part of the following case:—* The lady's reply was, "it may be possible, for I have been much subjected at times, to the pains you have described in the face, but the tic douloureux with which I suffered was an agitation and throbbing in the fingers, wrist, and arm:" finding my suspicions verified at every step of my patient's descriptive procédure, I begged, "if it lived in her memory," to state the particular progress of the attack, which was kindly thus described.

"The approach was always intimated by a numbness, and tingling sensation down the inside of my arm, (describing with her finger the course of the supinator longus muscle,) wrist, and hand, with a violent agitation of my little finger." "And was this of any long duration?" "Two or three minutes, and then the agitation of the finger ceased, and the sensations seemed to retrace their steps up the arm, in a regular reverse to their approach." "And thus, madam, happily ended your attack of tic douloureux?" "O yes, certainly, as far as regarded tic douloureux! but I cannot say happily, for, most remarkable, the attack I have described, was ever the precursor to a violent pain in the face!" at the same time placing her finger on her cheek, in the situation immediately occu-

* By Charles Bew. London, 1824.

pied by the bicuspis in question, and the first molaris, or large grinding-tooth.

I forbear to trouble the reader with any thing more on this subject. Facts enough have been adduced to remind us ever to attend to the teeth in painful affections of the face.

SECTION IX.

SYMPATHETIC HEAD-ACH, &C.

Violent head-achs are occasionally to be excited by diseased teeth, so much so as to have been a subject of notice for a great length of time—of which I subjoin a few cases. The first three from the work of Jourdain.

*In 1775, Madame de Maubreuil, living at Nantz, was afflicted with a very severe head-ach, and consulted, on this occasion, her physician and surgeon, who ordered her several remedies. This lady was bled and purged several times; but as her malady was not, in the least diminished, the gentleman ordered her the bath, and the application of leeches to the head: she executed punctually their orders. All the remedies which were applied, did not ease her in the least. This lady had two teeth decayed, which, long since, had given her pain, and hindered her from eating. This made her think that they might be the cause of all the pain she suffered. As I had the honour to be particularly known to her, she was resolved to come to me, at Angers, where I lived then. Having come to me, I examined her mouth, and found

*Fauchard, pages, 413, 414, 415, 416, 417.

she had two very carious molar teeth, one on the right side of the lower jaw, and the other on the left side of the same jaw. I judged that these two teeth were the only cause of her head-ach. I was determined, at length, to extract them, which was no sooner done, than this lady found herself entirely free of a pain which had tormented her for the space of six months. This lady, whom I have seen often since I have been established at Paris, has assured me she suffers no more with the head-ach."

"Madame, the Marquis of Jeans, living in Brittainy, was incommoded for a long time with a pain which occupied the whole head, consulted many regular physicians and surgeons who assured her that her head-ach was a rheumatism. Founded on this opinion, they had recourse to many remedies, from which she derived not the slightest ease. Her sorrowful situation made her resolve, four years ago, to visit the waters of Bourbon, which they ordered. In this design this lady came to Paris, where she consulted a celebrated physician, who gave her, at length, the same advice as the first, treating her malady as a rheumatism. The remedies he employed to cure her were useless. The lady always complained of the excessive pain she felt in the head and teeth. This physician conjectured at length, that the excessive pain in the head of which she complained, might be caused by the teeth; and upon this conjecture, he advised this lady to see a dentist. As I had the honour of being known to her for many years, I was called upon to see her. Having examined her teeth, I found a large molar tooth on the left side of the lower jaw, and two teeth of the upper jaw of the right side very carious. The gums of these three teeth were swelled, and inflamed. After having sounded these teeth, I told this lady that the caries had arrived at a certain point, which rendered it impossible to save them, and I had not the least doubt this caries was the sole cause of her head-ach: in fine, I thought she ought to have them extracted. She opposed my advice; but having observed it was in conformity to that of her physician, she permitted me, in consequence, to draw two. The pain was not entirely taken away by their extraction. She called upon me five days after to take out the third: this was the last great molar tooth of the upper jaw, which I extracted for her. The pain immediately left her, and since that time this lady has never felt any pain in the head or teeth."

*Inveterate Head-ach cured by the extraction of several roots of carious teeth.**

A lady was affected continually with a very cruel pain, which occupied the left side of the head: the violence of the pain being worse principally in cold and wet weather. She had used, by the advice of physicians, many different remedies, internally as well as externally, but always without success. At the last, I was called to her. I examined with care all the causes of her malady. I was apprised by her, that four years before, she had been afflicted for the space of six months, with a very severe pain of the teeth on the left jaw; since then this pain was a little dissipated, but then there was another, remaining of the head of the same side. I conjectured from what was said that the actual head-ach was caused by the roots of spoiled teeth. After having examined her jaw, I really found in the upper jaw, four corroded teeth, wherein the roots were deeply buried. I advised her to have them extracted: she readily consented. Then I prescribed the most convenient remedies. I purged her as much as was necessary. The day following the purgation, cupping glasses were applied to the nape of the neck

* Jourdain, Tome I, pages, 482, 483.

and shoulders; then I directed her an apozème, which she took, for the space of four days, in the morning; and the fifth day, while she was still fasting, I extirpated these roots. The following day, she took pills; and for the space of some days, there was applied warm to the painful part, twice a day, a fomentation of the flowers and leaves of bettony, the flowers of rosemary, of chamomile, melilot, of dried red roses, leaves of marjoram, of wormwood, aniseeds, the shavings of guaiacum that has been infused with heat in red wine. By these means the patient recovered her health.

I did not calculate on the virtues of the ingredients that composed the fomentation, but I believe that the extraction of the teeth, a temperate regimen, some purgatives, and a blister might prove sufficient.

*Head-ach dependent on the Teeth.**

"The late Madame the Princess of Condy, had confided to her physicians a person under her protection, to be cured of a head-ach she had for five years. She was bled twenty times, almost successively, both in the arm and foot. After that, having thought about bleeding her in the throat, the Princess begged M. Petit to do it. But as he had not seen the patient, he questioned her about her malady, and finding nothing which appeared to warrant so much bleeding, he examined her mouth, because the patient spoke of feeling a weight and stiffness of the lower jaw. M. Petit found some irregularity in the arrangement of the teeth. He counted them, and found eighteen instead of sixteen. The second molar tooth on each side appeared to him to have generated

* Jourdain, Tome I, page 483.

the others. He extracted these two, which cured this girl in twenty-four hours, of a malady that had continued for five years.

Concluding Remarks upon the Sympathy of the General System with Diseased Teeth, and the Agency of these in Producing General Disease.

I have already protracted the consideration of this subject much beyond what I at first anticipated, and yet I do not find myself at the end of it. Much more may be said than what has been said upon it, and many more cases might be adduced. As it is my desire to render this work of the first practical utility, and to present to the medical reader all that I have seen in my own practice, or have read upon it in the works of others, which may be useful, I still beg his attention to several observations and cases more.

Dr. Rush makes the following observations upon it:* "I have been made happy by discovering that I have only added to the observations of other physicians, in pointing out a connexion between the extraction of decayed and diseased teeth, and the cure of general diseases. Several cases of the efficiency of that remedy in relieving head-ach and vertigo, are mentioned by Dr. Darwin. Dr. Gater relates, that M. Petit, a celebrated French surgeon, had often cured intermittent fevers, which had resisted the bark for months, and even years, by this prescription; and he quotes from his work two cases, the one of consumption, the other of vertigo, both of long continuance, which were suddenly cured

* Koecker, pages 119, 120.

by the extraction of two decayed teeth in the former, and of two supernumerary teeth in the latter case."*

"In the second number of a late work entitled Bibliothèque Germanique Medico Chirurgicale, published in Paris, by Dr. Bluver and Dr. Delaroche, there is an account, by Dr. Siebold, of a young woman who had been affected for several months, with great inflammation, pain, and ulcers in her right upper and lower jaws at the usual time of the appearance of the catamenia, which, at that period, were always deficient in quantity. Upon inspecting the seats of those morbid affections, the doctor discovered several of the molares in both jaws to be decayed. He directed them to be drawn; in consequence of which, the woman was relieved of the monthly disease in her mouth, and afterwards had a regular discharge of her catamenia.

The dental nerves, as we have before said, are derived from the third branch of the fifth pair; and such is the intimate connexion of this pair directly, with many parts of the system, and indirectly, by means of the great pneumo gastric with the lungs, stomach, and several important organs, (as for instance, the uterus, from which cause the improper extraction of a pained tooth has produced immediate abortion,) and by means of the different ramifications of this pair, to the ear, tongue, the eye and its integuments, eye-lashes, to the integuments of the face, &c. &c. that we cannot for one instant wonder if diseased teeth, by means of these communications and connexions, should produce, under some states of the system, derangements and disease in every one of these organs.

---

* Recherches sur differens points de Physiologie, de Pathologie, et de Therapeutique, pp. 353, 354.

Dr. Darwin has made many useful and accurate observations upon the effects of diseased teeth upon different parts of the system. Speaking of ear-ache, he says, "Ear-ache sometimes may continue many days, without apparent inflammation, and is then frequently removed by filling the ear with laudanum, or with ether, or even with warm oil, or warm water. This pain of the ear, like hemicrania, is frequently the consequence of association with a diseased tooth; in that case, the ether shonld be applied to the cheek over the suspected tooth, or a grain of opium and as much camphor mixed together, and applied to the suspected tooth."*

Hemicrania sympathetic, sympathetic pain of one side of the head, is often occasioned by a diseased state of the teeth. Dr. Darwin, speaking of this subject, says, "This disease is attended with a cold skin, and hence whatever may be the remote cause, the immediate one seems to be, a want of stimulus, either of heat or distension, or of some other unknown stimulus in the painful part;. or in those with which it is associated. The membranes in their natural state are only irritable by distension; in their diseased state, they are sensible, like muscular fibres. Hence a diseased tooth may render the neighbouring membranes sensible, and is frequently the cause of this disease."†

I do not wish to be understood as entering into Dr. Darwin's theoretical views, but only introduce the subject so far as to have the facts understood He continues, "Mrs. ——, is frequently liable to hemicrania, with sickness, which is probably owing to a diseased tooth; the paroxysm occurs irregularly, but always after some previous fatigue, or other cause of debility. When it (the sympathetic head-ach) affects a small

---

* See Zoonomia, Vol. II. Classes 1, 2, 4, 13.

† See Zoonomia, Class IV, 2, 2, 8.

defined part on the parietal bone, or one side, it is generally termed clavus hystericus, and is always, I believe, owing to a diseased dens molaris. The tendons of the muscles, which serve the office of mastication, have been extended into pain at the same time that the membranous coverings of the roots have been compressed into pain, during the biting or mastication of hard bodies. Hence, when the membranes which cover the roots of the teeth become affected with pain, by a beginning decay, or perhaps, by the torpor or coldness of the dying part of the tooth, the tendons and membranous fascia of the muscles about the same side of the head, become affected with violent pain by their sensitive associations; and as soon as this associated pain takes place, the pain of the tooth entirely ceases.

The dens sapientia, or last tooth of the upper jaw frequently decays first, and gives hemicrania over on the same side. The first or second grinder in the upper jaw is liable to give violent pain about the middle of the parietal bone, or side of the head, on the same side, which is generally called clavus hystericus." He places hemicrania as a disease of association, and produced by diseased teeth in many cases. He continues,* "The last tooth, or dens sapientia, of the upper jaw, most frequently decays first, and is liable to produce pain over the eye and temple of that side. The last tooth of the under jaw is also liable to produce a similar hemicrania, when it begins to decay. When a tooth in the upper jaw is the cause of head-ach, a slighter pain is sometimes perceived on the cheek-bone. And when a tooth in the lower jaw is the canse of head-ach, a pain sometimes affects the muscles of the tendons of the neck, which are attached near the jaws. But the clavus hystericus, or pain about the middle

* Zoonomia, Section 35-2-1.

of the parietal bone on one side of the head, I have seen produced by the second of the molares, or grinders of the under jaw; of which I shall relate the following case:

"Mrs. ——, about 30 years of age, was seized with great pain about the middle of the right parietal bone, which had continued a whole day before I saw her, and was so violent as to threaten to occasion convulsions. Not being able to detect a decaying tooth, or a tender one, by examination with my eye, or by striking them with a tea-spoon, and fearing bad consequences from her tendency to convulsions, I advised her to extract the last tooth of the under jaw on the affected side; which was done without any good effect. She was then directed to lose blood, and to take a brisk cathartic; and after that had operated, about sixty drops of laudanum were given her, with large doses of bark; by which the pain was removed. In about a fortnight she took a cathartic medicine by ill advice, and the pain returned with greater violence in the same place; and before I could arrive, as she lived thirty miles from me, she suffered a paralytic stroke, which affected her limbs and her face on one side, and relieved the pain of her head. About a year afterwards, I was again called to her, on account of a pain as violent as before, exactly on the same part of the other parietal bone. On examining her mouth, I found the second molaris of the under jaw, on the side before affected, was now decayed, and concluded that this tooth had occasioned the stroke of the palsy, by the pain and consequent exertion it had caused. On this account I earnestly entreated her to allow the sound molaris of the same jaw opposite to the decayed one, to be extracted; which was forthwith done, and the pain of her head immediately ceased, to the astonishment of her attendants.

Here we have an undeniable case of hemicrania and palsy, produced by diseased teeth, after most violent and protracted suffering. I beg leave to continue a short extract more from Dr. Darwin on this subject. He says,* "Since the above was first published, I have seen two cases, which were very similar, and seem much to confirm the above theory of sympathetic hemicrania, being perhaps always owing to the sympathy of the membranes about the cranium, with those about diseased teeth. Lord M. and Mr. B. of Edingburgh, both of them about the middle of life, were afflicted with violent hemicrania for about two years; in the beginning of which time, they both assured me, that their teeth were perfectly sound, but on inspectng their mouths, I found all the molares were now so decayed as to have lost their crowns. After having suffered pain for sixteen or eighteen months almost incessantly, in different parts of their heads, they had each of them a hemiplegia, from which they gradually recovered, as much as paralytic affections generally do recover. All the stumps of their teeth, which were useless, were directed to be extracted; as the swallowing so much putrid matter from decaying bones, seemed to injure their digestion." Here are two more cases of palsy from diseased teeth. It may be asked, why have not other physicians than what I have mentioned, made observations of this kind? I believe the correct answer to this question would be, that the great body of physicians, have never paid any attention to the subject. From what cause arise the celebrity and fame of Rush, Hunter, Darwin, and many more I could mention? It was because they noted with the utmost care, almost every fact connected with both disease and health, and possessed a nice tact in discerning the causes of both.

---

* Zoonomia, Class iv. 2, 2, 8.

Dr. Darwin says more upon this subject than I have extracted, as I do not wish to weary the reader, or to protract the subject. I trust I have said enough to induce every medical man to consider the diseases of the teeth as at least worthy of attention; if he still doubts it, let him look at a correct delineation of the ramifications of the fifth pair of nerves, and consider that the dental nerves have at least a nervous association, by being a part of this pair, with almost all the principal organs of the animal system, and consequently, their diseases.

I would not dwell upon the teeth so long, or with so much earnestness, as to lead any person to suppose, that I consider them the most important organs of the system; still I would be understood as viewing them, as having been formed by the wisdom of a Creator, whose hand never swerves from perfection; and had they not have been necessary to the health, beauty or perfection of the animal, they would never have been formed: and if an all-wise Providence, has formed our systems so, that the teeth under some circumstances may be dispensed with; or, if he has given us that superior sagacity, by which we are all enabled when our teeth are lost to prepare our food, so as to compensate in some degree for the power of mastication, still this function can be viewed in no other light than of great importance.

Man obviates in some degree the consequence of the loss of his teeth, but in most animals, their loss or inability to use them, is followed by death.

Nor are we from the same causes to lightly esteem the diseases of the teeth, and because we do not every day notice probably injurious or fatal consequences resulting from them, to conclude that there is never any danger. A masked battery is to be dreaded. An insidious foe may plunge a dagger in our bosoms when least we expect it. The teeth form a link in a series of organs, whose united healthy functions are necessary to the health of the animal;—a link which, if struck, the whole chain vibrates—a link which, if weakened, the strength of the whole series is impaired.

We are not to contemn the diseases of the teeth because they seem insignificant. Many persons are formed of a fibre so fragile, as to be broken by the slightest shock;—of a stamina so delicate, as to be affected by the slightest impression. Disease in its steps at first is, at it were, soft and hesitating, weak in its powers, and slow in its progress. (Nunc, nunc, monstrum horrendum. Meda advertite.) But every instance of indulgence and each succeeding advantage gained, confirms its steps, increases its powers, and hastens its progress, and what but a moment ago seemed a thing too insignificant to mention, now rises a monster that derides human effort, and whose sting is the arrow of death.

Almost unappreciable are the beginnings of many fatal diseases; and could the grave reveal its secrets, I have not a doubt, when I consider the number of diseases produced by diseased teeth, but it would be found that thousands are there, in whom the first fatal impulse was given by a diseased state of these organs; and could I raise my voice so as to be heard by every medical man in America, I would say to him, attend to your patients' teeth, and if they are diseased, direct such remedies as shall restore them to health; and if in health, such means as will keep them so; and know for your satisfaction and pleasure, that you will always administer to the well-being and best interests of your patients, and may perhaps occasionally preserve a valuable life.

The Indian lightly esteems the rills he bestrides upon the mountains of the cloud-capt cordilleras; how little does he know that from these small beginnings, there swells the mighty Amazon.

I hardly need remind the man of science, from what slight causes in the natural, moral, and physical world, arise those tremendous agencies, which prove at once the fulcrum and the lever of Achimedes.

II

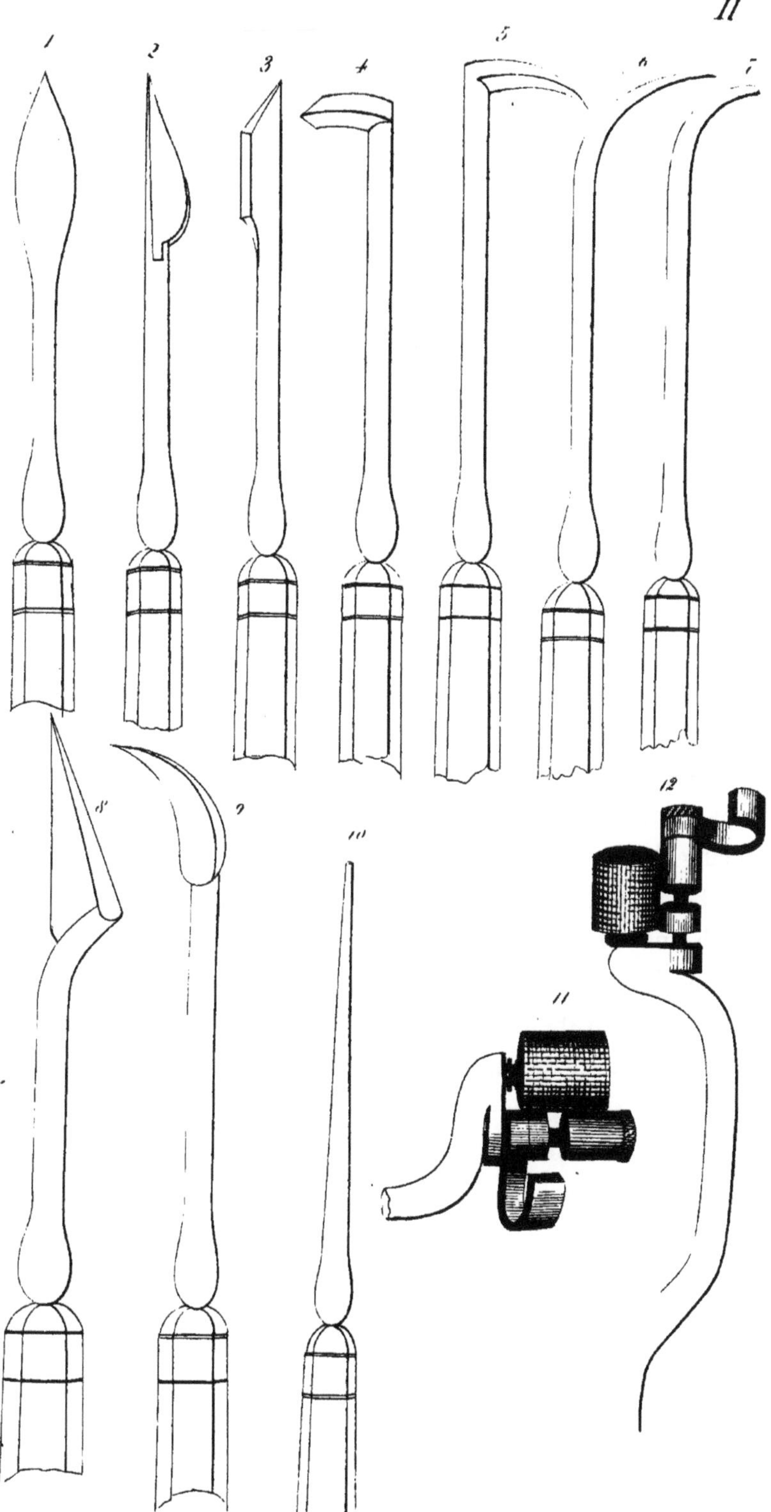

C. Bonnat lith.

PART II.

CHAPTER I.

OPERATIVE DENTAL SURGERY.

It is the object of the writer, in this part of our work, to present to the reader a faithful, and, as far as he can, in a correct and impartial manner, all that will be useful to him, that he has been able to collect upon this subject, either from his own experience and practice, or from his knowledge of the practice and writings of others; and he flatters himself that he shall be able to communicate so much, as that the medical man and the student of this art and science, will be fully enabled to understand in what consist the several operations performed by the surgeon-dentist, and how to perform them, either for the cure of diseased teeth, or for preserving the health and beauty of those which are not diseased. Also that they may know how to supply by art those which may be lost, and know how to direct the growth and position of the permanent teeth in such a manner, as to insure to their patients, perfect regularity, health and beauty of these organs. He cannot promise his reader any thing more than general principles illustrated by cases, for after all that can be said, still there is such a variety in different cases, that much must necessarily remain to be learned by the experience of the practitioner, and every case will call for the exertion of a correct judgment, to direct the proper course of treatment. Dental Surgery differs in some respects from every other kind of surgery. In the first place, our operations are mostly confined to organs that are liable to a loss of their substance, but in no instance, except perhaps in the very slightest degree, are they able to repair this loss; unlike the condition of many organs of the human body, which when by disease have lost some of their substance, are able by their own organic powers to restore it. In the second place, such is the small vitality of the teeth, that when a part of their substance is lost, they will allow it to be supplied by the presence of some foreign body, which I believe is not the case with any other bone of the body. In another respect the dental organs are distinct, they are duplicate, having one set which are deciduous, and when lost, are succeeded by another set. In this respect they differ from all the other organs of the animal system. It is on these principles, and one or two more I might mention, that dental operations are founded. Dental operations as far as regards the removal of useless, pernicious, or diseased teeth or stumps, and the preservation of the health of those which are or might be useful, may be reduced to the following:

First, Extraction.

Second, Removal of foreign matter from the teeth.

Third, Removal of carious portions from the teeth.

Fourth, Separation of crowded teeth.

Fifth, Supplying the loss of substance in a tooth, by a metallic substance; and,

Sixth, Excision of the crowns of the teeth, when we wish to preserve their stumps.

Each of these will receive a separate consideration.

SECTION I.

EXTRACTION OF THE TEETH.

This operation naturally divides itself into first, extraction of the infant teeth, and second, extraction of the adult teeth.

Extraction of the Infant Teeth.

The infant teeth are liable to be affected with caries, and in the progress of this disease to have their nerves exposed, and consequently, at times, are subject to tooth-ache, in the same manner as adults. It is recommended by almost every writer upon this subject, to have them extracted. This is a correct general rule, as regards carious deciduous teeth, when this has progressed to any considerable extent, or when they have become inflamed, so as to produce tooth-ache. A question arises, at what period ought deciduous teeth to be extracted? should we wait for them to become loose, or not? I consider these to be practical questions of great importance, because the judicious extraction of the deciduous teeth has a great influence in directing the regular growth of the permanent set. Whilst I consider, as a general rule, that the deciduous teeth, if considerably decayed, ought to be extracted; yet, if not diseased, or the gums, they should never be extracted, until they become loose, or some appearances or symptoms are present which denote the coming of the permanent teeth. I think this ought to become an axiom in dental surgery. Perhaps an exception may be found in some cases of diseased gums, but then these may become loose, and if they are firm, their extraction, perhaps, will rarely be the best mode to adopt in curing the gums. Peculiar circumstances may form other cases of exceptions to this rule: the exception proves the rule. Sometimes these teeth become very dirty, and considerably covered with tartar and other foreign and injurious matter; in this case, parents often ask the advice of the dentist, and, in many instances, their extraction is recommended, even if the teeth themselves are sound and firm. In these cases, I recommend to have the teeth carefully cleaned by the dentist, and direct a brush and some suitable tooth-powder to be used, so as to insure cleanliness of the child's teeth. The following case I will mention to illustrate the position.

A lady, in April 1827, sent her little daughter, aged three years and six months, to me, that I might extract her upper incisor teeth, which, the lady supposed, from their being very dark coloured and almost encrusted with tartar, were decayed. Upon examining them I found they were sound, and firm in their sockets. Instead of extracting them, I removed the tartar, and rendered her teeth very white and clean, and gave her nurse a soft brush and a box of tooth-powder, composed of myrrh, peruvian bark, &c., with directions to keep the child's teeth perfectly clean with the use of the brush and tooth-powder, and sent her home with her teeth in perfect order, much to the satisfaction of the mother. The child's gums, which were considerably inflamed, soon became very healthy, and she will, no doubt, have the use of her teeth two or three years.

Injurious consequences arising from the Premature Extraction of the Deciduous Teeth.

In the first place, the pain which attends the extraction of the infant teeth, when they are sound and firm in their sockets, is much greater than when they are allowed to remain until they have become spontaneously loose, or until the new teeth begin to appear, and the violence done to the surrounding parts is quadrupled. Nature by a beautiful process, in almost every instance, loosens the deciduous teeth, and seems to provide with great care for their removal, so as not to produce any injury to the surrounding parts. We generally find, when left to nature, and probably always, when a new tooth is coming in place of the deciduous one, that the fangs of the latter are taken away by a process of absorption, and the gum, which embraced the neck of the tooth, is also absorbed away, so that the tooth drops out; and often, from the absorption of the fangs, the dentist, upon extracting the tooth, thinks he has broken it; and it is only when they have become somewhat loose, or when this process is so tardy as not to allow the regular descent or ascent of the permanent teeth, and the other exceptions I have before mentioned, that we are to extract the deciduous teeth. In some cases, some of the permanent teeth are not formed; and in these cases, the deciduous teeth, which otherwise would have become loose, remain firm, and are of use to the individual for many years. It is but a few days since a lady, aged about twenty-eight, called on me to have some operations performed upon her teeth, and I found that she had never shed her deciduous molar teeth, nor had any of the bicuspids, which usually supply the place of the former, appeared. I but lately saw another case, when the individual, a gentleman, aged about twenty-one years, had had the infant molar teeth of the lower jaw extracted, but which had never been succeeded by any bicuspid teeth. In these cases we can see how peculiarly correct and proper it is for us to adopt a general rule not to extract these, unless they are diseased, or seem to divert the course, or impede the progress of the permanent teeth, or are loose: for when these last are wanting, the deciduous teeth may remain of use for some length of time. The permanent incisors do not, in some cases, appear. I lately saw a case, when one of the permanent upper lateral incisores had never appeared. Mr. Fox mentions having seen several instances of deficiencies of the permanent teeth. In one case, a lady, who never had but four permanent teeth.* In all these cases we can easily conceive how improper it would have been to have extracted the deciduous teeth, which, by being left, would compensate, in some degree, for the deficiency of the permanent teeth. Another injurious consequence resulting from a premature extraction of the deciduous teeth is, the injury which is often done to the permanent teeth. It must be always borne in mind that the permanent teeth are formed upon, or by pulps produced from the deciduous teeth; and consequently, if early violence is done to these last, the former are liable to be greatly injured by it: and this is the fact, in many cases. I lately witnessed an instance when a child had one of its molar teeth extracted, and the crown of the permanent tooth beneath it very soon came away. We noticed that the enamel of the tooth is formed upon a membrane which invests a pulp, and the pulp becomes the form of the bone of the tooth; and the form of the membrane, consequently, determines the form of the enamel. A knowledge of this anatomical and physiological fact enables us to explain the reason of a peculiar appearance of the teeth, or some of them, in a few cases, which is noticed by some writers.† They look as if a small round file had been passed across the en-

* Fox, Part I, page 41. †Hunter on the teeth, Part II, page 155.

amel so as to leave a round furrow upon the surface of the tooth: at times we notice several of these furrows on the teeth—sometimes one, two, or three teeth of a set will have this appearance; in other cases, the whole set with the exception of the dentes sapientia, or wisdom teeth, which I have never seen thus affected; still, I will not say they are never so situated. Mr. Hunter says it is a peculiar kind of decay, but not caused by any external agency, or, to use his own words, "not to depend on accident, way of life, constitution, or any particular management of the teeth," but that it is an original disease of the tooth. Others, I believe, have imputed it to an improper or excessive use of brushes, or tooth-powders, &c. &c.; but I think the true cause of this situation of the tooth is owing to some disturbance given to the membrane on which the enamel is deposited. If the membrane is ruffled the enamel will have this appearance. And this is further corroborated from this, that these furrows run either across, or length-ways, or diagonally on the tooth, not confined to any particular direction, although across is the usual direction which these furrows have. The enamel will generally be found as perfectly polished on this irregular surface as on perfectly formed teeth, which would not be the case if it proceeded from caries or the brush. I have seen several cases of it in persons who never used the brush to any extent in their lives. In one case of this kind, Mrs. W. of Frankfort, I saw a whole set of teeth, except the dentes sapientia, thus affected: every tooth appeared otherwise perfectly sound. This lady had never used a toothbrush more, she assured me, than a dozen times in her life: she could give no account of the extraction of her infant teeth. The following cases seemed to me to amount to a demonstration that this peculiar appearance of the teeth is owing to some disturbance of the membrane upon which the enamel is deposited; and the enamel being deposited on the ruffled membrane, had, necessarily, assumed the same shape. The cases occurred in the family of Mr. M—, a respectable mechanic from London. He extracted the teeth of his two oldest children (sons) when they were quite young, and the permanent teeth of both had the appearance I have mentioned. This induced him, at the suggestion of the mother, in the two succeeding children which he had, to leave their teeth to nature; consequently, he did not extract them until quite loose, and the result was, that the permanent teeth of the two last children were perfectly smooth and beautiful. This narration I had from several members of the family, who perfectly concurred in their statements of it. The deciduous teeth seem to serve, in some degree, as a guide to the growth of the permanent set, as these last are apt to be irregular if the first are extracted too soon; consequently, they should not be extracted, unless under the limitations before mentioned. It is of the greatest consequence that the person having the care of children should know precisely the order in which the permanent teeth appear, and what deciduous teeth should be removed to give place to the second set. Mr. Fox, speaking upon this subject says, "every thing depends upon a correct knowledge of the time when a tooth requires to be extracted, and also of the particular tooth; for often more injury is occasioned by the removal of a tooth too early, than if it be left a little too long: because a new tooth, which has too much room long before it is required, will sometimes take a direction more difficult to alter, than a slight irregularity occasioned by an obstruction of short duration. If an improper tooth be extracted irreparable mischief will ensue; as in the case when young permanent teeth have been removed instead of the obstructing temporary ones, which I have several times known to have been done." When the deciduous teeth have been removed by accident, or art, too soon, the permanent teeth are apt, in some cases, to be very late in making their appearance. I know a young lady, who, by accident, when she was three years old, lost her upper incisor teeth, and the new ones did not appear until her eleventh year. Of this I have noticed several cases.

Of the Manner in which the Deciduous Teeth should be extracted.

At first sight, one would suppose that no direction upon this part of the subject need be given; but as from caries of the deciduous teeth, proceeding so far as to expose their nerves, so as at times to produce tooth-ache, we are obliged to extract these teeth while yet quite firm, I deem it proper to give a few hints upon this subject. The instruments proper to be used, in almost every case, are the common extracting forceps; for these teeth extract much easier than the permanent ones, because the infant jaw is not so hard and perfectly ossified as the adult. There is but one rule in regard to the manner of extracting these teeth. They should be extracted with the utmost care: they should rather be solicited out, if I may use such an expression, than dragged out with that violence and butchery which is sometimes practised. Mrs. H——, a few months ago, called on me with her daughter, a child about eleven years old, and wished me to clean and perform some operations upon the daughter's teeth. One she wished extracted; and mentioned to me, that when her daughter was about six years old, she procured a dentist to extract one of her molar teeth, which he did in the most barbarous manner, mangling the gum and breaking the jaw, in the most shocking manner. A violent inflammation ensued, suppuration took place, a fistulous opening was formed passing outside the cheek, and several pieces of bone were discharged through the external opening, and the child did not recover from this state of her jaw and face, until about nine months had elapsed. An ill looking scar was left ever after upon the side of her lower jaw. If great care in extracting these teeth is not used by the dentist the most pernicious consequences are the result. The gum is apt to be torn, the jaw shattered in the most dangerous manner, so as often to destroy the rudiments of the young permanent teeth, and to lead to violent inflammation and suppuration. The tooth should be first loosened by carrying it to one side of its socket with some force, so as to break the attachments of the lining membrane, and then by a moderate effort, it is easily lifted out of the socket. If the tooth itself is not loose, the gum in general should be previously separated in the most perfect manner from the tooth by the use of a gum-lancet. If the tooth is loose, the gum need not be separated.

Extraction of the Adult Teeth.

This is an operation of very frequent occurrence as we seldom see a person arrived at twenty years of age, who has not been obliged to submit to it at one time or another. It is very important that its principles be well understood. This operation is performed by almost all country physicians, and many in the cities. It is to be regretted that many persons attempt the performance of it, who have not suitable instruments, and have no correct idea of the manner in which it ought to be performed, and consequently are guilty of the greatest mal-practice by their injudicious attempts to extract the teeth. It is very important that the student of this art should have correct views of the subject, before he attempts the operation; for after having imbibed an erroneous opinion respecting it, he is apt to carry this error into all his future practice.

Indications for Extracting these Teeth.

It is all-important that the physician or surgeon-dentist should know when he ought, and when he ought not to extract a tooth, for it is often the case that much more skill is shown in curing and preserving a valuable tooth than in extracting it. No practice can be more reprobated than that of the indiscriminate extraction of every tooth, which the physician or surgeon-dentist may be asked to extract; and yet it is a notorious fact, that there are many persons, possessing such an insatiable thirst for gain, as to extract every tooth that they might be asked to do, whether the teeth are sound or not, and whether the individuals asking for the operation be sane or not.

The following are the usual indications in correct dental surgery, for the extraction of the adult teeth:

First, It is proper, and often very necessary, to extract adult teeth, to remove or prevent irregularity, inconvenience, or deformity. If the teeth, especially at the time when they are first appearing, appear to be too much crowded, it is highly necessary to extract some of them; in this case, the first molar teeth on each side of the jaw, by being extracted, will often give room for all of the other teeth of the jaw to become regular; and if we extract for this purpose one of them, we must extract the other, for if we do not, all the teeth are apt to incline to the side which has lost one of these teeth. This is an important rule, and ought always to be remembered when operating upon either jaw. The front teeth not only become regular by this means, but the dentes sapientia and other molar teeth, which succeed, are apt to be much more perfect and large. In some cases, the canine teeth, or some of the other teeth, protrude either outwards or inwards; and in this case, the deformity or inconvenience is such, as that we are obliged, in some cases, though not in all, to extract the irregular teeth. Supernumerary teeth generally occasion deformity or inconvenience, and ought, if they do so, to be extracted.

Secondly, Those molar teeth which have no opposing teeth on the opposite jaw, and are in a considerable state of decay, or are loose, may with propriety be extracted; and if so far decayed as to be unable to support a plug in the decayed part, they should always be extracted.

Thirdly, When the nerve of an adult molar or bicuspid tooth, which otherwise ought to be preserved, is in a state of inflammation, and all our efforts have failed to relieve the pain, it should be extracted.

Fourthly, Teeth which are the cause of gum-boils whether externally decayed or not, should be extracted.

Fifthly, Teeth which are decayed, and yet could be preserved so as to be useful, but are the suspected causes of general nervous affections, &c. as mentioned when speaking upon that subject, should be extracted.

The front teeth, namely, the canine and incisor teeth, if regular, and are not the cause of gum-boils and nervous affections, &c. &c. should never be extracted; if painful, or to a considerable extent carious, they should be cut off, and the stump treated as I shall direct in the chapter on that subject. This is, and ought to be, a general rule in dental surgery. The reasons why it should be so, and the manner of performing the operation, together with the treatment of the nerve, and the treatment of the stump, will form the subject of a separate section to be considered hereafter.

These are the general rules which are to direct us in determining upon the extraction of the adult teeth, but such are the variations which will occur in practice, that our judgments will often be called into exercise, whether to pursue these rules or not. In all cases of pained teeth, we ought to use our efforts to preserve them, if they are useful, and would be so, if preserved. Often in this way the judicious surgeon-dentist will be able, and have the pleasure of preserving many valuable teeth, by which he will insure the gratitude of his patient, and feel the luxury of doing good. A case of this kind I will mention, which occurred in my practice. In the month of July last, Mrs. W——, a very respectable lady, living opposite the new market, in Second-street, called on me to ask my advice with regard to her teeth. She said, in consequence of taking cold, several of them were in pain, and had been so for three or four days. She said, she sent for a dentist to examine her teeth, and he instantly, and without regarding her feelings, advised their extraction. Disgusted with his want of feeling, and apparently slight consideration of her case, she declined his advice, or the extraction of the teeth, and immediately called on me. I found, upon examination, that the pained teeth were in a state of decay, but not so much so but what they could be preserved, and would be useful. The nerves of the teeth before mentioned were considerably exposed, and in a state of inflammation. I directed her to take a gentle aperient, with fomentations to her face, and gave suitable directions for the treatment of the teeth themselves, and in a few hours had the pleasure of entirely arresting the inflammation of the exposed nerves and teeth, and which has not recurred again. The nerves and teeth are now in a state of preparation for being plugged, which will perfectly complete their cure, and render them of use to the patient. In the section on the preservation of the nerves of teeth we wish to preserve and plug, will be found detailed directions for this purpose.

Instruments proper for the Extraction of the Adult Teeth.

It is not my intention to notice the great variety of instruments which have been proposed, and used in the extraction of the teeth; I only wish to mention those which are useful and generally used, and pass over the others in silence. The instruments at present used by the most judicious and respectable dentists of Europe and this country, are the dentist key, and the forceps. Of the former there are several kinds, of which the improved key of Mr. Fox, possesses the most advantages; it is constructed so that the book can be placed before the bolster, by which contrivance we can readily extract the dentes sapientia; it can be also carried behind the bolster, so as to avoid, if we choose, pressure upon a diseased and tender gum, opposite to the tooth we purpose to extract. An objection I have often made to the common keys is, that in general, the bolster is made too large and often quite flat, when a proper key should have a small bolster of an oval shape approaching to round, by which shape when the hook and bolster are brought to act upon the tooth, the latter by being oval will carry the tooth out of its socket, by pressing it up or down as the case may be; but if long and flat, it presses dead against the tooth without raising it at all, so that the tooth will be violently dragged out by the action of the hook alone. Mr. Koecker objects to the use of the key in nearly all cases, and recommends the forceps.* I concur

* See Koecker, page 341

with Mr. Koecker, that in a great many cases the forceps are preferable, but I believe every dentist will find cases, where the key will be indispensable, as Mr. Koecker acknowledges.

The forceps are the next instruments used after the key, and they ought to be used when the dentist can extract the tooth without the key. They should be made of different sizes, straight and curved at their acting ends, so that we may be able to apply them to any tooth we please, either the upper or lower, front or back.

MANNER OF EXTRACTING THE TEETH.

*Of Extracting the Tooth with the Key.**

The first step in every operation for extracting, is to divide the adhering gum to the very edge of the socket; this prevents a laceration of the gum, and much facilitates the operation. I need not describe the different gum-lancets used by dentists. They should be perfectly sharp, and made so as to divide the gum all round the tooth, consequently different shaped ones are required. The gum being divided, the patient seated in a firm chair, the key having the bolster covered with a piece of patent lint, sponge, or the corner of a pocket handkerchief, may be applied to the tooth, so as to firmly embrace it, when with a steady turn of the instrument we loosen the tooth; at this instant give the bolster of the key a perpendicular impulse, and the tooth instantly passes out of the socket. A proper key, and used in this manner, is, I think,

* See Fox, pages 165 to 168.

the best instrument we now have for the extraction of a considerable proportion of the teeth. It is now considered, as a general rule, proper to apply the hook so as to extract the teeth outside of the mouth, with the exception in some cases of the dentes sapientia, and the second grinder, which may be directed by the judgment of the practitioner, as may all the others. Great care should be used by the practitioner in applying the hook, not to allow it to infringe upon the neighboring teeth, as by this means he might loosen if not extract not only the tooth he intends to extract, but a tooth next to it. The perpendicular impulse given to the instrument, either up or down as the case may be, carries the tooth out of the socket, and prevents the breaking of it, or the sides of the socket, which from inattention to this is often done. I have been in the practice of extracting teeth for several years, and never since I have adopted this mode of using the key, have I had the misfortune to break or shatter the alveolus, except in the very slightest degree. Again, the movement of the instrument should be steady, and not hastily or with a jerk. This observation at first sight would seem superfluous, as it would hardly seem that any man of common sense would be in the habit of operating in this manner. But the fact is otherwise: there are dentists in this city who after applying the key, twitch upon the tooth with as sudden a jerk, as an angler would upon the bite of a trout. Accidents are the daily consequence of it. It is an old observation that all operations are performed sufficiently quick, which are performed well, and peculiarly so with regard to the extraction of a tooth. Mr. Fox mentions the case of a lady, who had one of the second bicuspides of the lower jaw extracted, and with a sudden jerk of the instrument: inflammation and suppuration took place in the socket, she lost the other bicuspis and two adjoining molar teeth and with the extraction of the last of the two molar teeth, came a piece of the jaw more than two inches long. From the time the first tooth was extracted, to coming away of the large piece of the jaw bone, and healing of the gum was six months, all of which time there was constant pain and discharge of pus.* The key should be provided with several hooks of different sizes, so as to be adapted to the size of different teeth with exactness, and the operator will seldom fail of success.

Of Extraction with the Forceps.

This operation performed with the forceps, when practicable, is much the most preferable mode, as by using the forceps, we very seldom break the tooth or shatter the alveolus. The operator should be provided with forceps of different sizes, that he may be able to select one which will readily fit the tooth intended to be extracted, so as to grasp it firmly in every case. In all, or nearly all cases, when we wish to extract irregular front teeth, as the canine or incisores, the forceps are the only instruments we can with propriety use. The key should never be applied to a canine or incisor tooth, for such is the great mechanical disadvantage with which the key acts upon these teeth, that in almost every case we shall either fail in the outset, break the tooth, shatter the alveolus, or contuse and lacerate the gums, so as to induce inflammation, swelling, and even suppuration. If we adopt the rule never to extract the regular front teeth, and we attempt the key upon irregular ones, we shall be very apt to loosen the regular teeth. The forceps are certainly the most proper instruments for extracting the front teeth, and such is the mechanical advantage with which we can apply and use

---

* See Fox, Part II. pages 167, 168.

them in the extraction of front teeth, that the judicious operator will seldom fail of success. When we have determined upon the use of the forceps, the patient seated, and the gums separated from the tooth as we have before mentioned and directed, we must apply a pair of forceps of a size which will readily hold and embrace the tooth, but not so large as to touch the neighboring teeth, when with a firm and steady motion, we must carry the tooth to the outside so far, as to loosen it from the membrane by which it is held in the socket, and then by carrying the foreceps in a perpendicular direction, we shall be able at once to pass the tooth out of the socket. We must remember not to embrace the tooth so tight as to crush it, which we are in danger of doing, if we are not aware that we are liable to this accident. In extracting the front teeth, especially irregular or supernumerary ones, we may give a slight rotatory motion to the tooth, by which means, as there is but one fang to these teeth, we shall loosen them, and at once be able to carry them out of their sockets.

Various instruments have been contrived to extract the teeth in a perpendicular direction, but none have been as yet invented, which on trial have been found applicable to common practice. Nearly all only tend to demonstrate the superiority of the key. In extracting the teeth of young children we need not in general divide the gums, as the laceration of their gums if the teeth are extracted with the forceps will be slight, and their fears are so excited upon having their gums lanced, that we often find it excedingly difficult to apply the instrument for the extraction of the teeth. The moment of deliberation with them should be the moment of extracting the tooth.

Extraction of Roots and Stumps of Teeth.

It should be a general rule with us never to allow any loose or useless stumps of teeth to remain in the mouth, but to extract them ; and for this purpose we require instruments entirely different from those used for the extraction of the teeth themselves. When the stump of a tooth is sufficiently long and firm to be taken hold of with the forceps, we may extract them with the forceps, but in a great many cases we cannot use them. It is extremely difficult to give any written description of the instruments used by dentists for the extraction of stumps and roots of teeth. There are two general shapes, one set having their ends bent like hooks, by which we are enabled to take hold of the stumps and extract them, and in many cases with the most perfect success. Another set have their ends, terminating in a pyramidal shape, like the "levier pyramidal" of M. La Forgue, and others of different shapes from these, like punches. Success in the use of these instruments, depends very much on the skill of the operator ; and the greatest care is required in performing the operations with these instruments, as, if they slip from the stump, and the operator is not on his guard, the tongue, lips, gums, or cheeks, are liable to be wounded, or injury may be done to the other teeth. These instruments should be made of well tempered steel, with sharp edges, but should not be so slender or hard as to break in using them. Previously to using these instruments, the gums should be separated from the roots or stumps, as we directed in extracting the teeth. In extracting the stumps of teeth, no certain direction can be given, whether we shall attempt to bring the stump into the mouth or outside ; all must depend upon the skill and judgment of the operator. The situation of the stump will usually determine us what mode to adopt. A correct judgment, and tolerably skilful tact with the use of these instruments will usually insure success. In concluding the subject of extraction of the teeth, I need not speak of the remedial effects upon the health of the individual, but refer the reader to the different diseases and morbid effects before mentioned, as produced by bad and diseased teeth, and let him make his own application of the subject.

The operator will often find it necessary to use considerable address in persuading his patients to submit to these operations, by allaying their fears and convincing them of the great benefits which will result from the operation. He should, by all means in his power, dissipate a dread of the operation, and when he performs it, render it as light and easy as possible. He should seldom or never use any deception in the performance of it, as this almost always excites very unpleasant feelings on the part of the patient, and does but little in advancing the permanent reputation of the operator. Satisfy your patients that the operation is for their best interests, and if they have any confidence in the operator they will rarely decline the operation. The operator should have that confidence in himself as never to evince any timidity in the presence of his patient.

SECTION II.

OF HÆMORRHAGE AFTER EXTRACTION OF THE TEETH.

During the time of extracting several teeth or stumps, and after, we may direct our patient to rinse the mouth with warm water until the hæmorrhage ceases in some degree, which it usually does in the course of ten to sixty minutes. In some rare cases, bleeding from the socket of a tooth continues for several hours, and in some instances, becomes alarming to the patient, and even dangerous; and our assistance is asked for to arrest the hæmorrhage. In general, all that is necessary to be done is to take a lock of cotton dipped in some astringent or stimulating liquor and applied so as to completely fill up the cavity from which the tooth was extracted, and then lay on more cotton, until it rises above the line of the other teeth, so that the patient, by closing his mouth, will press the cotton hard upon the bleeding surface or vessel. By adopting this measure we shall rarely fail in stopping the hæmorrhage at once. The cotton which we apply to the wound may be dipped in the tincture of galls, a solution of sulphate of copper, or in a tincture from brandy, myrrh and galls, or in brandy alone, or in spirits of turpentine, or some diluted acids. In some rare cases a strong solution of the argentum nitratum may be used, or the wound may be brushed over with a pencil of the caustic. In some cases the actual cautery. In some cases the cotton dipped in diluted acids, &c. has been used; but rarely, if ever, will the surgeon fail in stopping the hæmorrhage by the use of the cotton dipped in some of the preparations before mentioned, and applied so as be pressed firmly upon the bleeding vessel. We never need hesitate to extract any tooth on account of hæmorrhage, which may follow; as, in the first place, hæmorrhage very rarely occurs, and when it does, we can immediately stop it by the means before mentioned.

In some instances fatal hæmorrhages have followed extraction of a tooth, but these cases have usually been found complicated with some peculiarity of constitution—these are very rarely witnessed. In addition to what I have already directed, the alveolus from whence the blood usually issues, may be stopped with a piece of cork, or the tooth itself may be returned until a slight inflammation takes place, and then removed. Blisters may be applied to the angle of the jaw, or behind the ear, &c. I will present the reader with an account of a fatal case of this kind, taken from the Dentiste Observateur.

*A person living in Paris called upon me to extract a canine tooth for him. On examining his mouth, I thought that this man was attacked with the scurvy; but this did not seem to me sufficient to hinder the person from having his tooth extracted; much less would he have consented to it, on account of the pain which this tooth gave him. After the tooth was extracted, it did not appear to me that it bled more profusely than is customary to do after similar operations. In the mean while, the following night I was called upon to see the patient, who had continued to bleed ever since he left me. I employed for stopping this hæmorrhage, the agaric of the oak bark which I commonly used with success. The following day I was again sent for, the bleeding still continued. After having disburdened the mouth of all the lint pledgets which I used for making compression at the place where the blood appeared to come from, I made the patient take some mouthfuls of water to clean his mouth of all the clots of blood with which it was filled: I perceived then that the blood came no more from the place where I had extracted the tooth, but from the gums; there was not one single place in the whole mouth from whence blood did not issue. I called in then the physician, who ordered several bleedings in succession to each other, besides astrin-

* Le Dentiste Observateur, par H. G. Courtois, Paris, 1775.

gents, which were taken inwardly, and gargles were used of the same nature; but all these remedies, like all the others he took to give the blood more consistence, were all used to no purpose. It was not possible to stop this, hæmorrhāge. The patient died the ninth or tenth day after the extraction of his tooth.

Removal of Foreign Matter from the Teeth.

Having now spoken of the several operations for the extraction of useless, diseased, or irregular teeth, and for the removal of stumps of teeth, we now proceed to a particular consideration of those operations which are performed for the preservation of the health and beauty of the teeth, and for remedying defects or irregularities in them. The first of these operations, which I shall proceed to consider and describe, is that of the removal of foreign matter occasionally deposited on the teeth and their fangs. This operation has been termed scaling of the teeth; and its utility and mode of performance will be particularly considered.

SECTION III.

SCALING OF THE TEETH.

Its Utility.

This is one of the most useful operations in dental surgery. In the first part of this work I have very frequently referred to the injurious effects of tartar and other foreign matter deposited upon the teeth and pressing upon the gums and alveolar processes, as indirectly causing caries, and directly a diseased state of the gums. I mention the tartar and other foreign matter as being the principal agents in producing diseased gums, and consequently the reader will be prepared to hear me say, that the removal of this matter is indispensable in the cure and prevention of these diseases. This is the fact, as in almost every instance our efforts in the cure or prevention of them will be wholly unavailing, unless we perfectly remove the foreign matter, and prevent its accumulation.

Of the Foreign Matters lodged upon the Teeth.

In the course of our observations upon the teeth we notice four, apparently, different kinds of foreign matter deposited upon them.

First,—An orange-coloured substance, giving to the teeth a peculiarly yellow colour.

Second,—A dark brown, or nearly black substance.

Third,—A greenish substance, lodged more particularly on the flat surfaces of the incisores, and on the canini; noticed mostly on the teeth of children and young persons; and, as far as my observation extends, I have thought that this matter appears to be an exciting cause of caries. In examining the teeth of individuals, whenever I have noticed this greenish matter, I have most usually remarked the presence of caries.

Fourth,—Tartar, or Zufa. This substance, perhaps from a fancied analogy to the tartar of wine-barrels, has been termed Tartar. It is quite doubtful whether it is a directly exciting cause of caries, but indirectly, by causing disease in the soft parts upon which it impinges, and thereby vitiating the secretions of the mouth, it no doubt, causes the destruction of a vast many teeth. Various conjectures have been offered to account for the origin of the tartar, with which I do not wish to fatigue the reader. It is, no doubt, deposited from the juices of the mouth.

I will present the reader with an analysis of this substance made by Mr. Pepys, for Mr. Fox, in Dec. 1805.

*Analysis of the Tartar.**

Dear Sir,

The specimens of the tartar of the teeth, which I received from you, I have examined chemically. Previous to the analysis, I subjected a portion of them to the following experiments. I am Dear Sir,

Truly Yours,

W. H. Pepys.

Artillery Place, Finsbury, Dec. 1, 1805.
To Mr. Fox.

Tartar of the teeth is of a dirty white colour, inclining to brown, stained, in parts, yellow and green—spongy, porous texture, yet considerably hard; when it is detached in large pieces, exhibits the impression of the teeth on which it was deposited. The pieces which were examined were dry and free from smell. Specific gravity 1.5714.

Sulphuric acid, 1.85, is immediately blackened—the substance becomes spongy and soft, but no complete solution takes place.

Nitric acid, 1.12, acts in nearly a similar manner on this substance as on the teeth. A gas which has the negative

* Fox, Part II, pages, 111, 114.

property of nitrogen, is evolved in small bubbles, and a flocculent mass of the form of the piece immersed, is left.

Solution of potash, boiled for some time upon it, had but little action; the tartar became whiter, the solution yellow: upon the addition of nitric acid to the separated solution, the colour nearly disappeared without any precipitate being formed: ammonia reproduced the yellow colour.

The flocculent substance left by dilute nitric acid, after washing off the acid, being boiled with solution of potash, was not wholly dissolved; the solution became yellow. Nitric acid being added, discharged the colour, which ammonia reproduced.

Water, boiled for some time upon tartar, gave no precipitate or turbid appearance on the addition of solution of tannin.

Tartar exposed to a red heat, in a silver crucible, smokes, accompanied with a greasy smell; is blackened in a similar manner to bone, and becomes more easily soluble in nitric acid, leaving a carbonaceous residuum.

The solutions of potash which have been boiled on tartar being neutralized with nitric acid, gave no precipitate with solution of nitrate of barytes.

Analysis.

Fifty grains of tartar of the teeth were placed in 400 grains of nitric acid 1.12; nitrogen gas was slightly liberated: in twenty-four hours it was diluted with two ounces of distilled waters, and then filtered.

The solution was then precipitated by ammonia, and filtered; and, upon the addition of carbonate of ammonia, remained, clear, the precipitate produced, being dried at 212°, weighed 40 grains, and, when ignited, it weighed 35, which were again soluble in dilute nitric acid, giving a copious precipitate with solution of acetate of lead: this precipitate, washed, dried, and exposed to a flame urged by a blowpipe, fused into a globule, accompanied with a bright phosphorescent appearance, and was, therefore, phosphate of lead.

The substance not soluble in nitric acid, was washed and dried at 212°, weighed 9 grains.

The separated solution was of a yellow colour; the addition of nitric acid produced no precipitate, but lost colour, which was recovered by ammonia.

The 9 grains of residuum, after treatment of the potash, were placed in boiling concentrated nitric acid, by which they were completely dissolved; and by the test of tannin proved the cartilage to have been gelatinized.

Tartar of the teeth consists of,

Phosphate of lime, - - - - - - - - - -	35
Fibrina, or cartilage, - - - - - - - - - -	9
Animal fat, or oil, - - - - - - - - - -	3
Loss, - - - - - - - - - - - - - -	3
	50

Next to caries, nothing is more destructive to the health of the mouth than this substance. It is apt to be insinuated between the gums and teeth, passing upon the alveolar processes, producing irritation, inflammation, and suppuration of the former, and caries and absorption of the latter; and consequently, it causes the teeth to be loosened, and ultimately to fall out. This is the cause of the loss of the teeth in elderly persons, which otherwise were perfectly sound, of which I have spoken before. By causing a diseased state of the gums, it affects the breath, and causes it to be very offensive. By being deposited upon the teeth in quantity almost equal to the whole of the teeth, and being of a dark colour, it completely destroys the beauty of the teeth, and causes them to assume a dark and very repulsive, dirty, and offensive appearance. It is, no doubt, directly, and indirectly, one of the most efficient causes of the loss and destruction of the teeth. Many persons, upon breaking off pieces of this matter, are disposed to think they have broken off a portion of their teeth or tooth. Many persons disposed to calculous and gouty affections are liable to the abundant deposition of this matter. Females, during pregnancy, and confinement in particular, are very liable to it. Persons who are not cleanly with regard to their teeth are more liable to acumulation of it than those who regularly clean their teeth. It is usually, at first, deposited around the necks of the teeth, in the form of dark yellowish paste, mixed, more or less with mucus, and soon concretes and hardens into a substance like hardened mortar: it is often scaled off in pieces resembling the teeth around which it is deposited. It is deposited in greatest quantity around those teeth situated near the opening of the salivary ducts, and on the inside of the under incisors, and about those teeth which are not much used, as the use of the teeth in mastication usually brushes this substance off, more or less. The vitiated saliva deposits itself in the dark mucus and tartar, and is held by these in contact with the teeth, so as to act with violence upon the enamel. It is deposited about the necks of the teeth, in the interstices between them, and in the irregularities of the grinding surfaces of the large teeth. There are different idiosyncrasies in respect to the deposition of tartar; the teeth of some persons will have little of it deposited in many years, while some persons have as much in a few months. This substance is removed from the teeth by mechanical means, and is prevented from accumulating by the judicious use of suitable brushes, tooth-picks, and dentifrices. During sleep a viscid mucus is deposited around the teeth, and if not removed in the morning, or by mastication, is apt to leave a considerable quantity of tartar. The deposition of tartar in the saliva is an unavoidable circumstance, but its accumulation can be prevented, and thereby all the pernicious consequences resulting from its presence will be obviated.

Of the Instruments required in the Performance of this Operation.

The instruments usually employed in this operation, are made of steel, with fine sharp edges, and these edges are usually allowed to become dull, so that they will not cut the enamel of the teeth. Their cutting ends are usually bent into different shapes, some like very small chisels, others spear-pointed, or pyramidal-shaped; others, thin and flat, so as to be passed between the teeth, and remove all the tartar deposited on them; others are made to scrape the flat surfaces of the teeth. It is impossible to give a written description of these instruments, so as to be intelligible to the reader. They are generally known and put in sets. The surgeon-dentist should be provided with a sufficient number and variety of these instruments to be able to remove all foreign matter from the teeth in every possible place of deposit, for if he is not able to do so, his operations will be imperfect, and in consequence of being imperfectly done, will be of more injury to the patient than benefit.

Of the Manner of Performing this Operation.

Having provided ourselves with suitable instruments, the student or practitioner of this art, should consider that he is to operate upon organs which are injured, even to a considerable extent, even by slight violence, and consequently, that he must handle his instruments with care, so as neither to injure the teeth nor the gums. It is repugnant to the practice of any judicious surgeon-dentist, to injure the teeth or gums, or to occasion much pain during the operation. It is astonishing at times, to witness in what a brutal and butcher-like manner some persons operate upon the teeth; wounding or injuring the enamel, and loosening the teeth, and mangling the gums in the most unnecessary manner.

There is no need of any violence; but by the suitable application of different instruments to the different teeth, the tartar may be scaled off, so as to occasion little or no pain to the patient, nor any violence or injury to the teeth. The operator should persevere by gentle efforts, and the proper application of suitable instruments, until he has removed all the tartar from the teeth, and rendered them clean. He should be peculiarly careful to remove all the tartar adhering upon the teeth, beneath the gums and between the teeth, so that none will remain. In cases where the gums are very tender, and bleed considerably we are not often able to remove all the tartar at one sitting, but are obliged to defer the completion of the operation for some days, until the gums heal. Mr. Fox, in cases where there is a considerable accumulation of tartar, objects to removing it at once, but recommends its partial removal at first, and after an interim of one or two weeks, to remove the rest.* Because, he says, if all the tartar is

* See Fox, Part II, page 108.

removed at once, pain and tenderness of the teeth will be produced. Mr. Koecker says, this is an erroneous opinion, and that "instead of believing that the removal of all the tartar at the same time, can endanger the teeth by exposing them, it seems to me, that the sooner they are relieved from so pernicious a coating, the more we contribute to their preservation."*

I coincide with the last named gentleman in his opinion of the subject, and consider, that if we can remove all the tartar at once, it will be for the best interests of our patient; but as I before mentioned, the bleeding of the gums may not allow of our doing it at once, we may defer it from five to twelve days, when we ought to complete the operation. I never saw any pain or inconvenience arise from the complete removal of the tartar but in one case, and this was quickly relieved by holding a little brandy in the mouth for a few minutes. If any of the teeth are loose, and have tartar on them, which is often the case, we are to use great care in removing it, and support the tooth with our fingers, or some instrument, whilst we remove the tartar which adheres to it. This is an important direction and should be carefully adopted by every operator. During the operation, and after it is accomplished, until the bleeding entirely ceases, the patient should rinse the mouth frequently with warm water. After the bleeding ceases, some astringent lotion may be used if the gums are tender, which is not always the case. The astringent I prefer in this case, is the decoction of the oak-bark, or of galls, mentioned when speaking of the mode of treating scurvy of the gums. In using any astringent wash, we must direct our patients after using the astringent lotion and brushing the gums, so as to carry it completely over every part

* Koecker, Part II, page 291.

of the mouth and teeth, then to wash the mouth and teeth with water of a temperature which shall be agreeable to them, so as to make them clean, for the astringent is apt to dirty the teeth, or give them a dark colour, if not washed off in the most particular manner. To complete the cleaning of the teeth, and to render them clean and beautiful, they should be washed with a brush, and some tooth-powder possessing some mechanical properties, as for instance, a dentifrice having a little prepared chalk in it, &c. and rub the teeth with this and a soft piece of leather or brush, and you will render the teeth very clean, take off the peculiar yellow colour which is occasionally seen, and render them, in most cases, from being dark and repulsive to the observer, to be clean, white, and beautiful. The eye will rest upon them with pleasure. The acknowledgments of our patients, especially females, will be of the most flattering and agreeable nature. We shall not only receive their thanks and patronage, but have the pleasure of reflecting, that we have rendered them an essential service.

Of the Good Effects resulting from this Operation, and the Symptoms by which we know that it is effectually performed.

One of the first effects of the proper performance of this operation which we shall notice, will be a return of health to the gums: their inflamed, swollen, spongy, and bleeding condition will, in the course of from three to eight, or twelve days, with the use of the astringent wash, become entirely altered. The swelling and inflammation will immediately subside, and from an angry red colour we shall soon notice a mild florid appearance, and no pain or uneasiness will be perceived about them. From being spongy and ready to bleed upon the slightest touch, they will become hard and firm, and not inclined to bleed any more than when in perfect health. The gums, from having been pressed away from the teeth, and hanging loose around them, will immediately embrace them: if abandoned, in many instances grow to the tooth, and a perfectly healthy state of the gums will follow. If these effects do not take place, and the gums continue swollen and inflamed, and hang in a loose flabby manner around the teeth, we may be assured that the tartar is not all removed, or that some of the teeth have lost their vitality. In this case, we should examine the teeth in the most careful manner, and if any tartar is left, as generally we shall be able to detect some beneath the gum, pressing upon the alveoli, or between the teeth, upon the removal of which, the best effects follow. It should be remembered by every operator, that this operation, if properly and faithfully done, is one of the most useful in dental-surgery, but if not well performed is of little benefit, if not an injury to the patient.

SECTION IV.

REMOVAL OF CARIOUS PORTIONS FROM THE TEETH, AND THE SEPARATION OF THEM WHEN IN A CROWDED STATE, &C. &C.

We have before noticed and detailed the progress of caries in the first part of this work, and considered that in the great majority of cases, decay of the teeth proceeded from external agencies, and was produced by a vitiated state of the saliva, and that the decay usually commenced externally, and in those parts of the tooth where the enamel was thinnest; as for instance, in the depressions of the grinding surfaces of the molar teeth; upon the edges of those teeth which touch each other, or are crowded together, or overlap each other; and by not having room to grow, the enamel was thin; and also when the enamel began to be attenuated near the necks of the teeth, decay was apt to commence, especially when a part of the gums were lost, and in a majority of cases, as soon as the enamel was perforated by the progress of the decay, that the bony part of the tooth decayed very fast, and soon formed a considerable cavity. Caries of the teeth usually after penetrating the enamel, excites a chronic inflammation of the bony part; so much so, as to produce mortification of the inflamed part; by a constant continuance of the inflammation and mortification, the caries proceeds until it penetrates to the nerve of the tooth, and at last produces, if not arrested in its progress, the entire destruction of the crown and body of the tooth. In some cases as soon as the decay penetrates the enamel, the bone becomes inflamed and sets up a powerful barrier to the progress of the caries; the bone of the tooth at this particular spot becomes very tender, so as to hardly bear the touch of a brush, and seems in a great many cases to do much towards arresting the progress of the disease; and the caries instead of penetrating the tooth, spreads like an irregular patch over it. This state of caries when it takes place, is usually situated on the front flat surface of the incisors, and on the outside of the grinders and biscuspid teeth, and demonstrates in the clearest manner, how little the statements of those writers are to be credited, who assert that the teeth or at least their bony structure is almost extraneous, with regard to the rest of the system, and possessed of little or no vitality. For by disease it becomes quite as sensible as most of the fleshy organs of the system. When caries has proceeded so far as to penetrate the bony structure of the tooth, and can in any proper manner be made to receive and retain a plug, by which I always mean a metallic filling of the cavity, &c. we ought to make it an universal rule and not to be departed from, to fill the cavity with a metallic substance, as will be particularly described and detailed in a subsequent section on that subject. But many cases will occur, when the caries has merely penetrated the enamel, or acting upon it, and has not much affected the bony structure of the tooth, as is especially the case in those instances, when the caries excites so much sensibility of the bone, and is arrested in some degree, and then proceeds superficially upon the tooth. In this state of caries it becomes our duty to remove it; having previously however removed the tartar from the teeth, and by every dental operation required, placed the mouth in a healthy condition, so that no disease or cause of disease shall be present, save the caries which we are to operate upon, and then our operation will in most cases be successful in arresting the progress of the disease. But if we presume to operate upon the teeth in removing carious portions of them, without at the same time or before placing the gums and the other teeth in a healthy condition, we shall, instead of curing, aggravate the disease. We shall by denuding the bone of the tooth in order to remove the carious portion, expose it to be acted upon by all those destructive agents which I have before noticed, as being present in every unhealthy state of the teeth and gums, and consequently our operation adds by the irritation it induces to an already over inflamed and irritated state of the gums, jaws and teeth; and the caries in the teeth which are operated on, proceeds with increased violence to the complete destruction of the teeth. Very often under these circumstances, a tooth or two or more, in which caries had made but little progress, upon being operated on whilst the mouth is in an unhealthy state, are in a few months after entirely destroyed by the progress of the caries. It should be a rule never to be departed from, never to file the teeth, unless the the rest of the mouth, is in a healthy state.

Of the Instruments requisite for the performance of the operation of removing Carious Portions from Diseased Teeth.

The instruments required for this operation, are in the first place, different kinds of files, having different shapes, &c. so that we can operate upon the teeth under almost any circumstance; so that we may be able to file one tooth and not any others, or divide the teeth and cut a little from the two teeth in contact, or in other cases to merely separate them. The files required for dividing the teeth, or filing between the two teeth so as to remove a part of both, or to remove a portion of a tooth in contact with another, and not injure its fellow, must be thin and flat. The flat sides of some may be cut on both sides, and others on one side only; whilst others should be thin and smooth on both sides, having the edges cut, &c. Round files are in some very rare instances required, but very rarely. The files should be of fine cut, and immediately laid aside upon becoming dull, for the sharper they are, the less jarring and pain is experienced by the patient. We ought to have the instruments in such order as to make as little irritation as possible, and this is prevented in some degree, by having our files very sharp.

The next instrument we want, is one to cut away superficial caries upon the flat surfaces of the teeth, and outside of the grinders and bicuspids, &c. which I have before mentioned, as often being attended with so much tenderness and sensibility, a kind of fungus appears to be on it, or a slight pullulation of the blood-vessels of the part affected. The operator may have a set of instruments for this purpose exclusively, or he may use some one or more of his scaling instruments, kept sharp for the purpose. In dividing the front incisores, especially the upper ones, it is often desirable to remove more from the posterior side than the front, which may be done with a sharp knife made strong and like a gum lancet. The next instrument we require, is a pair or pairs of forceps, with which we may take hold of the tooth, upon which we intend to operate and hold it firmly. This is especially necessary if any of the teeth upon which we operate are loose, or of a delicate structure.

Indications for the Performance of this Operation.

I do not wish to enlarge upon this operation any more than is absolutely necessary, in order that the student may have the most definite views of the subject, and a correct knowledge of it. A crowded state of the teeth is considered by some practitioners as sufficient indication for their being divided with the file. It is observed by Mr. Fox,* that the incisores of the upper jaw are very liable to become carious, in consequence of being crowded, or pressed much against each other; and to prevent this taking place, it is advisable to make a separation of them with a very thin file, and the space ought not to be wider than to allow a piece of paper, or fine linen, to be passed between the teeth. If they have begun to be carious, a wider space should be made. The former direction of Mr. Fox to divide the teeth, when crowd-

---

* Fox, Part II. page 145.

ed merely, and not carious, has, by its injudicious adoption and indiscriminate performance, been productive, probably, of more injurious consequences than any mode of practice, or any direction ever given by any writer or practitioner of dental surgery. Almost every dentist who has read Mr. Fox, has adopted and followed this practice. The pernicious consequences of it are seen almost every day.

The enamel as we have before remarked, is the protection which nature has provided for the teeth, and consequently, if it is removed, they are rendered much less capable of defending themselves against those injurious agencies which we have before considered, and instead of preventing decay, this operation, in a vast many cases, becomes a powerful adjuvant in the progress of caries. By removing the enamel, especially when there are decayed teeth, or diseased gums present, the saliva vitiated by these last causes, acts upon those teeth which have been filed, with the most destructive certainty; and in fact, the file, as far as it goes, assists the progress of caries towards the lining membrane of the tooth, and removes that covering which the vitiated saliva might have acted upon for years without abrading. The separation in this case, is of very little moment, as the teeth, in many cases, immediately advance forward, and fill the spaces made by the file, and are soon in as close a state of contact as ever, and ten times as liable to decay as before. If the teeth are separated so much as never to become again in contact, the case is but little better; for so much of the substance of the tooth is taken away, as that it is ever after more or less tender, and liable to be affected by almost any cause, heat, cold, &c. &c. The appearance of filed teeth is, at least to me, far from being agreeable. I have seen many persons' teeth, which, although at the time of the operation, were perfectly sound, had been filed away so much as to destroy in a considerable degree, their natural shape and beauty, and made them resemble some forms of artificial teeth. I could mention many cases of the injurious effects resulting from the improper use of the file. I have seen cases when the individuals, subjects of the operation, assured me, that their teeth were perfectly sound at the time of being filed, and in the course of from two to three years, not only the filed teeth, but almost every tooth, in their mouths, were diseased, commencing with the filed teeth, and spreading to all the others in the mouth. I will mention the following case, with the subject of which I have been acquainted for some time: Mrs. A—— M——, a lady about 32 years of age, called on me in the month of April, 1827, with a view of having me examine her teeth, and to ascertain what could be done for their preservation, if any thing. The lady informed me, that some years ago, she was then residing in the town of Erie in this state, an itinerant dentist spent a few days in that village, and at the solicitation of the dentist and of some of her friends, in consequence of her teeth being somewhat crowded upon each other, although perfectly sound, she suffered the dentist to separate her teeth with the file. He divided the incisores of the upper jaw, and the first bicuspids and canine teeth of the under jaw. The lady assured me, that in less that three years she had scarcely a sound tooth in her mouth. She said, that in a few months caries commenced on those surfaces of the teeth which had been filed; from these it spread to her molar teeth, nearly all of which she had lost. At the time she called on me, her upper front incisores were in a complete state of decay; one of them had crumbled away and broken off, until nothing was left but its fang; the other was decayed to a mere shell. One of the lateral incisores had decayed and broken off, so that at this time every tooth of her upper jaw that remained was in a state of disease, and nearly all her under ones. Some of her teeth I extracted, and by cleaning the others which remained, and plugging those which admitted of it, I was enabled to put her mouth, teeth, and gums in a healthy condition, and after this I replaced her upper incisor teeth with a set of natural teeth. This is not an isolated case; I could mention many more of nearly the same kind, but I need not do it, as the reader at this time has only to take notice of this subject among the people, and he may see similar cases every day. From these facts I would lay it down as an established rule, and one from which I never deviate, never to file any tooth which is not carious, unless it might be to obviate or remove some deformity, or for artificial purposes. Never to apply the file merely to separate the teeth. If this is judged necessary, we may extract one of the bicuspid molar teeth on each side of the jaw, and the crowded teeth will fall back from each other, so as to be relieved from pressure, and the injurious consequences resulting from the use of the file will be obviated. In these cases, the loss of these teeth, either a bicuspid or a molar, (I prefer the latter one on each side of the jaw,) is of an advantage to the health of the others, and by the falling back of the front ones, and advance of the posterior, the cavity is soon filled up, and the teeth are greatly relieved from the bad consequences of pressure, and this without injuring or irritating the remaining teeth. This direction is one of more especial consequence in younger persons, whose teeth and alveoli possess more mobility than when older. At this time of life too, in a majority of cases, caries is apt to take place in those teeth which are filed, unless ever after the most rigid adherence to cleanliness is observed by the patient. I would not by any means advance an opinion, that the enamel cannot be removed, or the bone of the tooth exposed, without decay following; or that decay necessarily follows the loss of the enamel, or a part of it; but this I would be understood as meaning, that the removal of the enamel from the bone of the tooth renders the tooth much more susceptible of injurious impression from all those agencies I have before detailed as inducing caries, and that the separation of the teeth is much better and more effectually obtained by the judicious extraction of two or more, than by the file. The filing induces irritation; the extraction, if well performed, removes it. Extraction supports and strengthens the enamel of the remaining teeth, whilst filing removes it, and greatly weakens the teeth, by jarring them and removing their substance. Filing the teeth induces a state of tenderness in them which may remain during life. Extraction of the teeth, we have mentioned, never has this effect; but on the contrary, removes and obviates a disposition to irritability of the crowded teeth and the dental nerves. In crowded sets of teeth, the loss of two, as I have before said, is amply compensated to the individual by the healthy state it induces in the remaining teeth; and if done before the dentes sapientia are developed, these will grow much larger, and be much firmer,* and more perfect in their organization. I have dwelt much longer upon this subject than I at first intended, and still I feel reluctant to leave it. I consider it as one of vital consequence to the reputation of the dental practitioner, and of the utmost moment to the patient. I dwell upon it the more because it is often most pernicious to the teeth, and at this time is all the fashion, all the rage. Few persons now-a-days escape if they apply to a dentist (with the exception of a few well-informed among the profession) for his services in any respect, without having some of their teeth filed, whether they are carious or not; and a

* See Koecker.

most effectual mode it is of perpetuating the business of the dentist. I am now speaking of filing the teeth when they are sound, in order to separate them. There are states of the teeth, as when caries has commenced at their edges, in which it becomes our duty to use the file; and if we attend to the preceding directions, as respects the healthy state of the mouth, teeth, &c. and perform the operation judiciously, and oblige our patients to observe the most perfect cleanliness of their teeth ever after, we shall be able to arrest the progress of the caries. Whether to remove decay, or separate the teeth, the most perfect cleanliness must be observed by the patient ever after the operation, and if he does, filed teeth may never decay so long as kept clean. Many persons never keep their teeth clean, but suffer them to be dirty; in these, extraction, as before mentioned, is altogether better than to file their teeth. It is true, it may be said, that it is neither the fault of the operator or of the operation, if the patients do not keep their teeth clean. I admit it, yet still it is the duty of the surgeon-dentist to perform those operations, if possible, which shall leave the teeth as little susceptible to injury as may be, even if his patients are negligent, and do not endeavour to preserve their teeth. It was observed by Mr. Hunter,* that "we seldom or never see any person whose teeth begin to rot after the age of fifty years." This is to a certian extent true; but not in all cases, as they decay, in some instances, after that period. But the teeth of the young are much more irritable, and the enamel is weaker, than in old persons; consequently, caries in the young is more readily excited, and proceeds with much greater rapidity than in persons of advanced age. Caries, as I have before observed, appears to proceed and be excited in a ratio nearly,

* See Hunter, Part II. page 141.

if not exactly inversely with the age, and the mobility of the teeth follows the same rule; consequently extraction, to obviate a crowded state of the teeth, is, on every account, more indicated in the young, whilst the file is more admissible in persons of advanced years. But that same cleanliness, which is so absolutely necessary to preserve filed teeth from decay, will, in almost every instance, preserve crowded teeth from the same fate. When the enamel has been filed away to separate the teeth, and they have approximated so as to be nearly, or quite in contact again, they are far more liable to decay than they were before they were filed. We noticed that kind of superficial caries which attacks the enamel of the teeth on the flat surfaces of the incisores, and on the outside of the grinders and bicuspides. Would it not be just as proper to cut away the enamel on these parts, while sound, to prevent caries taking place, as to do the same to the edges of the teeth in contact with each other whilst they are sound? I consider that the expediency of filing or not filing the teeth ought to be a subject of serious deliberation on the part of the dental practitioner, and never, especially in young persons, perform the operation, unless obliged to do so to cure actual disease. I will now notice those situations in which this operation is necessary and proper.

First, To remove superficial caries, when it is not deep enough to receive and retain a pulg.

Second, To separate teeth which are carious so as to allow the dentist to introduce a plug.

Third, To separate teeth, between which we wish to pass the clasp of a spring in order to retain artificial teeth.

Fourth, To obviate irregularity, or to cut off teeth which are elongated.

Consequently, it will be seen, that I do not consider a crowded state of the teeth to be a positive indication for the use of the file. The same cleanliness which is indispensable after filing the teeth will keep them sound without it.

Of the Manner of Performing this Operation.

This operation requires a careful, gentle hand. The operator should remember that he is operating upon living organs, and that with at least a harsh and disagreeable instrument, which, if harshly handled, almost doubles the pain of the operation. It is surprising to notice of what roughness and violence some operators are guilty in filing the teeth; often breaking their files, and occasionally the teeth themselves. It is but this day, whilst writing this section, a lady called on me to have my advice respecting her teeth, and showed me one of her front upper incisores, having a large piece broken out of it by the dentist in filing it. Before applying the file to the teeth, examine them with the utmost care, and notice whether there is any checks or cracks in the enamel, which is sometimes the case; and if so, there will be great danger in using the file, as the jar and violence of it will very often break off the enamel which was before cracked. In these cases, the enamel will usually be found checked on the front flat surface of the incisores, and not on the posterior surface; as I do not remember as ever I saw a check of the enamel on the posterior side or surface. If, however, the tooth has strength to allow the use of the file, and we purpose to divide the teeth merely, then we may take a flat file, the patient's head supported against the head-piece of the chair, and apply it so as to cut equally upon each tooth, and by gentle strokes of the file, pass it between the teeth to the gum, keeping the file true, so that it shall not bind itself, or be confined before the operation is finished, as if it does become confined before the operation is finished, we are apt to strain the tooth and break the file ; should the file become much confined, we should substitute another file of a different thickness, and complete the operation. If superficial caries is present, we ought to file every particle of it away, until we arrive at the healthy part of the tooth. This, we ought ever to bear in mind, that if we do not remove the carious and inflamed part entirely, we shall do but little in arresting the disease. When we wish to file one tooth alone, and not its fellow, then we may use a file smooth on one of its surfaces, so as not to cut the tooth we wish to avoid. The tooth we operate on should be firmly supported by the forceps which I before mentioned for this purpose. In dividing the teeth in order to introduce a plug, we are often obliged to divide the bicuspid and molar teeth, and in this case, are apt to cut the cheek, which can be prevented by putting a soft piece of leather between the file and the cheek. We should notice the same when dividing the teeth to allow the passage of the clasp of a spring, when we wish to confiue artificial teeth. When we cut off elongated teeth we ought to support them, so as to prevent their being loosened by the action and jar of the file. It is worthy of notice that the diseased part of a tooth, when it has not reached the lining membrane, is much more sensible, and creates much more pain in filing it, in a great many instances, than the healthy bone of the tooth itself, so that the commencement of the operation is much more painful than the conclusion, which proves that caries, in most, if not all cases, proceeds by a chronic inflammation and subsequent mortification of the bony structure of the tooth, after the enamel has been abraded by mechanical or chemical causes. We ought, if possible, before we file any of the teeth, to put them in as healthy a condition as possible ; and, if in our power, prevent any irritable state of them, so as not to create much pain or irritation by the application of the file. This is often the case with elongated teeth, which are usually pushed up by a chronic enlargement and inflammation of the lining membrane of their sockets, and consequently these should not be operated on if their alveolar membranes are in a state ofchronic inflammation, or in a very irritable condition. It is impossible to give minute directions which will suit or apply to all cases in which the file may be used; but with the foregoing general principles, rules and directions, and the judgment of the judicious practitioner, the file will seldom be used to the injury or disadvantage of the teeth, or the reputation of the practitioner. Judiciously used, it is a valuable adjuvant in curing diseased teeth, and in facilitating and assisting dental operations.

In removing superficial caries upon the flat surface of the incisores, and on the outside of the grinders and bicuspid teeth, we may make use of the file, in some cases, to advantage; in others, we may use a sharp cutting instrument having a firm edge and attenuated to a point. Beginning at the very edge of the caries, which is often very sensible, we may cut down to the healthy bone, and having this for our level, we may scrape off the carious portion entirely, and without creating much pain to the patient; but if we attempt to carry our instrument over the tender surfaces at once, and not cut down to the healthy bone at one side, as before mentioned, the pain we shall occasion will be so great, as that our patients will oblige us to desist; but if we begin carefully at the very edge of the caries, and cut down to the healthy bone, we may remove every part of it, and in the most effectual manner, and without much pain to the patient; and by a strict observance of cleanliness adopted, the progress of the caries will be effectually prevented, and permanent health will be established in the tooth or teeth from which we have removed the carious portions. Perhaps I ought to remark that if we file between the teeth, we ought to preserve, as nearly as possible, the shape of the tooth, by carrying the file parallel with the edges of the sides of the teeth, and never gouge or cut out portions from the sides of the teeth with round files or three cornered ones; if we wish to remove a considerable of the tooth, the better way will be to file the front edge of the tooth, in a handsome manner, that is, straight, up and down; and if we wish to remove any more, to cut away the posterior plate of the enamel, and then, with the same instrument, remove all the carious bone of the tooth. In this way we shall preserve the beauty of the tooth, and at the same time remove the carious portion. I will mention the following case to show the want of correct views on this subject, which are occasionally seen. Mrs. S——, called on me in April 1827, with her daughter, an amiable young lady, aged about eleven years, and requested my advice respecting the daughter's teeth, and remarked that the incisores had been filed by a dentist of this city, in consequence of their being carious. I examined them, and found that the dentist, instead of attempting to preserve the shape and beauty of the teeth, had cut one of her lateral upper incisors nearly half off with a three cornered file, and other ways injured the teeth, by the improper use of this instrument. I restored the teeth to health by plugging them with gold, &c.

SECTION V.

OF RESTORING THE SUBSTANCE OF A DECAYED TOOTH WITH A METALIC SUBSTITUTE; COMMONLY CALLED PLUGGING THE TEETH.

This is an operation of great antiquity, which very naturally suggests itself to the mind of the practitioner of medicine, if he is acquainted with the structure and uses of the teeth. For his reason would at once teach him, if he found a cavity in a tooth, to fill it with some substance which would exclude injurious matter, and prevent the bad effects of cold air, &c. entering the tooth. Hence we learn that this operation was one of very early adoption, it is said to have been practised at an early period by the Greeks and Romans. If properly done, this is one of the most useful operations in dental surgery; and if practicable, it bears the preference to any other operation for the cure of diseased teeth. If well done, the preservation of the tooth will be in almost every instance complete. By excluding the presence of foreign matters from the exposed bony substance of the tooth or its nerve, that chronic inflammation and mortification upon which the progress of caries usually depends, is entirely cured and prevented. It should be an object of solicitude in every case when we are called upon to extract or file the teeth, to obviate both operations by plugging them, if in any way expedient or practicable.

Indications for the Performance of this Operation.

The indications for the performance of this operation are generally very clear and distinct. Yet there are cases in which we shall find that the operation is not practicable, without cutting away a considerable of the healthy substance of the tooth; and other cases when it is not expedient, either from the caries having progressed so far as to render the tooth so weak, that it will not retain a plug; or when a tooth is entirely useless or loose, or dead: in many instances of this kind, we should prefer extracting the tooth to plugging it, directed however in some degree by the feelings and wishes of our patients. In cases when the caries is very superficial, and extending superficially to a considerable extent, we shall find that it will be better to cut away the caries and let the tooth remain, than to cut away a large portion of the tooth, to make room for the plug and retain it.

There are two states in the progress of caries, which requires separate consideration, as our treatment will be different as regards the preparation of the tooth for receiving the plug. These two states are;

First, When the caries and chronic inflammation has affected the bony structure of the tooth, and not exposed its cavity lining membrane or nerve. This state of the decay, as before mentioned, is called Simple Caries.

The second state is, when the cavity and lining membrane and nerve are exposed; this is called Complicated Caries.

Treatment of Simple Caries.

All that we have to do in simple caries, is to clean out the cavity of its decayed and inflamed substance, and introduce our stopping at once as will be directed hereafter.

Treatment of Complicated Caries.

The treament of complicated caries, is a matter of considerable nicety, so as to preserve the tooth, and not by our operations excite pain and active inflammation of the nerve and lining membrane. For in a majority of cases, if we attempt operations upon a tooth whose nerve is exposed without a previous preparation of the nerve, we shall excite in it active inflammation, and be compelled to extract the tooth. There are three ways in which the lining membrane of a tooth when exposed, is now treated by surgeon-dentists. The first consists in destroying the vitality of the nerve and lining membrane, by the use of some of the concentrated acids, or caustics, or the actual cautery, (red-hot iron) as for instance, the nitric, sulphuric, or muriatic acids, the caustic potash, or the argentum nitratum, (lunar caustic) and some of the essential oils, &c. &c. These are introduced into the tooth, and applied to the nerve, so as to destroy its vitality. But as it was observed by Mr. Hunter, page 149, these very often fail, and the dentists have then at times, used the actual cautery, introducing into the tooth a piece of platina or iron wire heated to redness: but this also often fails.

Attempts to destroy the inflamed nerves of teeth, especially the molar and bicuspid, are not only very painful; but most usually ineffectual. If we succeed in destroying the nerve, the tooth is often rendered almost useless.

I here subjoin a case of an unsuccessful attempt to destroy the nerves of a diseased tooth, which came under the observation of my friend Mr. Eleazar Parmly of New-York, who referring to the subject remarks*: "In a front tooth

* Parmly. Disorders and Treatment of the Teeth. Pages 52, 53, 54, 55.

the nerve is most commonly destroyed by a single operation, because the fang is single, and has the advantage of being more perpendicular than in a tooth with divaricating fangs. But it is an erroneous idea, that a diseased tooth, if it has more than a single fang, may be rendered useful and free from pain by destroying its nerves. The practice has only served to expose the emptiness of the theory, since most of those who have undergone the operation, which can be termed little less than martyrdom, have barely found that they have been made to forget the usual pain of tooth-ache in the unutterable agony of the operation. But this is not all the objection; for where the operator is so fortunate as partially to destroy the nerves of double teeth, as even this is very rarely the case, the membranes are apt to become diseased by inflammatory action, and the tooth requires to be extracted in a very short time afterwards. It cannot therefore be too strongly urged, that where a double tooth is painful, and has become so much decayed as not to be capable of being saved by the operation of stopping, it should, in order to prevent all unpleasant consequences, be extractcd immediately. In evidence of the fallacy of the attempts of destroying the nerves of back teeth, I shall adduce a single instance, which came under my own observation.

A gentleman possessing highly organised teeth, having twice suffered very serious lacerations of the bone from extraction, and having even been threatened with lock-jaw, submitted to have the fangs of the first lower molaris, which had long been a source of torture drilled, with the hope of thus eradicating its nerves. The operation, after excruciating agonies, proved within a few hours, to have been useless; the cavity of the tooth was then filled with a compound metallic stopping; but the pain returned with such violence, that it was necessary to remove it. The patient continued during many months to make every application, and adopt every measure, which the most experienced medical practitioners could suggest, but in vain. His protracted sufferings brought on a low fever, accompanied by frequent delirium. Efforts were again and again made at extraction; but at the first touch of an instrument, the patient was always seized with convulsions, and the operation could not be effected. Having thus lingered on for six months, the tooth was fortunately extracted during a period of insensibility, the result of intense suffering: but, although the expected local relief was thus obtained, several months elapsed before he regained his former health and vigour. The tooth was examined after extraction, when it appeared that very trifling portions of nerve had been destroyed; that one fang contained a large and vigorous nerve, sending off five branches at its point: the other fang a large nerve equally unaltered, sending off six branches around its point."

All these modes of destroying the nerve occasion great pain to the patient, in most cases; and what is still more objectionable, by destroying the nerve, the rest of the vitality of the crown and body of the tooth is soon lost, and, at any rate, these parts change their colour, and often incline to produce a diseased state of the gums and remaining teeth; although bad consequences may arise to the patient from this cause, still, in some cases, from the desire of the patient, or our own inclination, we may do it in preference to extracting the tooth.* After destroying the nerve we should immediately plug the tooth and leave it to nature. It should be our object, in all praticable cases, to treat the nerve in such a manner as to preserve its vitality, and that of the tooth, and at the same time to plug the tooth, so as to preserve its vitality

* See Case, Part III.

and prevent farther decay. There are two ways of doing this. The first is, by covering the exposed nerve with a thin piece of leaf lead, and completing the operation by the introduction of gold leaf, so as to fill the cavity entirely, and in the most perfect manner. This mode of treating the exposed nerve is recommended by Mr. Koecker* with considerable earnestness. The reason why he applies lead to the nerve is, because this metal has the least irritating effect upon the nerve or living parts of the system of any metallic substance with which we are acquainted. I have adopted this practice, in some cases, with the most perfect success, and in others it has entirely failed.

The second mode of treating the nerve in order to preserve its vitality is, to apply some powerful astringent substance to the exposed nerve, and confine it there by first placing a piece of the astringent in the bottom of the cavity upon the nerve, and complete the filling of the cavity with wax, or some other substance of the kind, so as to retain the astringent upon the nerve for some time; and the astringent may be changed occasionally for fresh material, and worn in this manner for some months, if necessary. The effect of this is to gradually reduce the sensibility of the nerve, until it will, without irritation, admit the presence and pressure of a plug. This is the practice which I think will be found to succeed better than any other; indeed I do not think it will ever fail, or, at least, very rarely, if proper substances are used, and persevered in. In the chapter upon the extraction of the adult teeth, I mentioned the case of Mrs. W——, who called upon me with several of her teeth having their nerves exposed, and in an inflamed state; her teeth I treated as I shall now mention. There are several different astringent

* Koecker, page 437.

substances which may be used to apply to the nerve ; among which, I will mention alum, borax, &c. &c., or the soft part of the gall. This last is what I use, and prefer to any thing I have tried. We should select, for this purpose, the best fresh Alleppo galls, break the nut, and with the point of a knife, take out some of the soft part, put a small piece of this in the cavity of the tooth, having the nerve exposed, then fill the cavity with bees-wax, so as to retain the gall, and exclude the air. If this is not displaced of itself as often as we wish, it may be taken out and the gall renewed once in ten or fifteen days, and replaced with fresh gall, as before. In this way, with almost a certainty of success, and with little pain or inconvenience to the patient, the sensibility of the nerve and lining membrane may be so much reduced as to allow, after a few weeks or months, the safe introduction of a plug, so as to complete the cure of the tooth. Either of these three modes of treating the exposed nerves of carious teeth may be adopted by the dentist. The first is, on most accounts, very objectionable, as it should be an object of the utmost solicitude to preserve the vitality of the teeth we suffer to remain in the mouth. Either of the two last methods may be used, and I think the best practice will be, and is, to unite both, as I am in the habit of doing, which is to use the astringent for some time, and then to cover the nerve with a leaf of lead, and complete the filling of the cavity with gold. I could mention numerous cases of the complete success of this practice, but do not wish to tire my reader with cases, sensible that if he adopts the practice he will very seldom fail of complete success in his operations. The last mode of treating exposed nerves which I have mentioned, I believe was originally introduced by Mr. Harrington, a highly respectable dentist of this city. Mr. Murphy mentions that the nut-gall has cured tooth-ache, but I am not aware that it was ever applied to reducing the sensibility of the nerves so as to allow of the reception of a plug, until the practice was adopted by Mr. Harrington. I consider from its easy application, and almost certain good effect, that it is a discovery of great consequence, and places the name of Mr. Harrington amongst the foremost of those whose labours and discoveries have contributed to the advancement and perfection of this part of medical science.

Of the Instruments required in Plugging the Teeth.

There are two kinds of instruments used in this operation, and required, in order to perform it in a proper manner. The first are those with which we clean out the cavity which is formed by the progress of the caries, of all putrid foreign or dead matter. These consist of small bent instruments, made of steel, with pearl, ivory, bone or wooden handles, or many of them to fit one handle with which to scrape out the cavity; others are a kind of hard drills, having the ends, instead of terminating flat, like the common drill, terminating in a small bur or chevy, as it is termed by mechanics; this bur may be cut so as to have four or six edges, and with this we may drill the tooth, and take away all the dead and inflamed matter, and shape the cavity so that it will receive and retain a plug. Every operator should have a considerable variety of these instruments, so as to adapt them to every case. The instruments he rquires for forcing in the metallic substance should be made of steel or iron, having their points blunt, and attenuated to different sizes, and bent in different shapes as well as straight, so as to fit them to the size and situation of the different cavities which are to be filled. He may likewise have a handle, to which he can fit different pieces of iron or steel wire, and which he can readily adapt to every possible variety of shape and situation of the cavities, by filing or bending them, &c. The operator should be prepared with a sufficient number and variety of them, so as not to be prevented from plugging a cavity in a tooth, from its situation or peculiar shape. Resolution and ingenuity will, in most cases, overcome any obstacles which may present by the assistance of a tolerable variety of instruments.

Of the Substances proper for Filling the Cavities of the Teeth.

It would seem superfluous to speak particularly upon this subject. One would suppose that the common sense and discrimination of men and practioners in particular, would determine this point, after the years of experience that have elapsed since plugging the teeth has been practised. But such is the ignorance or cupidity of some dentists at this period, that there are not wanting men who will assert to their patients, that lead or tin is better than gold, and thereby impose in the grossest manner upon their patients and the public in general. Of this, as an illustration, I will mention the following case: Two young gentlemen, who were preparing for the Christian ministry, called on me in May, 1827, to consult me respecting their teeth. I found in both, that their teeth were in a very bad condition. The front incisores of both were in a state of decay. I advised a course of dental operations which would place their teeth and gums in a state of health, and that the carious front teeth should be plugged with gold; and more especially so, because they were intending to become public speakers, in whom the health and beauty of the teeth are indispensable to a cleanly appearance of their mouths, and perfect enunciation of language. They both went away, saying, if they concluded to have their teeth operated on, they would call soon. One of them called in two or three days, and by a judicious course of operations on the principles before detailed, and which will be hereafter, I rendered his teeth perfectly healthy. The upper incisors, two or three, I plugged with gold, in a very perfect manner, so that I saw him the next November, and his teeth were all in fine order and health. While plugging his teeth, he told me, that his friend who came with him at first to ask my advice, had called upon another dentist, who persuaded him, that tin foil was far better than gold for plugging the teeth, that it was retained longer; and was in all respects quite preferable to gold; and so little was the young gentleman acquainted with the subject, that he suffered the dentist to plug his teeth with tin foil, and two or three of his incisores, one of which he said was so far decayed, that he thought best to leave it to ultimate destruction. Now, any person can see the result of this case; a gradual oxidation, to a certain extent, of the tin immediately commences, which gives the substance of the tooth, opposite the plug, a dark and repulsive appearance, and what is far worse, beyond comparison, that by the gradual oxidation of the tin, the caries of the tooth is suffered to go on, favoured by the oxidizing metal, and ultimate destruction of the tooth is the inevitable consequence; whilst those, as in the first case, plugged with gold, will remain in all probability, external caries excepted, during the life of the patient, precisely as when first introduced. It is but a few weeks since I saw the front incisor shown me by a young lady, which had been plugged about two years and with lead, in which the lead was almost completely oxidated, and the caries had proceeded so far as to entirely destroy the vitality, and almost the substance of the tooth; so much so, that I could pass a probe directly through the front surface of the tooth, which was black and a mere shell. She told me, that when the tooth was plugged it was but little decayed. Cases of this kind are seen every day, and yet some dentists have the hardihood to assert, that tin and lead are as proper for plugging the teeth as gold, although be it said, to the credit of the profession, that very few respectable dentists are guilty of this abominable ignorance or dishonesty. Lead may be applied, as we have before mentioned, to cover the nerve of the tooth, and the filling completed with gold. Tin foil, if pure, may be used, in some cases, for plugging the grinding-teeth, if the patients are not able to pay for gold, or if the gold cannot be obtained. But gold in purity is the substance which we ought to use. Gold, without alloy, is a substance which may be retained a century in the mouth without oxidating.* It reposes upon the living substance of a tooth, and excludes all foreign natures of every kind; the saliva, the food, decayed portions of other teeth, cold air, &c. &c. and at the same time gives firmness and strength to the tooth, whilst itself remains unchanged. When pure, and beaten into thin and suitable leaves, it is extremely malleable, and it is adapted to the cavity of the tooth to be filled, with the utmost facility, and may be pressed into the tooth until it is perfectly compact, like a solid piece of the metal. The expense of the gold should never deter the dentist from its use. I remarked that tin might be used in plugging the molar teeth, if we could not consistently use the gold. But the incisores and canine teeth I never plug with any metal but gold. I always rather divide the expense with my patients, if necessary, than to use tin, lead, or silver in plugging these teeth, as their loss is deplorable to the patient; and if the caries is arrested, by a plugging of these metals, still in many instan-

---

* See Koecker.

ces, the dark colour of the plug formed of any of them is seen through the enamel of the tooth. I could say a great deal more upon this subject than I have, and detail a great many cases, but I do not wish to swell this volume with matter that must be self-evident to every reflecting mind. I will just mention a composition which has been proposed to be used in plugging the teeth. This is the fusible mixture spoken of by Mr. Fox, formed by uniting bismuth, eight parts, lead, five parts, and tin, three parts, which melts at the temperature of boiling water. This in a state of fusion, has been recommended after cleaning out the cavity, to pour a drop of it into the cavity, so as to fill it. But this metal is as objectionable as lead or tin, and at the temperature required it is apt to injure the tooth, and lead either to farther decay or to active inflammation of the membrane; consequently, the practice has been found pernicious, and is, as far as I know, entirely rejected by the profession. Gum mastick, &c. has been used.

Of the manner of Performing the Operation of Plugging the Teeth.

The first step previously to performing this operation is to clean out the cavity to be plugged, so that every particle of decayed or diseased matter shall be removed, and a shape given to the cavity, larger within or at the bottom than the external opening, so that the metal may be confined within, like a dove-tail in a mortise, if but slightly, so the plug may be retained, or if the cavity is not smaller within than the external opening, but if this is reversed and the external opening is larger than the internal, and all the way so, a plug cannot be retained. To clean and shape the cavity, the scraping instruments and our pointed drills described before, should be used, especially the drills to shape the cavity.

Different sizes should be had by the dentist, so as never to much enlarge the external opening, only so far as barely to remove the external caries. This should be done with great care and nicety, for upon its proper performance the success of the operation considerably depends. If the nerve is exposed, the utmost care must be used not to wound it, and at the same time to remove all the caries near it. I will here mention a very objectionable mode of preparing the cavity for the plug, and also a most injurious manner of introducing or compacting the metal. It is by using a common drill, turned with a bow and string, to prepare the cavity and fit it for the plug, and then to introduce the metal and farther compact it by using a hammer and punch. The most pernicious consequences often follow this practice: in the cavity not being often perfectly cleared of the carious matter, and of the inflamed and diseased part, which is absolutely necessary to the proper performance of the operation; in the next place, the heat and irritation arising from the use of the drill, often excites an irritable and inflamed state of the bony substance of the tooth, if not of the nerve and lining membrane. The hammer and punch when used to drive in the plug, cause great pain in the operation and injure the tooth. I lately saw the front incisor tooth shown me by a lady residing in this city, which she had plugged some time since. The plug was introduced on the front surface, near the middle of the tooth, close to the gum. The operation was conducted as I have before mentioned, and in hammering in the plug, the enamel of the tooth was split from the edge of the gum, to the very lower cutting edge of the tooth. I could mention several more cases I have seen of the injury resulting from this practice, but I do not think it necessary, as I am persuaded that no judicious surgeon dentist, will ever adopt this very objectionable mode of performing the operation. After we have cleaned out all the carious portion, and shaped the cavity as we wish it, then we should fill it with a lock of cotton dipped in warm water, so as to completely wash out of it every particle of dust and dead matter, minnute pieces of the bone, &c. This done we should dry the cavity with a piece of dry cotton, introduced into it, and repeated until it is perfectly dry; then if the nerve is not exposed, or the sound bony part not irritable or very tender, we may introduce the gold leaf, and with a punch of a suitable size, shape, &c. so as to apply perfectly to the cavity, pass in the gold so as to fill the cavity in the most perfect manner and by firm pressure upon the gold render it perfectly compact, so as to completely apply to any part of the cavity, and be quite as impermeable to any foreign agent, as the solid gold itself. After we have done this, we cut off the projecting part of the gold, and conclude the operation by burnishing the surface of the gold, so as to make it perfectly smooth, and not projecting in the least above or outside of the substance of the tooth; by so doing we shall prevent the gold from being seen, and also prevent it's being acted upon by any thing which might loosen it or push it out. When the substance of the tooth is irritable and the nerve and lining membrane are not exposed, we may in some cases if we choose, with a camels-hair pencil, touch over the internal surface of the cavity with the brush of the pencil previously dipped in a saturated solution of the argentum nitratum, and then plug the tooth as before directed. When the nerve and lining membrane are exposed, and we have prepared them as before directed, with an astringent, or not, as we choose, or when we cauterize the nerve, we should cover it with a plate of leaf lead, and finish the plugging with gold, remembering to keep the lead perfectly dry, and the two metals attached to each other in a perfectly dry state; for if not dry, it will be very difficult to press them together, so that they will be retained in perfect union, not to mention the oxidation of the lead which might take place, or the galvanic action, which might result from moisture between the two metals. It should be a general rule with us never to suffer our stopping, if we can avoid it, to be exposed to view, and yet we should never because we find that the gold will be seen, hesitate to perform this operation, and thereby preserve a valuable tooth. For it is far better to preserve a valuable tooth having a plug which may be seen when the lips are open, than to suffer the tooth to decay. In some cases we detect caries between two teeth, and in order to plug them, we are obliged to file them apart, so as to allow room for the cleaning out of the cavity, and for proper introduction of the plug. At times the practitioner is at a loss to determine whether he should attempt to remove caries with a file, or whether he shall plug the tooth. His guide in this case, is to clean out the carious portion from the tooth, and if so situated or shaped as to be in any way practicable to plug the cavity, he should do so, if not, he should remove all the carious portion with the file; and if it occurs in the lateral parts of the incisores, so as by being all cut away to very considerably injure the appearance of the teeth, he should separate them with the file, and remove the posterior plate of enamel with a knife, and all the caries, and leave the front plate of the enamel uninjured. I have now spoken in very general terms of the several particulars respecting the operation of plugging the teeth, &c. But a great deal more may be said of it, and a great many cases adduced of its utility, were I disposed to protract this section. I shall, however, content myself with leaving the subject with what has been already said, to direct the practitioner to the correct and judicious performance of the operation, assisted by his own ingenuity and a ready tact for adapting means to ends. I will in this place make one general remark that I have often hinted at, which is of the first consequence, and should be noticed by every operating dentist. When we operate upon the teeth, we should remember that they are living organs, and that all our operations ought to be performed with care and tenderness, and not with that butchery and violence which is occasionally witnessed, to the disgrace of the operator, to the injury of the patient, and the disrepute of the profession.

SECTION VI.

OF THE ORDER IN WHICH DENTAL OPERATIONS SHOULD BE PERFORMED.

Having now passed over, in detail, the several operations required for the removal of the teeth, for the preservation of their regularity, and for the cure of their diseases, and for the cure of diseased gums, I now deem it necessary and proper, for the complete elucidation of the subject, and to enable the surgeon-dentist so to direct the order of his operations as to insure a return of perfect and permanent health to the teeth, to mention the order in which these several operations should be performed, in order to insure the grand object for which they are performed, which is to completely eradicate disease from the teeth, and their appendages. When our patients call upon us for our professional advice or services, the first step is, to examine, in a critical manner, the state of the teeth and gums, noticing whether there are any dead or useless teeth or stumps—whether any of the teeth are irregular, carious, or have foreign matter lodged upon them; and observing the state of the gums, whether in health, or not. The use of a small reflecting glass, or mirror, will greatly facilitate the examination of the upper teeth and gums, &c., of which the dentist may have several, of different sizes.

Having completed our examination of the teeth, gums, &c. which should be done with delicacy and with the utmost urbanity and politeness withal, we shall be able to form our opinion of the dental operations required, if any, for the health of the teeth, &c. Our advice should be given unequivocally and without reserve. If dental operations are concluded upon, this is the order in which, if circumstances permit, we should conduct them. Firstly, however, noticing the general health of the patient; if a febrile and inflammatory state of the general system is present (unless occasioned by diseased teeth, &c.) some operations, as a general principle, cannot, with propriety, be performed; as, for instance, plugging and filing the teeth; if so, direct antifebrile remedies, and when the patient is better, perform the operations. But if we find no objection of this kind, our first operation should be to remove all the dead or loose and useless teeth, and stumps of teeth, the manner of which has been before pointed out. The bleeding should be favoured by drinking warm water until it spontaneously ceases. Our patients may now be dismissed, and directed to observe a little precaution not to expose themselves to take cold, as inflammation of the jaw and swelling of integuments sometimes follow. They should be requested to call again as soon as their gums are well, which will usually be in the course of from six to fifteen days. At the second call we may remove all the tartar and other foreign matter from the teeth. We should endeavour to remove it all if circumstances will permit, our time, state of the gums, &c. In some cases, when there are no teeth to be extracted, or but one or two, we may remove the tartar and then extract the one or two teeth, at the same sitting. If the gums are much swollen and do not bleed much after the extraction and removing the tartar, we may, in some cases, scarify them, and give our patients an astringent wash for the gums, with cautions as to taking cold, &c. with directions to call as the state of the gums may be, in about one week, when we may remove any remaining tartar, if any is still retained upon the tooth. At the third sitting, generally, we may commence the operation of plugging what teeth we find require it in order to be rendered sound. As a general principle, we should not plug more than two or three teeth at one sitting. Our patient should then be dismissed, to call again in about a week, and so continue the course of operations until all the teeth requiring it are plugged. If the nerves of any we wish to preserve are exposed, we should, as before directed, put them in a course of preparation, that they may, eventually, be plugged. After having restored the teeth and gums to perfect health, with, perhaps, the exception of those which are in a state of preparation, and may be considered in health and soundness, and removed all vestige of unhealthy irritability from the gums and lining membranes of the sockets and of the teeth, we may proceed cautiously with the file and cutters to remove the superficial caries from the teeth, if there is any present. This too should be done at intervals, and with the utmost care, so as not to excite an irritable state of the teeth and gums by the injudicious use of the file. With the complete removal of the superficial caries, if properly and judiciously done, will the health of our patient's teeth and gums be completely restored. If, after any of these operations, as, for instance, plugging any of the teeth, inflammation of the lining membrane or nerve follows, we should direct an aperient, as some of the saline cathartics, &c. with fomentation or poultice to the face, or perhaps a blister, and, at the same time, perhaps, remove the plug from the inflamed tooth, and direct the application of the gall retained with wax, &c., as mentioned when speaking of that subject. With proper prudence, on the part of the patient, and a faithful performance of the foregoing directions, inflammation of any of the teeth, or their membranes and nerves, or of the lining membranes of the sockets will very rarely take place. If a disordered state of the general system is present whilst these operations are going on, it should be remedied, as far as possible. By observing the foregoing order of performing the dental operations, and if performed judiciously, the surgeon-dentist will have the pleasure, at the expiration of from twelve days to four or six months, as the case may be, of seeing his patient's teeth, the sockets and gums, restored to perfect and permanent health, which, with proper attention to cleanliness, may be preserved so, in most instances, during the life of the patient. Suitable dentifrices and brushes, and mode of use, &c. should be directed, and the patients dismissed. Every person can easily conceive that in the great variety of cases with which we meet, that great variety, as to the different operations, will be noticed. A great many circumstances may occur to prevent our adopting this practice to its full extent. We should, however, do it as far as is practicable. If but two of these operations are to be performed, let them be done in the order and manner I have directed, and they will very rarely fail of perfect success. As, first, extraction, if required; then cleaning the teeth; next, plugging; and, lastly, filing or cutting away the carious portions, if required, &c. I consider it is of great importance that the filing, &c. should be done last, as then the other teeth, gums, &c. will be in health, and the living bone of the tooth exposed by the file, without any protection from the enamel, will not be liable to decay, as it would if done before every other part of the mouth was in health.

SECTION VII.

THE TREATMENT TO REMEDY IRREGULARITIES OF THE TEETH, &c. &c.

We have frequently adverted to the fact, that irregularities of the teeth often occur, and from a variety of causes. The period at which these are apt to take place, or from which they nearly all date their commencement, is during the second dentition. Irregularity is very rarely seen in the first teeth, but if these are retained too long, they generally prevent the permanent teeth from taking their situations in a regular manner. In other cases, we find irregularity to arise from a disproportion between the jaw and teeth, the former being unusually small or pointed, and the latter more than ordinarily large. Too early an extraction of the deciduous teeth, in some instances, inclines them to take an unfavourable situation. I will here give Mr. Fox's directions for remedying irregularity of the teeth. However, just reminding the reader to note what has been said respecting the mobility of the alveoli, and that if he wishes to enlarge the ellipsis of the jaw, the crowns of the teeth are to be carried out, and vice versa, if we wish to reduce the ellipsis, press the teeth inwards.

Mr. Fox observes,* "The mode of treatment prescribed

---

* Natural History of the Teeth, by J. Fox, pages 57 to 69, London, 1814

in the preceding chapter, is not always had recourse to, at a time when every irregularity might be easily obviated. Parents most commonly wait, until by an irregular growth of their children's teeth, a manifest deformity is produced, ere they perceive the necessity of advice.

In all cases of irregularity during the shedding of the teeth, the treatment to be observed is to remove the obstructing temporary teeth, and then to apply pressure in the most convenient manner upon the irregular tooth, in order to direct it into its proper situation. I will now describe the different states of irregularity, and to avoid confusion, take each jaw separately.

In the under jaw, when the growth of the permanent central incisores has exceeded the absorption of the temporary ones, they grow up immediately behind them, in a direction towards the tongue. These two new teeth are generally so broad as nearly to cover the inner surface of the four temporary incisores. It will therefore be necessary, in order to obtain room for these teeth, that the four temporary incisores be extracted. The teeth will then gradually come forward, in which they will naturally be assisted by the pressure of the tongue of the child, and may be occasionally helped by the fingers of the parent or nurse.

If the temporary central incisores have loosened, and come out previous to the appearance of the permanent teeth, the space is seldom sufficiently wide, and the new teeth will either grow up with their sides turned forward, or one will be placed before the other. In this case, the two lateral incisores must be taken out.

When the permanent central incisores have completely grown up, they occupy full two thirds of the space, which contained the four temporary incisores; therefore, when the permanent lateral incisores appear, they are placed partly behind the central incisores and the temporary cuspidati; or they grow up with one corner turned forwards, and the other pointing backwards. In either of these cases the temporary cuspidati must be removed to give room.

The four permanent incisores take up nearly the whole of the space of the temporary incisores and cuspidati. The permanent cuspidati are large teeth, and when they have not sufficient room they occasion very great irregularity. Sometimes they come through on the inside, but most commonly they cut the gum on the outside, and project very much out of the circular line from the temporary incisores to the temporary molares. In this case, the necessity of the removal of the first temporary molares is obvious.

It is not very common that the bicuspides of the lower jaw are irregular, because the temporary molares are generally removed before they appear; but when this is not the case, they always come through the gums on the inside, pointing towards the tongue, in which case the temporary molares must be removed, that the bicuspides may rise into their proper situations.*

In the upper jaw, the permanent central incisores sometimes pass through the gums behind the temporary ones; when this happens, the four temporary incisores must be extracted, and frequent pressure by the thumb should be applied to the new teeth, in order to bring them forward as soon as possible, and prevent one of the cases of irregularity most difficult to be remedied.

When the temporary central incisores have come out, the space is generally too narrow for the permanent ones, and hence they are pressed into some shape of distortion. Their edges do not assume the regular curve, but stand obliquely,

---

* Fig. 6.

or even sometimes one before the other. Cases of this kind require the removal of the temporary lateral incisores.*

The permanent central incisores are very broad; they occupy the greater part of the space of the four temporary ones, and leave scarcely any room for the permanent lateral incisores; on which account these latter teeth must grow very irregularly; they generally pass through behind, being forced considerably backwards by the resistance of the central incisores and the temporary cuspidati. Sometimes they pass through edgeways, and now and then they project forwards. In any of these cases, the removal of the temporary cuspidati is absolutely necessary, and unless the operation be timely performed, the irregularity is with difficulty remedied.

The greatest deformity is generally occasioned by the want of room for the lateral incisores and the cuspidati, and when too long neglected usually becomes permanent.

When the permanent cuspidati make their appearance, they generally project very much forwards, and not only disfigure the mouth, but are very dangerous. I have known several instances, where, from the accident of a blow, the upper lip has been cut through. Whenever the cuspidati are growing thus, the first temporary molares ought to be extracted.

When the bicuspides appear before the temporary molares have been extracted, they pierce the gums above the shedding teeth, and may be seen by raising the cheek and upper lip. The removal of the temporary molares immediately permits them to come down into their right situation.

In almost all the cases of irregularity which occur in the

* Plate XI., fig. 7.

under jaw, nothing more is necessary after the removal of the obstructing tooth, than to apply the frequent pressure of the finger, in such a manner as to direct the irregular tooth into its proper place. It will assist the natural tendency of the teeth to form a regular circle, and to take up as large a space as possible. But in the upper jaw, when the irregularity has been suffered to remain for any length of time, it cannot be obviated without having recourse to other assistance.

Irregularity is often occasioned by the teeth being much too large for the space allotted them, and then it will be necessary to remove one or more of the permanent teeth.

When the incisores are perfectly regular, and the bicuspides have appeared before the cuspidati, there is so little space left, that the cuspidati are thrust too far forward.

It has been the common practice to admit the cuspidati to grow down to a certain length, and them to extract them. This operation certainly removes the deformity of projecting teeth, but it destroys the symmetry of the mouth, and takes away two teeth of great importance. The cuspidati are exceedingly strong: they form the support of the front of the mouth, and in the advanced periods of life, to those persons who have the misfortune to lose the incisores, they furnish an excellent means of fixing artificial teeth.

On these accounts they should be preserved, and therefore it will be right to extract the first bicuspis on each side. The cuspidati will then fall into the circle, and if there should be any vacant space, it will be so far back, that no defect will be perceived. This is often the case in the under jaw, as well as in the upper, and the same practice ought to be adopted.

The first permanent molares often become carious soon after they appear; when this is the case, and the other teeth have not proper room, considerable advantage always attends their extraction. Their removal permits the bicuspides to fall back, and gives way to the regular position of the cuspidati.

The removal of these teeth, when decayed, ought always to be recommended, although they may not occasion pain, or there be no irregularity in the front teeth; diseased teeth always affect others, and therefore ought never to remain in the mouths of children.

If they be extracted before the second permanent molares appear, in a short time they will not be missed, because the bicuspides will go back, and the second and third molares will come forward, so that no space will be left.

The front teeth may even derive much benefit from this gain of room, as there will probably be left a small space between them, which will tend to their preservation; for it is observed when the teeth are situated so close as to press hard upon each other, they almost always fall into a state of decay.

Sometimes the upper jaw is too narrow from side to side, the teeth in the fore part are thrown forwards, and project very much over the teeth of the lower jaw, they also push out the upper lip. In this case the first bicuspis on each side should be extracted, which will permit the teeth to fall into a more regular curve.

When the permanent incisores of the upper jaw have cut the gum behind the temporary teeth, and have been suffered to remain until considerably advanced in growth, they always stand so much inwards, that when the mouth is shut, the incisores of the under jaw stand before them, which is always an obstacle to their acquiring regularity, and occasions a great deformity.

There are four states of this kind of irregularity. The first, when one central incisor is turned in, and the under teeth come before it, whilst the other central incisor keeps its proper place, standing before the under teeth.

The second is, when both the incisores are turned in, and go behind the under teeth; but the lateral incisores stand out before the under teeth.

The third variety is, when the central incisores are placed properly, but the lateral incisores stand very much in; and when the mouth is shut, the under teeth project before them and keep them backward.

The fourth is, when all the incisores of the upper jaw are turned in, and those of the under jaw shut before them. This is sometimes occasioned by too great a length of the under jaw, in consequence of which it projects considerably forwarder than the upper jaw. But the majority of such cases originate entirely from neglect, and may be completely remedied by early assistance.

The time to affect any material alteration in the position of the teeth, is before thirteen or fourteen years of age, and as much earlier as possible; for after that time the sockets of the teeth acquire a degree of strength, and the teeth are so fixed that they cannot be moved without much difficulty. If the irregularity be left to a much later period, it becomes a great deal more difficult to produce any alteration, and frequently all attempts are fruitless.

To remove the kind of irregularity above mentioned, two objects must be accomplished; one, to apply a force which shall act constantly upon the irregular tooth, and bring it forward; the other to remove that obstruction which the under teeth, by coming before the upper, always occasion.

The first of these objects may be attained by the application of an instrument adapted to the arch of the mouth, which, being attached to some strong teeth on each side, will furnish a fixed point in front, to which a ligature previously fastened on the irregular tooth may be applied, and thus, by occasionally renewing it, a constant pressure is preserved, and the tooth may be drawn forward.

The second object, that of romoving the resistance of the under teeth, must be attained by placing some intervening substance between the teeth of the upper and under jaws, so as to prevent them from completely closing, and be an obstruction to the coming forwards of the irregular tooth.

This instrument may be made of gold or silver: it should be so strong as not easily to bend; if about the sixteenth of an inch in breadth, and of a proportionate thickness, it will be sufficiently firm. This bar of gold must be bent to the form of the mouth, and should be long enough to reach to the temporary molares, which are the teeth to which it is to be tied. Holes are to be drilled in it at those places where ligatures are required, which will be on the parts opposed to the teeth designed to be the fixed points, and also at the parts opposite to the place where the irregular tooth or teeth are situated. Then to the bar a small square piece of ivory is to be connected, by means of a little piece of gold, which may be fastened to the ivory and the bar by two rivets. This piece of ivory passes under the grinding surfaces of the upper teeth, is kept there fixed, and prevents the teeth from closing, and consequently takes off all obstruction in front.

The bar is to be attached by a strong silk ligature to the teeth at the sides, so that if possible it may remain tight as long as it is required; a ligature is then to be tied around the irregular tooth, and the ends being brought through the holes in the bar, are to be tied in a firm knot. In two or three days this ligature must be removed and a new one applied: the tooth will soon be perceived to move. A fresh ligature must be used every three or four days, in order to keep up a constant pressure, sufficiently powerful to bring the tooth into a line with the others.

The same mode of treatment is to be observed whether there be one, two, or three teeth, growing in a similar manner. The teeth are usually brought forwards in about a month or five weeks, and as soon as they are so much advanced as to allow the under teeth to pass on the inside, the piece of ivory may be removed, and the bar only be retained for a few days, until the teeth are perfectly firm, which will prevent the accident of the teeth again receding.

In cases where the irregularity has been suffered to continue too long, no success can be expected to follow attempts to remove it; we must content ourselves in the treatment of these cases in adults, with taking away the most irregular teeth, and thus, as much as possible, lessen the deformity.

Mr. Fox does not mention an effect of irregular teeth which is occasionally noticed, and it is when an irregular tooth presses upon or is pressed upon by a regular tooth; so much so, as to occasion irritation, inflammation, and formation of matter at the roots of one or both of these which so impinge upon each other.

It is but a few days since a respectable clergyman called upon me to ask my advice, respecting the upper lateral incisors of the right side. Upon examining it, I found that by the irregular growth of the under cuspidatus of that side when the mouth was closed, the incisor before mentioned was thrust directly out, which by carrying it out of the circle of the upper teeth, occasioned considerable deformity, and had induced an inflammation and discharge of matter from the socket of the incisor. By filing away the projecting part of the irregular cuspidatus its irregularity was obviated, and in a very short time I was enabled to restore the incisor to its proper situation; and consequently perfect symmetry was restored to the upper teeth. By these means the discharge of matter from the root of the incisor was entirely cured, which saved the tooth from total destruction.

I am acquainted with an eminent physician of this city, who had a similar discharge of matter from the fangs of one of his molar teeth, which continued two years and baffled the skill of all the dentists of this city, either to explain its cause or effect its cure. The doctor finally discovered that the tooth was elevated above the level of the other teeth, so that when the jaw was closed, the whole force of both jaws rested upon this one tooth, which forced the fangs of the irregular tooth with some degree of violence into their sockets, so as to occasion inflammation and suppuration of the membrane covering the fangs and lining the alveoli. By filing away the irregular part of the tooth, so as to bring it to a level with the other teeth, the discharge of matter was entirely cured. In some instances irregular teeth not only prevent a perfect symmetry of the teeth, but of the face itself. As for instance, we occasionally notice the lower jaw turned to one side, so that the nose and chin will not be in their usual natural and symmetrical line with each other. In other instances we shall notice the under jaw thrust forward, so as to cover the upper jaw. This last may not always be occasioned by irregular growth of the teeth, although it often is. Whenever we notice any unnatural position of the lower jaw, especially in children and young persons, we ought to examine, and if any of them are irregular, correct the irregularity by judicious operations, which have been before sufficiently detailed.

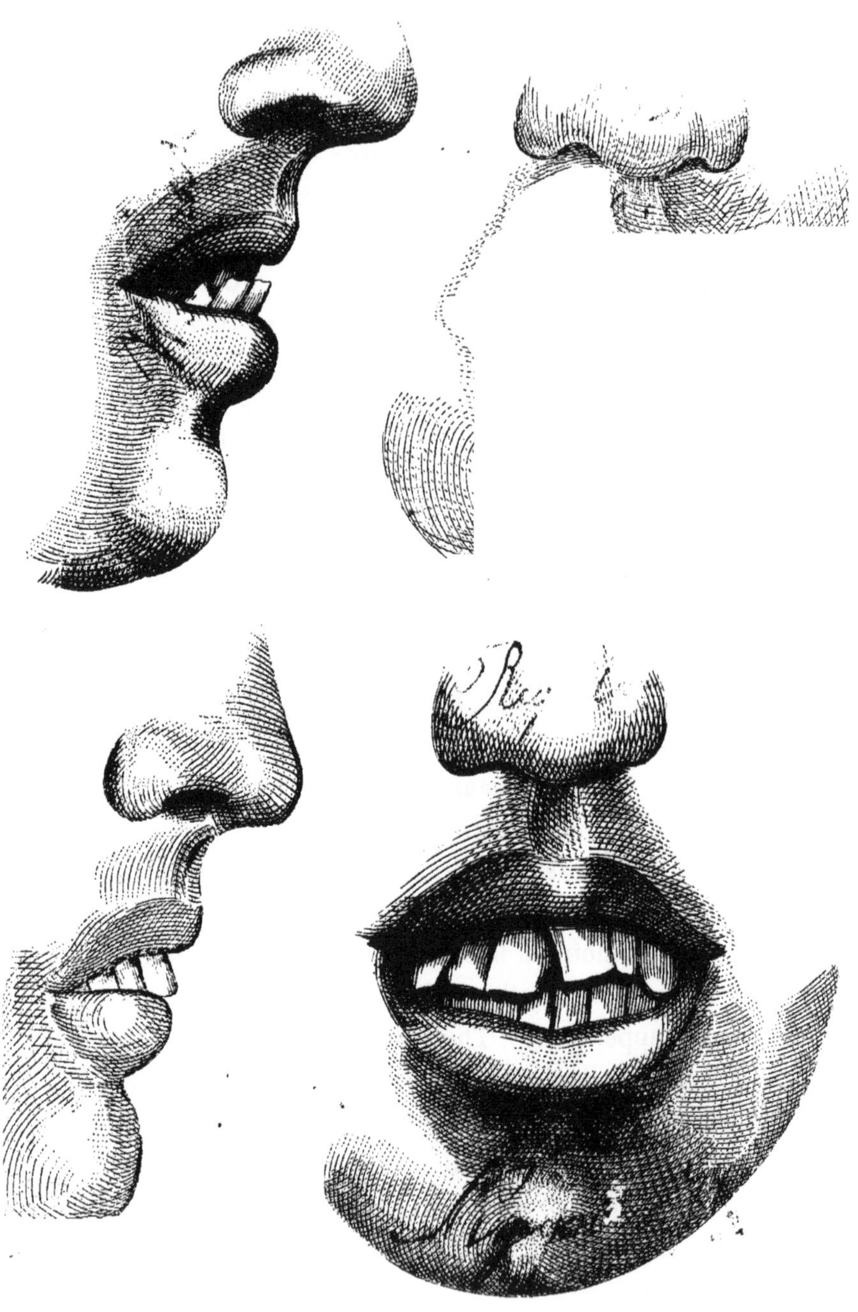

Irregularities of the Teeth, which may be obviated and reduced to symmetry, by the judicious Dentist —

Eng^{d} by C. Tippun

SECTION VIII.

OF THE MANNER OF PRESERVING THE HEALTH AND BEAUTY OF THE TEETH.

Having now spoken of the several operations for the cure of diseased teeth, the removal of useless and pernicious ones, and for the prevention and obviation of irregularity in them, I now deem it profitable to suggest the proper course to be pursued by the patient, in order to preserve the health and beauty of the teeth, if either in health by nature, or rendered so by judicious dental operations. It is an impression generally abroad in the minds of medical men and philosophers, that the decay and loss of the teeth, is a necessary consequence of advanced years, but I humbly conceive that no mistake is greater. The universality of the fact is not a positive proof, that it is a necessary consequence of age, for there are numerous instances of persons who have not attained the middle periods of life, and yet have lost all their teeth. It only proves this, that those destructive agents which we have before mentioned, as being the exciting causes of disease in the teeth, gums and alveoli, are implacable and persevering foes to the health of these parts, which if not as perseveringly opposed, baffled or removed, will pursue the health and vitality of the teeth, until they have eradicated these noble, useful, and beautiful organs from the mouth. Had the all-wise Author of Nature intended that the teeth of man should be lost in his declining years, and this be a necessary consequence of age, it would be always the case, and an old man with teeth would be a lusus natura. But this is not the case, a vast many aged persons go down to the grave, possessing sound and beautiful teeth. It should be always remembered that the teeth fail only in the same ratio as the other organs of the system, and that their local diseases are not the natural consequence of age, but of other causes, and if prevented and perseveringly obviated, that it is in the power of every individual, by an early, judicious, and persevering attention to his teeth, to preserve them to an advanced age, and that their powers will only decline with the decline of all the system. The rules for this purpose are few and simple. If irregularity or disease is actually present in the teeth or their appendages, or if foreign matter is lodged upon them which cannot be moved by the use of the brush or dentifrices, then the assistance of the judicious dentist will be required to perform such operations as will remedy and cure all disease or cause of disease in them; after which the patient may, by the most persevering attention to cleanliness, preserve the health of his teeth, and gums, &c. In order to preserve the health of sound teeth, they should be kept perfectly clean, which is readily effected by cleaning them at least once or more a day with one or more tooth-brushes, so made as to enable the person to clean them on the inside and out, so as to remove all the thickened mucus from them and the gums and from between the teeth. If the brush alone will not do this, he may use some suitable dentifrice, as for example, charcoal and peruvian bark, or some of the bolar earths mixed with a little prepared chalk, or some of the several preparations which will be found in the pharmaceutical part of this work, adapting the properties of the powder to the state of his teeth and gums. If the latter are tender, he should use those which have an astringent in their composition. If the dark coloured tartar and greenish mucus are apt to collect on the teeth, let the tooth-powder have more mechanical properties, as for example, the union of prepared chalk, and some of the barks, &c. Some of these he can find in the pharmaceutical part. If the mouth is in rather an unhealthy state, and ready to be loaded with mucus, or the patient's breath is offensive, use some of the alkaline mixtures, or a very weak solution of the argentum nitratum, &c. We should caution the patient never to use any of the acids to remove the tartar, &c. from his teeth, as this practice will most assuredly destroy the enamel of the teeth.

I would not recommend using the acids in any state of dilution, or form of exhibition. Nor should he use any metalic tooth-picks. The best of these are formed from the common goose quill, born, or turtle shell, ivory, &c. Nor should he be in the habit of scraping his teeth with rough or sharp metallic instruments. And, in fine, he should never use any thing which will, either chemically or mechanically, injure or remove the enamel or substance of the teeth. He should keep the teeth clean, but not injure their substance. In using the brush, he should carry it across the surface of the teeth, and perpendicularly up and down, lengthways of the teeth, so as to remove all mucus from between the gums and teeth; and he may have such brushes as will enable him to clean his teeth on the inside, and between them. The brush used for cleaning on the inside may be made much harder than that used to clean the outside of the teeth, as the gums on the inside, from the constant action of the tongue upon them, are rendered much harder than those on the outside. In proof of what cleanliness will do in preserving the health and beauty of the teeth, we are only to remark the difference in the different parts of the teeth, in their disposition to decay. The teeth on the outside, between them, and in the pits of the grinding surfaces, from the disposition, in most cases, of the vitiated saliva, and other matters to be retained and to rest long in contact with these parts, decay here, in almost every case, first begins, whilst on the inside of the teeth which is kept clean, or the saliva constantly changed by the action of the tongue, they rarely commence a decay, if regular, so that the tongue constantly acts upon them. During a period of sickness, or the exhibition of medicine, especially in inflammatory diseases, these directions become of momentary consequence. No portion of medicine of any consequence should pass through the mouth without afterwards rinsing it with warm water, or cold, as the case may be. The brush should be freely used, so as to remove all the clammy mucus and saliva, which is generally vitiated by disease, or the exhibition of medicine, especially mercurials. It is often proper and necessary to rinse the mouth very frequently, and to use the brush, at least, twice a day. In inflammatory diseases the teeth suffer as much as the other organs, in general, and as the vital powers of the crowns and bodies of the teeth are, perhaps, less than any other organs, consequently they must suffer greatly in disease. It is here that the kind and attentive physician will prove himself truly so by strictly noticing his patient's teeth, and enforcing towards them the strictest cleanliness. I once knew a beautiful little girl, who, when sick of a typhoid fever and comatose for several days, had a large portion of calomel mixed up with molasses introduced into her mouth as she lay, nearly, or quite insensible, upon her side, in bed, and such was the abominable and unpardonable stupidity and negligence of the physician and nurses, that instead of seeing that the calomel was swallowed, and her mouth rinsed clean with water, they entirely neglected to notice her mouth. The consequence, in this case, was, that the calomel was not swallowed, but passed with the molasses in which it was mixed down upon the inside of the cheek of the side upon which she rested. The calomel lay upon the cheek, teeth, and gums of that side, pages 430-434 and Plate IV missing

these united properties in the degree in which they are possessed by the human teeth. If sound good teeth, they are perfectly congenial to the remaining teeth and to the gums; they rest upon the latter without exciting any irritation in them, or causing them to be absorbed away. Their colour and form are nature itself; and if the mouth is in order, if kept clean, they retain their colour and form unchanged, either by absorbing the saliva of the mouth, or by decay, for many years. There is a considerable difference in the quality of the natural teeth which the dentist is able to procure; consequently there will be a difference in the length of time which they last in the mouth, depending on the quality of the tooth, and the health of the mouth. I have known artificial natural teeth, which had been worn in a tolerably healthy mouth for eighteen years, with but a slight change of colour, and which from perfect correspondence with the other teeth, would elude the closest scrutiny of the dentist himself in detecting it. No other substance with which we are at present acquainted, possesses these united properties in the same degree, and as far as I have been able to learn, the natural artificial teeth at present are preferred to any others, as a general principle, both in Europe and this country. But as we are not able, in all cases, to procure natural teeth, and as there are persons who are not able to pay the high price for them, which their scarcity and value demand, other substances are used, some of which approximate in value considerably to the natural teeth.

The second material we propose to notice is,

The Animal Teeth.

I wish my reader will bear in mind those united properties which I have before mentioned as being desirable, and in part, indispensable to the formation of proper artificial teeth, which were first a congeniality between the living teeth, the gums, and the artificial teeth, so as that the latter shall not injure the two former. In the second place, there should be an exact similarity, as far as may be, in colour and form; and third, that the substance should retain these properties; and fourth, they should not be liable to take up the saliva, and thereby become offensive to the patient. These properties are possessed, to a very eminent degree, by the teeth of old neat cattle, &c. They are very congenial to the living teeth and gums. They can be rendered of a perfectly natural shape. They retain their form and colour unchanged for a great many years in a healthy mouth. They do not absorb the liquors of the mouth but in the slightest degree. There is one point of difference btween them and the natural teeth, which, if obviated, they would be nearly equal to the latter. Their enamel is very beautiful, and has an animated appearance, which is found in no other substance, except the natural teeth. The point of difference from the latter is, that their enamel is generally of a shade lighter in colour in most cases, and they are not so strong. As they are, they form a very valuable substitute for natural teeth; when properly prepared and inserted, as will be hereafter directed, and next after the natural, perhaps unite as many advantages and properties, especially for single teeth, which we have before mentioned, as any substance with which we are at present acquainted.

The third material for artificial teeth which I propose to mention, is the ivory from the tooth of the Hippopotamus, (sea horse) and also from the Vacca Manina, (sea cow.) This kind of ivory is much more expensive than animal teeth. It can be cut and worked into very elegant artificial teeth; but they are very deficient in those properties which we have mentioned as desirable, and to a degree necessary, for artificial teeth. In the first place, their substance is soft, much more than the human teeth, or animal teeth. They have not the peculiar enamel which is possessed by the two latter. Although their colour is, at first, nearly like the natural teeth, it is very soon lost. They at first become yellow, then of a dark dingy colour: they have nothing like animation in their appearance. Besides losing their colour, in some cases, I have seen them decayed. They are apt to contract a most offensive, filthy smell. This last is an objection which, if there was no other, is sufficiently weighty to banish this substance forever from the list of materials used for artificial teeth. To those who have never taken notice of this subject, it would be astonishing to observe how even two, three, or four of these teeth do pollute the mouth and breath of the person wearing them, even when they are kept as clean as circumstances will allow; and when persons are not cleanly with them, they become insufferably offensive, in most cases. Individual exceptions are found, but rarely, to these observations. So much do these facts weigh with me that I never use the sea horse ivory for any purpose about the mouth. And very frequently, I take out these teeth and replace them with natural or animal teeth, and to the great satisfaction of my patients. I need not mention the injurious consequences resulting from the use of such teeth, for every injury resulting from a vitiated state of the saliva is produced by these. They vitiate the former to a great degree. I could mention numerous instances of the kind, but do not, in the least, think it necessary. If any one doubts it, I would refer them to any person who wears these teeth, and he will find my observations verified in ninety cases out of a hundred. I will not deny if the sea horse ivory is good, and principally the enamel, and the individual particularly cleanly, they may be preserved in a good state for some time.

Transplanting of the teeth.

The fourth mode of replacing the teeth which I think of mentioning is, by extracting a sound, healthy tooth from the jaw of one person and transplanting it to that of another; at the same time we are to extract the diseased tooth or stump which we wish to replace, and into its socket pass the warm fang of the new and living tooth. In some cases, a dead tooth was put in the socket and allowed to remain, and, as Mr. Hunter asserts, in a great many cases, he had seen these grow. When a living tooth is thus transplanted, in many cases, it will grow sound and be firm, and continue so for many years; in others, there will be no union at all. I have only introduced this subject in order to inform the reader that such a case has occurred, and such a mode of restoring lost teeth has been practiced, but not with a view of ever recommending it. This practice was a favourite one with Mr. John Hunter, and had been suggested and practiced a great many years before.* That teeth may be transplanted and grow firm in their new situations, there is not a doubt, as it has been often done. But such are the dangerous cousequences resulting from this practice, that it is now almost wholly abandoned; and, as Mr. Fox observes, it involves a moral principle, for it seems contrary to the laws of every just principle, to mutilate one person to perfect another. But this is not all; the most dangerous diseases are liable to be propagated along with the new tooth, and, from this rea-

---

* See Fauchard, vol. I, page 383.

son, the practice has fallen into disuse, almost entirely, and very justly so. Syphilitic, and other most dangerous diseases have been propagated this way, even when the individuals from whom the scion tooth had been extracted were in apparently perfect health. I will give one case of this kind, to show the reader what consequences may arise from this cause, believing that, in this country, this operation will rarely, if ever, be performed. This case was drawn up by Dr. Watson, and inserted in the Medical Transactions, Vol. III. Art. XX.

*Case.**

"An incisor tooth of the upper jaw, from an unknown cause becoming carious, in a young unmarried lady about twenty-one years of age, it was extracted; and its place very dexterously supplied by a like tooth from another young woman, who, upon examination for the purpose, appeared to be in good health. The scion very rapidly took firm hold, and soon bid fair to be of great service and ornament. In about a month, however, the mouth became painful; the gums inflamed, discoloured and ulcerated. The ulceration spread very fast, the gums of the upper jaw were corroded, and the alveoli left bare. Before the end of another month the ulceration stretched outwardly under the upper lip and nose, and inwardly to the cheeks and throat, which were corroded by large, deep, and fetid ulcers. The alveoli soon became carious; several of the teeth gradually dropped out, and, at length, the transplanted tooth, which had hitherto remained firm in its place. About this time, blotches appeared in

*As quoted by J. M. Good, Study of Med. vol. I, page 44.

the face, neck, and various parts of the body; several of which became painful and extensive ulcers; a considerable degree of fever, apparently hectic, was excited; a copious and fetid discharge flowed from the mouth and throat, which impeded sleep, and the soreness of the fauces prevented a sufficiency of nourishment from being swallowed. An antisceptic course of bark and other tonics were first tried and persevered in, till found to be of no service whatever, and calomel pills, in alterative proportion were then had recourse to in their stead. This plan was found to soften every symptom, and totally to eradicate many; but the bowels were soon affected with severe pain and purging, and the calomel was exchanged for strong mercurial ointment, which, from the present debility of the patient soon produced a like effect, and an effect that could not be corrected by opium. The venomous taint or putrescent tendency, though occasionally driven back, as often rallied, and at length prevailed; and the patient fell a victim to it, in the greatest distress and misery. The person from whom the tooth had been taken, had, in the mean time, continued in perfect health; and upon a minute inspection, as well of the sexual organs as of the mouth, evinced not the slightest syphilitic affection." Many similar cases could be produced, but enough in this one case is told to prove that the performance of this operation is most fearfully pregnant with bad and fatal consequences. This mode of replacing lost teeth is one which cannot be too much deprecated nor too pertinaciously avoided. It is a truth that the blood of one person, in apparent health, will prove a poison to another; as I have witnessed in cases when a physician has suffered his lancet to become bloody, and, without cleaning it, to bleed another person. I have known two cases of this kind, when the persons barely escaped with their lives; and how much more, when a warm, living tooth from one person's jaw has been passed in the socket in the jaw of another. I have said enough upon this subject; the practice has fallen into just disrepute, and probably will never again be revived.

Our fifth material for replacing the teeth, or for making artificial ones is,

The Porcelain Teeth.

In this place, I only wish to discuss the merits of these teeth, and take a short view of their history, whilst a detailed method of making them will be found in another place. It is to the ingenuity of the French dentists that we are indebted for the first intimation of the propriety of using the same substances for making artificial teeth, as are used in the manufacture of porcelain. According to Mr. Audibran, who has probably written the best work now extant upon this subject,* the manufacture of these teeth was suggested, if not practised by Mr. Fauchard, as early as the year 1728, and it is probable, says Mr. Audibran, that the first suggestion, or at least that in this respect he had profited by the experience of the celebrated Reaumer, who contributed so powerfully to the establishment of the royal manufactory of porcelain at Sevres.† The suggestions of Fauchard do not appear to have been much noticed for many years, or were entirely forgotten. An apothecary of St. Germain, says Mr. Audibran, by the name of Duchateau, was the first in modern times who made porcelain teeth.

---

* See Traité, Historique et pratique sur les Dents artificielles incorruptibles, contenant les procédés de fabrication et d'application, par Joseph Audibran, Chirurgien Dentiste, brevite du Roi, Paris 1821.

† See Le Chirurgien Dentiste, Tom. II. page 283, et suiv, Chap. XIV. par Fauchard.

Duchateau communicated his discovery to the Academy of Surgery, in the year 1776. Duchateau and his successors kept a knowledge of the mode of fabrication a secret. M. Dubois Chement carried the art to England. The mode of their fabrication was finally made public by M. Dubois Foucou, who contributed powerfully to the propagation of this new mode of making artificial teeth. M. Fonzi made some very handsome improvements upon these teeth, as they had been previously made by M.M. Duchateau, Dubois Chement, and Dubois Foucou, for which the Atheneum of Arts, in Paris, after a strict examination of them, decreed him a medal and crown; according to the terms of the report of a commission appointed for the purpose of examining these teeth, and which was the maximum of their recompenses. This was done, March 14, 1808.—(*See Audibran, page* 47.)

M. Fonzi, encouraged by the favourable report of the Atheneum of Arts, submitted his invention, or rather mode of making these teeth, to the Academy of Medicine, who after after an examination of them, confirmed the report of the Atheneum of Arts. The Society of Medicine of Paris, in the year 1812, decreed a medal to any one who would give correct answers to the five following questions, proposed by the society.*

"Question 1st. What are the motives of preference which the porcelain merits over the different animal materials for the construction of teeth.?

---

* Audibran, page 49, and following.

Ire. Question. Quels sont les motifs de préférence que la porcelaine mérite sur les différentes matières animales pour la construction des dents.

"Question 2d. What are the most simple and economical means to employ for the composition and colouring of the paste, and also of the enamel, and for the baking of the materials?

"Question 3d. Is the purple precipitate of cassius (oxide of gold, precipitated by the muriate of tin) preferable to any other substance for colouring the gums when they are required? What is the manner of using it?

"Question 4th. Platina; does it possess properties which render it more suitable than any other metal, so that when placed in the teeth it readily unites with them in the baking?

"Question 5th. What are the mechanical means most advantageous for mounting the teeth, and adjusting them in the mouth, without injuring the firmness of the natural teeth?"

To resolve these questions, two memoirs were addressed to the Society of Medicine; one by Meggidro, of Nantz, the other by M. Cornelia, of Turin. The former was honourably noticed, but the society decided that the questions had not been clearly resolved; consequently, the society at that time, found no person upon whom, for a clear elucidation

---

IIme Question. Quels sont les moyens les plus simples et les plus économiques à employer pour composer et colorer la pate ainsi que l'émail et pour les cuire.

IIIme. Question. Le précipité pourpre de cassius (oxide d'or précipité par muriate d'étain) est-il préférable à toute autre substance pour colorer les gencives au besoin? Quelle est la maniere de l'employer.

IVme. Question. Le platine jouit il des propriétés, qui le rendent plus apte que les autres métaux, à disposer les dents de manière à pouvoir être facilement réunies entrelles apres la cuisson?

Vme. Question Quels sont les moyens méchaniques les plus avantaguex pour monter les dents. et les ajuster dans la bouche, sans nuire à la solidité des dents naturelles.

and satisfactory answer to these questions, they could bestow their honourable reward.

It appears at this time, that the attention of the learned French societies was directed somewhat to this subject, and as correct answers to the questions proposed by the society of medicine had not been given, so as to affirm them, M. Fonzi again presented to the Atheneum of Arts a specimen of his incorruptible teeth, in order to obtain their approbation. At the same time M. Dubois Foucou submitted to the same society a pamphlet, in which he indicated the means of making the composition teeth. Commissioners were named by the society to examine and report upon these teeth, with the manner of their fabrication, as detailed by M. Dubois Foucou. M. Fonzi, and M. Dubois Foucou were at this time unquestionably at the head of those who practised this part of the profession. But the approbation of the society in favour of these teeth could not be obtained. The commission appointed to examine them reported unfavourably of their merits, and declared in their report, that they were defective in those properties which rendered artificial teeth useful, agreeable, and satisfactory to the patient; and in fine, that they did not sufficiently imitate nature.* Afterwards in the year 1821, Mr. Audibran presented to the same society some specimens of these teeth, with a volume detailing the mode of fabrication. They were examined by the society, and received their approbation. I have given this hasty sketch of the history of these teeth in order to give the reader a knowledge of them, and likewise to inform him, that they have had their vicissitudes in public favour.

I now wish to present a fair and impartial statement of their good and bad properties. The following are their ad-

---

* See Audibran, page 51. (1) note.

vantages which they enjoy, in a greater degree than any other artificial teeth.

First, They do not change, except perhaps very slightly, upon being worn in the mouth.

Secondly, They do not absorb the saliva or any juices of the mouth, so as thereby to offend the taste or contaminate the breath.

These two advantages are very considerable, and they have been and continue to be the only ones which can be urged in their favor over other substances.

I will now mention the disadvantages attached to these teeth, and which caused them to be more than once rejected as unworthy of the approbation of the Society of Medicine, &c. of Paris: and the reader will bear in mind, that when the Society of Medicine gave their approbation of these teeth, they did not by so doing disapprove of the other substances, but merely that porcelain might be used. The disadvantages of these teeth are the following.

First, There is no congeniality between them and the gums, against which they are placed. They are a complete foreign body. Animal or natural teeth when properly mounted and inserted in the mouth, will repose upon the gums for years, without much change taking place in them after being worn a few weeks; and in all cases the alveoli, after a tooth is extracted, are absorbed away, and if any teeth are inserted previously to this time, the jaw will change in some degree its shape. But putting these exceptions out of the way, the animal and natural teeth may be worn for years with little or no change taking place. It is otherwise with porcelain teeth; there is no fellowship between them and the gums, the remaining teeth, the lips or the tongue. The gums are constantly disposed to retire from the contact of these teeth, and in this respect we may notice that one of their great advantages, which is of not changing, is immediately rendered of little avail; because if they do not change themselves, the gums upon which they repose change, and consequently these teeth must be renewed in a few years, in order to be adapted to the situation and condition of the gums.

The second disadvantage of these teeth is, that they are far greater conductors of caloric than natural or animal teeth. They immediately become cold when exposed to cold air, as when a person is conversing with another when the air is cold, or upon walking in the cold wind, or upon taking them out to clean them, if done in a cold room or with cold water, they become very cold, and communicate a very cold sensation to the patient upon replacing them. To such a degree do they have this effect more than animal substances, that if there are many of them, a chill will be felt by the patient upon their being exposed to cold, and from this cause they are liable to produce pain in the living teeth which they touch. We very often experience pain in our teeth, upon taking a glass of very cold water in our mouths, and in this way porcelain teeth often affect the living teeth when they become cold, as we have before mentioned. This objection may seem somewhat trivial but it is not so. It should be a prime object with every dentist to place such artificial teeth in the mouth, and so insert them that they shall be perfectly comfortable and agreeable to the patient; and if so, after a very short time, he will be hardly conscious of having any thing like artificial teeth in his mouth; and if convinced that they cannot be detected by the common observer, he will be perfectly satisfied with them, will open his mouth without being abashed at the thought of his artificial teeth's being detected; and indeed he will rarely think of them: but if every time he opens his mouth, his teeth become cold and thereby disagreeable to him, he will be constantly reminded of them. He will not only think of them himself, but will be constantly harassed with the idea, that every body else notices them, which to say the least is a disagreeable state of things.

The third objection which I notice as applicable to these teeth, is their weight. They are much heavier than animal or natural teeth of the same size, thickness, &c.; so much so, that they are ready upon every occasion to fall down. If several of them are placed upon a gold spring or plate, which is the only way any tooth should ever be inserted, except upon the stump, unless the spring is very strong, and the living teeth to which it is attached very firm in their sockets, they will in most cases fall down, and the disposition to fall down is still farther increased by their having no fellowship with the gums.

The fourth objection is, that they are very brittle, and ready to be broken upon any slight cause. If made thick to prevent this, then they are two heavy; so then there are four objections to these teeth, which art cannot remedy. Their want of congenialty to the tongue, gums, lips and the other teeth; secondly, their disposition to become cold and unpleasant in the mouth of the patient; thirdly, their weight; and fourthly their fragility, brittleness, &c. These objections arise from the nature of the substance, and I cannot believe that they can ever be obviated. Another objection to these teeth, is their aspect and colour. Mr. Audibran who appears to possess the greatest partiality to the porcelain teeth, acknowledges himself, that in colour, the natural teeth far surpass the porcelain teeth.* He says, "The true superiority of

* La véritable supériorité des dents naturelles consiste principalément dans leur couleur qui se marie parfaitement avec celle des autres dents auxquelles on les a aggrégées, lorsque toutefois on les a bien choisies. Page, 66.

the natural teeth consists principally in their *colour*, by which they perfectly join themselves to those living teeth with which they are aggregated, when nevertheless, they have been well selected." Page, 56. This frank declaration of Mr. Audibran, I believe will be reciprocated by every person, who has ever noticed porcelain teeth. Their aspect is perfectly dead. There is a certain animation in the aspect and appearance of the living tooth, which is not seen in any dead substance used to replace them. A dead natural tooth when artificially inserted possesses, especially if a good tooth, a considerable of this animation. Animal teeth in consequence of their beautiful enamel, possess a considerable of it, but the porcelain teeth when in the mouth, have not the least animation in their aspect, but appear perfectly dull and dead. I have never seen any porcelain teeth, which possessed to any great extent a natural colour and aspect like the natural teeth, or as much so as the animal teeth. Mr. Audibran dwells with considerable emphasis upon the impenetrability of these teeth, and their not taking up any of the juices of the mouth, food, &c. This is indeed a very valuable property, and one which gives a principal value to these *teeth*. We have before noticed that no artificial tooth whatever, should be inserted, until the mouth and all the other teeth, if any remain, had been rendered perfectly healthy. Because if inserted in a diseased mouth, or when any of the teeth are diseased, it aggravates all the other complaints. If this rule is adopted, (and any thing short of it is incompatable to every principle of correct practice,) then we may insert the animal and natural teeth in the mouth so as to be very useful, comfortable, natural and agreeable to the patient; and if strict cleanliness is observed, they will remain clean and without contracting any bad smell for many years, and also retain their colour and good appearance. When we take into consideration how much the gums and alveoli are apt to change, and especially the former, upon the contact of porcelain teeth, our own reason and observation will at once teach us, that the latter will, before any great length of time, from the change in the jaw and the teeth to which they are attached, become out of fit, or not adapted to the shape of the jaw; and consequently become useless, and new ones will have to be substituted; so that natural and animal teeth if good, and properly inserted, and rigid cleanliness is observed by the patient, will, besides all their other advantages over porcelain teeth, add this, of being useful to the patient nearly as long as the latter.

When porcelain teeth are inserted upon the stump, the objection, as regards the retiring of the gums, is mostly obviated. But another difficulty arises: the porcelain teeth are so brittle and ready to break, that they cannot be fastened with that firmness which animal or natural teeth may be. I have now several sets of porcelain teeth, which I have taken out, and inserted either animal or natural teeth in their places. I do not wish to deviate from the strictest candor in the discussion of this matter, knowing that truth will ever remain, whilst every deviation from it will, like the darkness of night, be dispelled by the rise and progress of the sun of science and observation. It is too often the case that views of interest, will often prevent us from taking a comprehensive view of any subject. This appears to me to be the case with many of the advocates of porcelain teeth; who in many instances stoutly assert that they are superior to every other substance whatever for the construction of artificial teeth. When we consider that almost coeval with the first dawning of Dental Surgery as a science or an art, these teeth were known, that they have been known about one hundred years, (for Fauchard at least hinted at them in the year 1728,) and as yet, they have made but very little progress in public favour, either in Europe or this country, which they most assuredly would have done, had they possessed those advantages which some interested individuals have ascribed to them, we must infer some bad properties attached to them, whilst the use of the natural, and animal, and ivory teeth has been extended to almost every part of Europe and this country.

In concluding the subject of porcelain teeth I will remark, that having some insurmountable objections in the nature of their substance, their reputation has ever depended, in a great degree, upon the ingenuity of their fabricators. My own individual opinion of them is, that for single teeth, or a few in contact with others, they are much surpassed by natural teeth; but for whole sets, if well and ingeniously executed, and perfectly adapted to the mouth, they possess high advantages, and are nearly, if not quite equal, to those formed of other substances, natural teeth, &c. I will conclude the subject by giving the opinion of M. Delabarre, one of the most ingenious mechanical dentists in Paris. He remarks,* "The composition teeth, placed in the mouth, along side of the others, are nearly always illy matched with the other teeth; there is something about them that does not appear natural, that shocks a delicate eye, and which at length detects the mystery.

"In the mean while, until making them is brought to perfection, I think the preference ought to be given to natural teeth, where one is to be replaced here and there; but if a complete set of teeth is wanted, porcelain is preferable, because the person being without teeth, there can exist nothing by which a comparison can be made."

---

* Odontologie sur les Dents Humaines, par M. Delabarre, page 67. Paris.

SECTION II.

MANNER OF PREPARING ARTIFICIAL TEETH PREVIOUSLY TO THEIR BEING MOUNTED FOR INSERTION IN THE MOUTH.

We have now considered the several materials of which artificial teeth are made. I now wish to detail the mode of preparing these materials previously to their being mounted upon springs or pivots for insertion in the mouth.

Natural teeth are extremely liable to crack and split, when they are, or have become dry; consequently, to remedy this, and to render them perfectly clean, they should be constantly kept in alcohol or water, and should be rendered perfectly clean by scraping them, and often renewing the water in which they are macerated. It should be a general rule never to insert one in the mouth, unless perfectly clean and free from every impurity.

There is a great difference in the quality of natural teeth, as regards their colour, shape, and exemption from defects, which always modifies the price of them, and should be understood by the dentist.

Animal teeth should be selected of a handsome shape, with a fine, smooth enamel, free from any inequalities on their surface, &c. The teeth of neat cattle I prefer to any I have ever used. They should be boiled in water, or soaked for a long time: their fangs should be sawed off, and their crowns kept in water, in the same way as we remarked of natural teeth, as they are equally as liable to split upon becoming dry for any time. As their principal objection is of being of too white a colour, we should select those which are as yellow as we can find them.

Ivory from the Tooth of the Hippopotamus.

We should select this, if we intend to use it, which has a large proportion of enamel, and is of a fine clear colour, and of a close, dense, compact structure, with a fine grain, not coarse or cracked, and checked through its substance. It does not require any particular preparation before working it, nor is it necessary to put it in water, as it is not apt to split when dry, or upon working it, if carefully managed.

Transplanting Teeth, &c.

I have already said all that I wish to say upon this subject. Those who wish for directions upon it, can consult Mr. Hunter's remarks and directions upon transplanting teeth, &c.*

SECTION III.

OF THE MANNER IN WHICH ARTIFICIAL TEETH SHOULD BE INSERTED IN THE MOUTH.

There are various modes of inserting artificial teeth in the mouth; some of which are very pernicious, and others very useful and proper. Of these I shall mention but four, to wit:

Firstly, with Ligatures.

Secondly, with Springs and Clasps.

Thirdly, with Pivots.

Fourthly, with Clasps alone.

---

* See Hunter, Part II. pages 217 to 232.

Ligatures.

These are made of silk, or fine gold or silver wire, and are passed through the tooth or teeth which we wish to fasten in the mouth. When the artificial tooth or teeth are placed in the situation we wish them, the ligatures are carried around the two adjoining living teeth and tied so as to be firm in their places.

The following are the inconveniences which result from dependence upon this mode of fastening the teeth. In the first place we cannot always use ligatures; for very often we wish to insert six or eight teeth in the front of the mouth, and perhaps are obliged to fasten them to the posterior grinders, in consequence of there being no other nearer. In this case, we should have to continue our block of teeth to the last molar tooth, or not be able to use a ligature, and should we do so, a ligature would not confine such a large block of teeth as firmly as they ought to be. In the next place, if made of silk, &c. they are extremely apt to contract an unpleasant taste and smell, become dirty, and the patient is obliged to change them very often. If made of gold or silver wire, then the patient will be troubled to untie them, so as to take out the teeth to clean them, as he will desire to do occasionally, and he will be troubled to tie them in again. In the third place, they never give that firmness to the new teeth which we desire, and the teeth are constantly moved by the tongue. The fourth and last objection I would mention to ligatures, and one which, if we could pass by all the others, would for ever, in most cases, forbid their use altogether, is the injurious effects which the ligatures suspending the teeth have upon those living teeth to which they are tied. Their first bad effect is to pull those teeth out to which they are tied; which they generally do, sooner or later, or else they cut the tooth off, as I have seen done in repeated instances. I could mention a most numerous list of cases in illustration of these positions and facts. These effects are most noticed when applied to the upper teeth. If to the under, our three first objections come in with force. I will mention but two cases of the injurious effects of ligatures, when applied to the upper jaw, and these cases will be found to be a common effect.

Case I.

Mrs. A——, residing in the south part of this city, lost one of the front upper incisores, which was extracted. She applied to a dentist, who inserted a tooth in place of the lost incisor, and confined it to the lateral and remaining front incisor. In the course of four or five years, the other front incisor tooth, otherwise perfectly sound, was loosened and pulled out by the ligature and weight of the inserted tooth. She then had two artificial teeth inserted in the same way, and fastened with the ligature. Then the lateral incisor, to which the first tooth was fastened, became loose and came out. Then she had three inserted, in the same way, tied to the eye tooth and the remaining lateral incisor, which soon caused the other lateral incisor to drop out. She then had four inserted, and tied to the two canine teeth, which was followed by the loss of the canine tooth to which the last set, having three teeth, was tied. Then she had lost four front upper teeth by the use of the ligatures, to wit, the three front incisores, and one canine tooth, and the other canine tooth was useless by being almost drawn out, and very loose, so as to appear, from its unnatural length, very disgusting. In consequence of disease, no doubt, in a great measure, induced by these bad artificial teeth, which were of sea horse ivory, she had now lost both of the bicuspids and the first molar tooth of the side upon which she had lost the canine tooth, so that she was placed in precisely the predicament which I mentioned in my first objection to ligatures. *See the preceding objection to these,* &c. As her dentist's skill seemed to be somewhat at an end, as there were no more teeth to which a ligature might be tied, he applied to me to know what could be done to replace her teeth. I found her last set of four teeth tied to the remaining canine; of course on one side only, whilst the other was not fastened at all; consequently, whenever she spoke, her teeth moved as well as her tongue; which, to say the least, was a most unpleasant state of things, and rather bordering on the ludicrous. I took out this last set of teeth, which were tied in, and replaced six elegant animal teeth, mounted upon a fine gold plate, with gold springs and clasps, carried back so as to embrace the molar teeth, which the lady has since worn with the utmost pleasure and satisfaction. Cases when ligatures tied to the upper teeth, and having this effect, are seen every day. I will mention a part of the following case.

Case II.

Mrs. O——, living in the south part of this city, called upon me last spring, in great trouble. She had had several sets of teeth placed in her mouth at different times, as in the case of Mrs. A——; and like her, disease, probably induced or aggravated by her artificial teeth, had destroyed nearly all her back teeth, and the artificial ones had done the same for most of her front teeth, nearly as in case of Mrs. A——. But in that of Mrs. O——, the canine teeth were very firmly placed in their sockets, so as not to be readily moved by the weight of the other teeth; and the ligatures, instead of pulling them out, cut them off. At the time when her last set of artificial teeth were inserted, she had lost all of her upper teeth except the right canine tooth. The left canine tooth had been cut off by the ligatures of the set preceding these last, and to the stump of this tooth a silver screw was fastened, and to this screw and the right canine tooth the last set of artificials was fastened by ligatures. When she called on me, the ligature had cut off the right canine tooth; and the set dropped out. This is a brief history of objections to ligatures, and of their bad effects. We are obliged to carry them up close to the gum where the enamel of the tooth becomes attenuated; and, in almost every instance, they cut upon, and through the enamel, inducing pain in the tooth, and frequently exposing the nerve, if the tooth does not soon fall out. We can easily conceive how much this effect is increased when porcelain teeth are inserted in this manner, on account of their being heavier than other teeth. I think the objections to ligatures and the bad consequences resulting from their use, are sufficient reasons to forbid their being used in any case whatever to fasten artificial teeth to the upper living teeth. I could dwell much longer upon this subject, but I think I have said enough to induce the judicious practitioner, as a general rule, never to use ligatures to fasten artificial teeth.

Of Clasps for Fastening Artificial Teeth.

This mode of fastening artificial teeth is often adopted. The tooth, or, if more than one, they are united so as to form an entire block, which are placed in the mouth so as to perfectly fill the space of the lost teeth, and having a clasp on each side, which are carried around the two teeth adjoining, one on each side. This mode is preferable to the use of ligatures, inasmuch that the flat surface of the clasps does not cut or injure the teeth to which they are attached, and they may be taken out at pleasure. But the inconvenience arising from them is, that they in some degree pull down the other teeth, and they cannot be used in all cases. And if only one, two, or three teeth are inserted, as for instance the front incisores, they are apt to be exposed to view. As the clasp must pass nearly around the tooth, by their acting almost vertically upon the teeth they support, those which they clasp, they are apt in many cases to pull down. Yet this is prevented considerably by the ingenuity of the operator. They are probably in every point of view, much better than ligatures. Clasps are made of silver and of gold. In my observations upon the substances proper for plugging the teeth, I then discussed the merits of the different metals, and gave a decided preference to gold for any purpose, when we wish to have the metal retained in the mouth. I prefer gold for clasps, plates, springs, &c. much before any other substance, if we except platina, which is not at this time much used, although a highly proper substance for dental purposes.

Of Plates, Springs, and Clasps, for fastening Artificial Teeth.

The third mode of fastening artificial teeth, and which I prefer to any other I have yet noticed, is with plates, springs, and clasps, which I will now describe. Having obtained the size of the vacuity in the circle of teeth, made by the lost ones, we cut a plate of gold, rolled to the thickness of a wafer, to the size of the vacuity; we then solder this plate upon a spring of gold, which is bent so as to completely fit against the inner circle of the teeth and jaw, and is carried back and terminates in clasps, which pass around the molar or bicuspid teeth, and are not exposed to view when the patient opens his mouth. The teeth which we wish to insert, are sawed so as to be put upon the gold plate, and are riveted upon it with gold rivets, which keep them perfectly firm. The springs, by being carried back, so that the clasps shall embrace a posterior tooth, cause these last to act upon the tooth it embraces in a horizontal direction, and do not pull it out or loosen it. Plates, springs, and clasps made in this way, may be adapted to every circumstance of the teeth, and be firmly fastened if there are not more than two teeth on the jaw, or if there is one tooth and the stump of a tooth which is firm. They have none of those inconveniences or bad consequences, arising from the use of ligatures or clasps. They will be always perfectly neat, and, if made of gold, will last during the life of the patient. A considerable neatness is required in fitting them, but this done, and they are worn with the greatest comfort and satisfaction.

The plates instead of having the teeth fastened to them by sawing a groove into the teeth, are often prepared so as to rest in perfect opposition to the gum, and to the under side of the plate the artificial teeth are fastened. This is an excellent mode of mounting and inserting artificial teeth. Whole sets of teeth are prepared in this way, and confined to their places by spiral springs of gold or platina, passing on each side from the upper to the lower set.

Of Pivots.

This is the fourth mode of fastening individual artificial teeth, and is, without any doubt, the best mode, in which artificial teeth can ever be fastened in the mouth. The pivots are passed into the stumps of teeth, having the crown of a tooth attached to them, and may be done in this way so as to be perfectly firm, and remain useful to the patient many years. We sometimes fasten several teeth united in a block upon one or two stumps. The advantages of this mode over every other, is, I believe, now generally admitted. Clasps, springs, and plates united, may be worn with the greatest pleasure, but the stump is the better mode if sound and firm; if not, pivots should never be fastened in them.

Of the Materials for Pivots.

Pivots are made of gold, silver, and of wood. The metallic pivots are far better than any other, and their only objection is, that they are apt to wear the tooth which is placed upon them, and the stump in which they are inserted; and so much so do they have this effect, that we are induced to use pivots of wood. This last has the advantage, if perfectly seasoned, of swelling in the stump, by the moisture which they absorb, and in this way become very firm. The advantages and disadvantages of the two kinds, are perhaps nearly balanced. If we choose to use wood, the best seasoned hickory is what is now used, when wood is used at all. The wood has the advantage of being fastened to a much weaker stump than the metallic pivot. The decision in individual cases must depend on circumstances, and be determined by the judicious dentist. Metallic pivots are usually formed into screws by a screw plate, &c.

SECTION IV.

OF THE MANNER OF TAKING THE SHAPE AND FIGURE OF THE MOUTH.

It is necessary in order to know exactly the shape and size of the mouth, so as to enable us to form artificial teeth perfectly adapted to the gum and mouth, for us to take a cast of the teeth, and gums, &c. This we do by taking a piece of wax (bees-wax is usually employed) and softening it in warm water or by a fire, and then pressing it upon the gum and teeth, which will give the exact impression of the cavity, gum, remaining teeth, &c. We then, after suffering the wax to harden, pour upon it a paste of the sulphate of lime, gypsum, plaister of paris, and suffer this to harden; then melt the wax from the plaister, and we have an exact model of the mouth, if every part of our manipulations have been correctly done. It requires practice to perform this part of our art well. When we wish to insert whole jaws of teeth, it is necessary to take a cast of both jaws. After having obtained our model, we shall be enabled to form our artificial teeth by it, so that they will be easily adapted to the mouth of the patient. Much depends upon the nicety and exact correctness of our model, and great care is required in taking it. The plaister should be calcined before using it, and sifted so as to be clean, free from sticks, &c.

For whole sets, brass castings are taken from the models, so as to shape the gold plate on the brass models.

SECTION V.

PHYSIOLOGICAL OBSERVATIONS UPON STUMPS OF TEETH, AND THE MANNER OF PREPARING THEM FOR INSERTION OF ARTIFICIAL TEETH UPON THEM.

In the first part of this work, I noticed that the teeth were possessed of two sources of support. The body and crown of the tooth are supported by the blood-vessels, nerve, &c., which occupy the cavity in the interior of the tooth, whilst the fang, root, or stump, receives a share of its support from its external membrane, which covers it and lines the alveolus. The cortex striatus or enamel of the tooth, is, as regards the sanguinious circulation, entirely extraneous, having no sensibility whatever, and can be operated upon without the least pain being perceived in it. It has the same relation to the body of the tooth, that the cuticle has to the cutis, or the epidermis to the dermoid tissue: the latter is much thicker on parts which are subject to the application of pressure or hard substances, as the soles of the feet, and palms of the hands. But the enamel is formed at first perfectly adequate to sustain the pressure which falls upon it in mastication, and, under all ordinary circumstances, it completely protects the bony substance of the tooth from the contact of injurious substances. The cuticle, if removed, may be, and is reproduced from the vessels of the cutis, but the cortex striatus, or enamel of the tooth, is formed from a membrane, investing, as we have before said, the substance of the tooth, which, as its retention upon the tooth would be incompatible to the function of the tooth, is, after the perfect formation of the enamel, entirely absorbed away, leaving the enamel perfectly and beautifully formed, and attached to the substance of the tooth. Consequently as the membrane from which the enamel is derived is absorbed away, so, after that event, the enamel can never again be produced by nature or art. It is from not having a correct anatomical and physiological knowledge of the teeth, &c. that authors and writers upon these subjects, have fallen into the greatest, and, in many cases, most dangerous mistakes, in their remarks and observations upon the teeth, and in their mode of treating them, both in health and disease. Mr. Hunter considered the substance of the teeth, as regards the circulation through its substance, as almost an extraneous body.* Mr. Koecker asserts that the vitality of the teeth depends entirely upon the membrane lining their cavities, and that the tooth and fang were dead, and became noxious bodies, as soon as the lining membrane was destroyed.† Mr. Hunter in noticing the progress of caries, remarks, "That after the loss of the crown, the canal in the fang of the tooth is more slowly affected; the scooping process appears to stop there, for we seldom know a fang become very hollow to its point when in the form of a stump, and it sometimes appears sound even when the body of the tooth is almost destroyed; hence I conclude, that the fang of the tooth has *greater living powers than* the *body*, by which the progress of the disease is retarded."‡ This observation of Mr. Hunter, as regards the vitality of the stump, is no doubt correct; and Mr. Koecker's observation, that the fangs die with the internal membrane, is not true. Mr. Charles Bew in his observations upon the teeth, advances an idea with respect to the circulation of blood in the teeth, which, if true, would, upon the destruction

---

* See Hunter, Part II. page 39. † See Koecker, pages 254—5—6, 427.
‡ See Hunter, Part I. page 138.

of the lining membrane, leave the stumps entirely dead. He says, "I will suppose myself correct in the assumption, that as in the body's circulation a great portion of the blood is returned by the superficial veins, so, it is just to take for granted, that through each tubified fang of the teeth, which the most sceptical observer, anatomist or no anatomist, may distinctly discern, the blood is anteriorly thrown to the interior of the tooth, and there, following a due course of beautifully organized circulation through the osseous part, is (si interim nihil interfual) quietly returned by the periosteum of the exterior.*" This opinion of Mr. Bew, and the remarks of Mr. Koecker, are both incorrect and contrary to facts, and the most correct analogical observations. We find that in all hollow bones, of which the fangs of the teeth are a good example, that they have an external and internal periosteum, and that the bone has an internal and external pestiors which, in their circulation, depend mostly upon these membranes: if the external dies, a part of the external bone dies, but no farther than the circulation depended on the dead membrane; and, vice versa, when the internal periosteum is diseased or loses its vitality, &c. So it is with the fangs of the teeth, if the internal membrane dies, a part of the bone of the fang dies, but a much greater part, attached to the socket, and supported by the external periosteum, lives and may retain its vitality for a great many years. It is upon these principles that I have predicated my practice, as regards the stumps of teeth. I think I have demonstrated to every candid reader, that a stump of a tooth may possess vitality, and the internal membrane be dead. Whenever the external periosteum becomes inflamed so as to lose its

---

* See Bew on the Teeth, pages 64 and 65.

vitality, then the fang becomes dead if the internal membrane is or had been destroyed. In operating upon stumps of teeth, for the insertion of artificial ones, in cases when the internal lining membrane had long been destroyed, I have witnessed excessive inflammation to arise, in consequence of cutting upon the sound part of the stump; and this fact, a few times noticed, led me to make these observations and conclusions upon the fangs and stumps of the teeth. In my observations upon the extraction of adult teeth, I remarked, that the front teeth should never be extracted, unless very loose and wholly dead; but if all our endeavours to arrest inflammation in them fails, then we should cut off the crown and part of the body of the tooth, destroy the internal nerve and membrane, and thereby suffer the stump to remain, upon which we may engraft a new tooth; or, if the patient does not choose to have new teeth engrafted on the stumps, they will still be very useful by preserving the shape of the anterior part of the jaws, and not suffer the lips to fall in, or allow the jaws to lose their alveoli, and thereby allow the nose and chin to approximate, as they do in persons who have lost their front teeth, &c. I have repeatedly adopted this mode when persons wished me to extract their front teeth, and always to their great pleasure and satisfaction. The stumps, treated as I shall hereafter direct, if the individual does not choose to have new teeth engrafted, will still be very useful, by preserving the shape of the mouth, and in the mastication of soft food.

Mode of Performing the Operation, Instruments, &c.

The instruments required are a pair of sharp cutting forceps, like extracting forceps, only attenuated to sharp edges, and well tempered. These should be placed upon the tooth to be excised, and carried close to the gum, and even raise the gum a little, or depress it, as the case may be, when, with a steady deliberate pressure upon the handles of the forceps, the tooth is instantly cut off: then, with a pointed instrument like a probe, of the size of the internal canal of the fang, we make pressure upon the nerve, and carry the probe up the canal of the fang near to its termination. This will destroy the nerve and lining membrane, and prevent their subsequent inflammation. Having done this, if we wish to engraft a new tooth upon the stump, we may drill out the stump as much as will be necessary for the reception of a pivot; but we must not at this time insert the tooth, instead of which, we must put a small lead pivot in the fang, so firmly that it will not drop out; we may then dismiss our patient for at least one week, with directions to avoid taking cold, or heating himself much during that time. At the expiration of seven or eight days, if little or no inflammation has appeared, we may take out the lead pivot, and engraft the new tooth. In cases where the tooth is so far decayed, or crumbled away, as not to require much cutting away, and where the lining membrane and nerve are dead, if we wish to engraft a tooth upon the stump, we may drill it out as much as we wish to, and then insert our leaden pivot, as before directed; for if we neglect this precaution, inflammation, in a great many instances, will take place, so as often to compel us to remove the engrafted tooth, or, at any rate, it will greatly weaken the stump, and occasion much suffering to the patient. It should be our earnest endeavour, to save pain to our patients as much as possible, which will be done, to a great degree, by pursuing the practice I have here detailed. I claim it as my own, and consider it a very great improvement in this part of dental-surgery. The many cases of most violent inflammation and extreme suffering, occasioned

59

by the mode of inserting teeth upon stumps, without their being prepared, (so much so, in many cases, as to almost destroy the constitution and health of the patients,) has often thrown this part of dental-surgery into great disrepute, and has been a standing opprobrium to the profession. These wretched effects, in every case when I have followed this plan, have been completely prevented; and the whole course of operation has not produced as much pain as the extraction of the tooth or stump would have done. Other modes of preparing stumps have been practised, but I prefer this to any other. If the patients do not wish a new tooth to be engrafted, then we need not drill the fang, but fill the internal cavity with a piece of soft pure lead wire, so firmly introduced as that it will not come out, unless done so by art. Little or no pain will ensue, and the patient's mouth will retain its form. The first impulse of the instrument upon the nerve seems to paralyze it to its extremity, and very little pain is subsequently felt. The practitioner should have several of these probes, of different sizes, so as to accurately fill the cavity, and carry all the nerve before it, and not so small as to prick and partially lacerate it, or so large as to greatly strain the stump. I believe that this plan of treating the front teeth, and of preparing stumps of teeth for insertion of artificial teeth, is founded upon the most correct surgical principles; and if generally adopted, will disarm this part of dental-surgery of nearly all its terrors. We should, before inserting a new tooth upon a stump, cut away the end of the stump, so that the end of the new tooth shall pass completely within the gum, and firmly against the end of the stump. When so done, this is the best mode of inserting artificial teeth with which we are at present acquainted.

In concluding this subject, and that of artificial teeth, I cannot do justice to myself without remarking, that it is practice and the personal instructions of the judicious and ingenious dentist, which alone will convey just ideas of this subject: written description cannot do it. On this subject, see the work of Delabàrre on the "Partie Mechanique du Dentiste."

SECTION VI.

MANNER OF MAKING PORCELAIN TEETH.

As Mr. Audibran has given the best work extant upon this subject, I shall present to the reader the entire section devoted by him to the description of the manner of making porcelain teeth, remarking that in his formulæ of ingredients will be seen the names of many provincial earths, which, perhaps, may not be obtained in this country. Enough is developed to determine the general principles which should govern us in their manufacture, and the perseverance of the ingenious artist will surmount every obstacle.

Description given of the Proceedings for making Incorruptible teeth.—By Joseph Audibran, *Sec. III., pages* 64 to 126.

We know of the pamphlet of M. Dubois Foucou, in which we find a description of the means employed for making incorruptible teeth; but in rendering justice to the merit and views of this disinterested practician, we have already remarked, that the means which he employs are insufficient and less certain. It is sometimes very difficult to procure most of the ingredients which he makes use of, such as the red earth of Dourdan, &c.* In one word, M. Dubois Foucou is too enlightened and too impartial to not be agreeable, and of the service which he will never cease to render to the invention of the teeth made with porcelain, by propagating and calling upon the attention of other dentists, he has in the mean time, himself gathered but few fruits of the efforts of his multiplied essays, and without doubt, very expensive; because the success, in these sorts of enterprizes, depends very much on a variety of circumstances, which it is not in our power to control. In making haste to publish the proceedings which he believes useful, in making them known to all the world, in offering them generously to society, M. Dubois Foucou has been indifferently censured an egotist, who has since seen in this means of general-utility, wherein he finds a source of profit which he makes use of as a means of exclusive monopoly.

I could then, without offending his modesty affirm, that this third section of my work is altogether new; that fails essentially, and we need not be much astonished, that so necessary a part of the art of the dentist has never before been treated to the same extent by any author; and that which ought to inspire some confidence is, because it is not the only proceeding, among those that I have drawn. I have had myself much experience; and one may perceive that I do not omit a single detail in the process of fabrication. I enter also, in this regard, upon the most minute explanations on the choice of ingredients, and the manner of combining them, &c.

The principal merit in descriptions of this kind, consists in

* Since the publication of this pamphlet, entitled, New method of making Artificial Teeth, called Composition, I begged the person in vain, to procure me some of this earth, who furnished it for M. Dubois Foucou.

their exactness and perspicuity. I repeat, that I do not scruple to return to explanatory details as often as it shall appear to be necessary to a perfect understanding of the proceedings.

General Considerations on the different Substances which enter into the Composition of Incorruptible Teeth.

It would be a long time, without doubt, before the public would have been in possession of all the advantages which present themselves in the manufacture of incorruptible teeth, if the dentists had not made known, that there were so many difficulties to surmount.

If so little success has been made in this work, they ought not to charge it to the want of zeal, nor their less knowledge of chemistry, but uniformly to the absolute silence of the treatises of chemistry, which are silent, or give absolutely wrong information about the ingredients which it is necessary to know.

Every dentist that would make incorruptible teeth, begins by consulting the works of the most celebrated chemists, such as those of Lavoisier, Fourcroy, and Thènard, and finally draw up exact ideas on the work which they would undertake. We can say with regret, they draw from the reading of these works much general erudition, and but few hints upon making incorruptible teeth; in the mean time they are led into error, in hoping for what can never be realized. Indeed, who could hope to succeed in his work, when he sees in all the treatises which we have cited, that such an oxide makes a red, that such a one, a blue, that such another, finally in its result, a yellow; who does expect, I say, to attain the method of making incorruptible teeth, by using the oxides in the order in which they are mentioned? Well!

this is precisely the moment they believe they have arrived at the goal they aspire to, when in truth they find themselves at the greatest distance from it; because these different oxides, instead of giving such and such a colour, give quite the contrary; above all it is the yellow colour which it is difficult to obtain, because it is that which is most wanted to colour incorruptible teeth.

They have not only consulted the treatises on chemistry, of existing authors, who have equally indicated the means to be employed, but, it must be confessed they have not been specially occupied in this particular; they consequently have given incorrect information.

I have in my hands the note of a celebrated chemist, which proves he was solicitous for the interest of the public, but did not think proper to occupy himself with this branch of chemistry, which furnishes dentists with the means of perfecting a very important part of their art.

From what we have just said, it follows that the study of chemical works has not furnished, and cannot furnish, in effect, to the dentist but general ideas on the combination and manipulation of the earths and oxides; to succeed they must make numberless attempts, and must have sufficient knowledge of chemistry to make them profitable; without that, he ought not to expect to make incorruptible teeth of the proper kind.

How much trouble have I not had to arrive at one hopeful point! how many fruitless trials have I not made! but the more obstacles I had to surmount, the more the reader may have confidence in the formulas I present him. In effect, there is not one which does not give, in its result, the colour which I speak of; if it is not so, the fault will be in the bad quality of the substances employed. The kaolin and pétunzè sometimes contain foreign substances, which change very often the colour of the oxides. It is here necessary to be observed that these two substances are not always equally good and pure; but how shall we know it? There are not many who analyze these earths by which their principles are known; but with us, it is in using them we have known them. But what must be done to purify them? This is what chemistry does not teach us, but what it is indispensable to know.

The oxides themselves are more or less well prepared, which clearly explains the variations in their results: to have such as are good, they must be always taken from a laboratory well known to possess merited confidence; mine, I obtain from that of M. Vauquelin, and I believe they may be there procured of the proper kind.

In the following paragraphs, we shall occupy ourselves in enumerating all the objects which are indispensable in the fabrication of teeth, the properties of each substance in particular, then the different combinations to each which we have mutually submitted.

Incorruptible teeth, like human teeth, are composed of two substances; one, which is the paste or body of the tooth, hard and opaque; the other, vitrifiable, slightly transparent, in imitation of the living tooth, called enamel.

To commence, the following articles must be procured.

1st.—A very true scale, with which it is possible to weigh fourths and eighteenths of a grain.

2d.—A porphyry table, of a foot and a half square, and more.*

---

* I for a long time used glass for grinding my substances, but without success; the teeth were more or less cut by it, and their tints were not such as I wished.

3d.—A porcelain muller, which is to grind the different substances, of which we shall presently speak.

4th.—A whalebone knife, and not a steel, to avoid oxidation, to serve for tempering the enamel.

5th.—The argillaceous earth of Limoges, known by the name of Kaolin.

6th.—The earth of Vanvres, already baked.

7th.—Pètunzè, or flint stone of Limoges, which serves as a colour to the porcelain.

8th.—The oxide of Titanium.

9th.—The oxide of Zinc.

10th.—The oxide of Uranium.

11th.—The oxide of Manganese.

12th.—The oxide of Gold.

13th.—The muriate of ammonia of Platina.

14th.—The filings of Gold.

15th.—The filings of Platina.

These oxides and metals are sufficient for the composition of all the different shades, by beginning with the whitest, and then with those of deeper colour.

The colour of the natural teeth is ordinarily of a yellowish white; this tint is preferable, the teeth of this colour were always sound and good. Those wherein the yellow predominates less, and are as white as alabaster, joined to a kind of transparency, are very inferior, although the finest in appearance: physiologists have regarded them as signs indicative of an infirm constitution. It does not come within our province to examine this question, which we shall treat on another occasion, in a work in which we are at present engaged.

The colour of a whitish yellow, like all the others, is susceptible of alterations which all our organs undergo in time, whether from accidents, or diseases: of all the ornaments of nature there is not one more frail and fugitive, in general, than the colours with which objects are shaded. "Nimium ne crede colori,"—"Boast not of the lustre of your colours," said the prince of Latin poets, in speaking to a young nymph who had a young child: these words might be equally applied to the colour of our teeth! they fade and tarnish in proportion as we advance in age; the enamel becomes of a yellowish hue by a diversity of causes which contributes to make it thin, and by the successive addition of calcareous phosphate which it continually receives. When we wish to change, by replacing a natural tooth for a porcelain tooth, we must begin by giving it a hue like that of the others; and even choose it of rather deeper colour, and see that its colour becomes lighter in passing through the fire.

For this effect the shades are sufficient of which I have indicated the composition. I could obtain a great number, vary, and multiply them without end, although I have not done it, because I did not think it useful; but in attending these compositions at different degrees of heat, they themselves present a multitude of variations, which increase considerably, the number of shades.

The formulas which I have composed give shades sufficient to suit every mouth: it might be easy for those who would thus occupy themselves, to create new shades to suit the necessity of the cases. The principal thing is to know the oxides and other ingredients which are necessary for this operation. I have named them, and I wish that my brethren may use them.

We shall treat in a succinct manner, the properties of all the substances we have just enumerated.

§ I.—*Of the Porcelain Earth, or Kaolin.*

Kaolin is a very argillaceous earth, serving for the base of the different substances which enter into the composition of the paste proper for making the teeth.

It has the property of separating itself in water, and of making a very unctuous paste, which can be moulded into the most delicate objects, and gives them, at the same time, the advantage of preserving the shapes with which they are stamped.

It acquires, by baking, an extreme hardness and a smooth surface ; nor will the most penetrating liquids act upon it.

This earth, employed alone, shrinks in the fire, and supports with difficulty the sudden passage from heat to cold; but this inconvenience may be remedied, by mixing a small portion of the earth of Vanvres, as well as the oxides and metals in fine filings, which may be seen in the different formulas.

The fluid caloric is then more equally circulated through the mass, and the article is heated to a higher degree without cracking, which is indispensable in the soldering incorruptible teeth.

Kaolin may be obtained from all the manufacturers of porcelain, and particularly from Mad. Crèmière, Menie Montant-street, No. 48.

§ II.—*Of the Earth of Vanvres.*

The earth of Vanvres is very argillaceous; it is employed in the manufactories for making the circles on which porcelain is baked.

After being baked, it is of a shining rusty colour ; supports with impunity the highest degree of heat, and the most sudden transitions of heat and cold: it was this that determined me to enter it into the composition of my teeth, to make them more susceptible of the action of fire in the operation of soldering.

I consider this earth as an excellent conductor of caloric; and also the teeth with which it is combined are harder and less brittle: its colour does not oppose the colouring principle of the oxides with which I combine it; on the contrary, it combines very well with them, and produces the most satisfactory result.

I use only that which has been subjected to the first baking in the potter's furnace, and it is from him I procure it.

§ III.—*Of Pètunzè, or the Flint-stone of Limoges.*

Pètunzè is a flint-stone reduced to a very fine powder, which serves as a covering for porcelain.* It is used only for enamelling kaolin, but dentists have made use of it for the base of oxides, to serve as a colouring for the teeth which they make.

It is very fusible, and its fusibility and transparency must be checked, by the addition of a proper quantity of kaolin.

§ IV.—*Of the Oxide of Titanium.*

The oxide of Titanium ought to be considered the first for colouring incorruptible teeth; used by itself in different pro-

* It is said the manufacturers of porcelain put other materials with pètunzè to make their enamel, but that is of no importance to us; it is sufficient to know what furnishes enamel that answers the best for the fabrication of incorruptible teeth.

portions, it makes the greatest varieties of yellow; and mixed with other oxides, it contributes to give the teeth the most natural tints.

§ v.—*Of the Oxide of Zinc.*

The oxide of Zinc is very fusible in the fire, and becomes yellow: it gives this colour to enamel; but if submitted too long to a high degree of heat, the yellow colour becomes light, and sometimes altogether disappears. Nevertheless, it is useful to use it alone or mixed with with other oxides; for my part, I only employ it in uniting it to the oxides of gold and titanium.

§ vi.—*Of the Oxide of Uranium.*

The oxide of uranium is like cobalt, it makes a blue colour; it differs merely from the latter in the blue colour that it gives bordering a little on the green: it was for this reason I preferred it to cobalt, because I remarked that this shade united better with those of the other oxides. Combined with the oxides of gold and titanium, it gives an agreeable colour.

It is with the enamels with which they combine it, that they obtain teeth of a bluish tint, which are often obliged to be replaced. In this manner uranium is very useful; but it is wrong to suppose we may obtain yellow tints with this oxide; the experience to which we have submitted it, authorises us to consider as erroneous the assertions giving it the properties of making this colour.

Its colouring principle is very strong; so much so, that it cannot be used but in very small proportions.

§ VII.—*Of the Oxide of Manganese.*

The oxide of manganese is used in the fabrication of incorruptible teeth, by nearly all the dentists who have been engaged therein. M. Dubois Foucou himself, in his pamphlet recommends it, and it is in his work a principal auxiliary.

M. Chaptal, in his chemisty applied to the arts,* says that in the glass manufactories it is used to change the colour of glass, and for this reason, it is known by the name of soap of the glass-makers. In another place he says it is used to give glass a violet colour; and agam in another passage,† he prescribes it for making a yellow-coloured enamel. Considering the different properties attributed to this oxide by M. Chaptal, it appears to be a very convenient substance in the fabrication of incorruptible teeth; at least one would think so, after having read what this learned chemist has said about its properties.

In the mean time we would here observe, that after having submitted the oxide of manganese to numberless trials, we remain convinced it is less fit for this purpose when used by itself; being so extremely subject to change, that it seldom or never produces twice the same tint; it cannot be incorporated by itself in clay nor in enamel, and to make its colouring principle a little more fixed, it is necessary to mix it with other oxides, for without that, we must renounce obtaining from it the yellow colour, which it is pretended it gives, because so uncertain in result.

The oxides of manganese, of antimony, and of iron, were the colourings I used for my first trials; and I can say, with-

---

* Chimie appliquée aux arts, Tome III. page 385.

† Tome II. page 256.

out the fear of contradiction from those who, like me, have tried them, and who may perhaps use them again, they are so seldom to be depended upon that I was obliged to abandon many of them: the reader may then suppose that before having done so, I submitted them to numberless trials, for the sole purpose of ascertaining the use of each. In the mean time the oxide of manganese is then an ingredient, a substance which might be well used in an emergency for the fabrication of incorruptible teeth; and if I admitted it into two of my formulas, it was to prove that my aim was directed to all the useful substances in the manufacture in which we are engaged.

The oxide of manganese mixed with those of titanium and gold, produces the most natural tints, but it is necessary, where they may be seen by the formularies, No. 17 and 18, to employ them in larger proportions.

§ VIII.—*Of the Oxide of Gold.*

The oxide of gold is, perhaps, of all the oxides, that in which the colouring principle is the strongest and most active: it is used in very small proportions, and frequently colours too much the paste and enamel into which it enters.

To perfectly understand what I have here just said, about the inconvenience attached to the use of this oxide, it is proper to recollect that our teeth, although they appear to be of a stony and inert substance, are, notwithstanding, not the less animated with the principle of life.

The circulation of the blood takes place in the interior of our teeth, as in other parts of the body, by means of ramifications, which penetrate all their bony substance; inasmuch, if a tooth is broken, the blood may be seen oozing from the middle of the bone.

It follows from this circulation, that the colour of the living tooth, has some life and animation in it; a light red colour, which properly speaking, the dead tooth does not possess. The oxide of gold has the property of communicating to the substances into which it enters, a certain life and animation, without which, the colour of the incorruptible tooth would appear like a dull unpolished thing: but as excess is a failing, it is to be moderately mixed according to certain limits and the vivifying property of this colouring principle given it.

It will be wanted to colour the gum of certain pieces, which it is sometimes necessary to make.

§ IX.—*Of the Ammoniated Muriate of Platina.*

The muriate of platina like the oxide of gold, possesses a most active colouring principle: it is very fixed in the fire, and its result almost always the same. It can be used but in extremely small proportions, without which it will predominate over those of the other oxides with which, being mixed, it combines very well.

Used by itself, it produces a dark brown colour, and united to the oxides of titanium and gold, it produces very delicate greyish tinges. Combined in various proportions, it produces the most natural colours.

§ X.—*Of Platina.*

Platina is, of all the metals, the only one which resists the different chemical re-agents; the only one that is capable of supporting the greatest degrees of heat without melting. It cannot be fused without joining with a solvent; this infusibility, which distinguishes it from the other metals, has given it the preference for incorruptible teeth, by permitting us to introduce into their interior, the minute portions, whether thread like, or screw-like, without the heat, to which the teeth are submitting in baking ever altering it.*

No other metal, with the exception of fine gold, can be substituted for it, for here it incorporates itself into the porcelain tooth very soon to such a depth, so that the platina will resist the degree of heat which is required for the baking of porcelain.

Although it is difficult to fuse, this metal is remarkable for its great ductility; for when it is well prepared, it equals that of fine gold. The only inconvenience which it has, if it has any, it is in being heavier than gold; but this difference is not sufficient to make it preferable for artificial work; meanwhile, no other would suit for the mountings of incorruptible teeth.

Fine gold unites very well with platina, makes a well combined solder; but standard gold must be used.

The dentist is mistaken who supposes that platina is first used in the dental process. From whence arose the controversy upon the nature of incorruptible teeth in 1808, between two practitioners pretending each to have had the idea? M. Fonzi assures us, in a prospectus, it was he who first introduced it in making porcelain teeth; which M. Dubois Foucou was no sooner apprized of, than he assured us, that he was the first among the dentists whose name was inserted in the register of M. Janety, who prepared it at Paris.

This assertion of M. Fonzi is by no means convincing, nor is it sufficient to secure to this dentist the merit of a proceeding that well belongs to M. Dubois Foucou, who, in a pam-

* There are certain oxides which combine with platina, which change and make it brittle; I have frequently proved it in my essays.

phlet published before this date, a pamphlet which we have already cited, speaks of platina too, as serving for the union of sets of teeth; and likewise, in discoveries, the invention belongs always to him who makes it public. M. Dubois Foucou is considered, without doubt, as having been the first who used platina for this incorruptible work.

For my part, I remember long before 1808, having seen artificial teeth lined with this metal, belonging to a lady, a friend of the widow Bourdet, and I am certain they were never made by M. Fonzi, who at that time did not exercise his art in the capital.

Whoever was the first practitioner who first used it, it is certain, that platina is of great utility for dental purposes, because it always preserves its natural colour; the salivary mucus scarcely changes it, and when by chance it becomes tarnished, the least cleaning is sufficient to restore it to its natural colour. *See the manner of polishing, Section V. paragraph* 10.*

The platina filings, incorporated in the clay used for making incorruptible teeth, gives to it this hard consistence, so necessary for the purposes for which it is intended; it permits the teeth to be heated to the highest degree of heat, and prevents their cracking; it contributes to diminish the effects of loss during the baking, and it prevents the warping of a set of teeth.

Its grayish colour does not darken the other colouring principles, with which it combines very well; its utility is well demonstrated; the teeth into which it does not enter

---

* Dentists make use of platina in plates of different thickness, in thread and in fine filings.

M. Janety's son, Colombier-street, No. 11, at Paris, prepares it in any way we desire it.

are more brittle, and do not maintain so well the sudden transitions of heat and cold; their brittleness is increased on account of the different degrees of heat to which they must be submitted.

This is so true, that all those which have no platina, or the filings of gold, in their composition, are so very brittle, that it is almost impossible to work them. It would be easy for me to point out here the dentists who do not combine platina with the clay with which the teeth are made, but we think they will do so when they learn it is very useful.

§ XI.—*Of Standard Gold in Filings.**

I think that standard gold gives permanently yellow tints which will resist the action of the most intense heat; the different trials to which I have submitted it, justify my saying so. Used by itself, it gives to the enamel of the tooth a yellow red colour, a little too lively, but which may be weakened with the oxide of titanium; then it renders the enamel of a very natural colour. I am ignorant whether those, who, like me, make incorruptible teeth, have had recourse to this means, but it is certain that it is one of the best colouring principles.

To grind gold fine, we begin by filing it with a very fine file, or a file of the finest kind; it is in filings it is weighed,

---

* It is easy to make gold fine enough by filing it with a very fine file, grinding it immediately with the other substances which enter into the composition of incorruptible teeth, it divides perfectly well; it is in this way that I have for a long time used it: but if it is wanted in very fine powder, the gold-beaters can furnish it; that which I have had for some time was obtained from them. Up to the present time I have myself filed the platina, but it would be better to have it prepared by a gold-beater, after the same means they employ for reducing gold to powder.

and then it is mixed with the other ingredients. It is very necessary to grind very carefully the enamel into which it enters; it is besides very useful for diminishing the brittleness of the teeth, and its colour never changes in the operation of soldering.

Necessary Observations for the Preparation and Mixing of Earths and Oxides.

The kaolin, which is procured at the manufactories of porcelain, is not always in a sufficiently pure state. It frequently contains much of the oxide of iron, and then it cracks, is very hard, and badly maintains the transitions of heat and cold.* Whatever be the purity of the substances employed, the result is always in subordination to what is used for their preparation, as well as to the degree of heat to which the objects are submitted.

The best ingredients, improperly prepared, give results altogether different from that which we look for; this is so true, that all the defaults of the teeth proceed from their wrong preparation.

It is not less important to use pure water for softening the clay; that of rain is preferable.

As clay succeeds still better, the older and better tempered it is, it is more convenient to have prepared a certain quantity before-hand, kept in the cellar, in vessels of porcelain,

* What confidence may be placed in the formulas into which the oxide of iron enters? I also have coloured teeth with these oxides mixed with others; but I ought to declare they were of a certain brittleness, which I renounced a long time from my essays: that which authorizes me at this time to proscribe the oxides which I have renounced as not being fit for this work.

and to always keep it moist; it then becomes softer and easier to work.

The enamel requires a still more exact preparation, for without it the teeth will appear rough on their exterior surface.

If, on the contrary, the preparation has been perfect, the enamel will be of a very homogeneous finish, without which it does not imitate nature.

Neither must this enamel be too vitreous so as to make a bad contrast with the natural teeth; it is prevented from becoming too opaque, by the addition of a proper quantity of kaolin.

Incorruptible teeth cannot be baked but imperfectly in the furnaces which we use; to obtain its vitrification it requires a considerable degree of heat; and we are obliged to have it baked in the furnaces used for the baking of porcelain.

It is put in crucibles,* very carefully stopped, and it should always be recommended to the potter to take them in charge,† because if the teeth are brought too near the fire, the colouring principles become sensibly weaker, and even sometimes, (if the heat be too great,) it destroys them altogether.

It is from this cause that the variations are to be attributed, which are seen in the results. It must here be said, that the same formulas rarely give twice in succession the same tints.

---

* The crucibles in which incorruptible teeth are baked, are made with very argillaceous common earth; they are of all sizes at the manufactories of porcelain, and will answer for containing the largest, as well as the most delicate objects which are submitted to the baking process.

† It is understood by placing to the charge, in putting the caskets in places that are farthest off from the fire, so that eventually the teeth receive but a moderate degree of heat, experience having proved, that it was most advantageous to the developement and preservation of the colouring principle of oxides.

The same principle is perceived, but there is a difference, which is sometimes very sensible, and this difference is owing to the strength of the heat, and its greater or less duration. It would be very advantageous in a large city like Paris, if a manufacturer of porcelain would establish a furnace specially intended for the work of dentists. Then results would be obtained more satisfactory and certain, because the patterns to be tried could be put in and taken out at pleasure, which would indicate the moment it is necessary to stop the heat.

If incorruptible teeth should come to a degree of perfection, which leaves them nothing more to hope for, and their usage becomes more general, some manufacturer of porcelain, will, without doubt, one day accomplish the suggestions I give here.

Whatever be the formula for the clay, an essential condition to its good preparation, is in mixing intimately, and pulverizing perfectly, the substances which enter into its compositiou. In general, the beauty of the clay depends on the manner in which it has been ground. This is so true, that when this operation is imperfect, the small particles of the oxide form little spots on the exterior.

The colour of the paste ought always to be like that of the enamel;* the tooth must certainly be, in every part of it, perfectly homogeneous; it is for this reason that the same colouring principles which enter into the clay, enter into the enamel also.

---

* All the dentists who make incorruptible teeth, make their paste almost white; this is a great mistake; the teeth being much better which contain large proportions of the oxides.

Series of Clays and Enamels used for the Fabrication of Incorruptible Teeth, in the Order of their Tints.

Paste, No. 1.

Kaolin - - -	6 Ounces.
Earth of Vanvres -	1 Ounce 4 drachms.
Oxide of Titanium -	1-2 drachm, 4 grains.
Oxide of gold - -	1-8 grain, exact weight.*
Filings of Platina -	2 grains.

Put the earth of Vanvres on a plate, and grind it with the muller; add the oxides and filings of platina and grind again; at length, when these ingredients are fine and well amalgamated, add, by little and little, the kaolin; continue to grind, until they are all exactly mixed, and make a very fine and very unctuous clay.

At length, when the substances are sufficiently divided and mixed, which may be known when the particles can be felt no longer under the muller, and of an extreme fineness, this clay is put in a vessel of porcelain, for which a whalebone knife is to be used.

It is advantageous, as we have already remarked, to keep the clay in a cellar, which considerably improves it.

I believe it my duty to make known, that to make a quantity of paste or enamel, it takes a workman one day's work.

---

* I understand by exact, that the two plates of the scale remain in equilibrium, and by good weight, that in which the oxide is in bears down the other, which is indicated by the weight.

Enamel, No 1.

Pètunzè,	- - -	7 ounces.
Kaolin,	- - -	3 drachms.
Oxide of titanium	-	1-2 drachm 4 grains.
Oxide of gold,	- -	1-8 grain, exact weight.

Put the oxides and the kaolin on the plate, and grind intimately; at length, when these ingredients are mixed, and very fine, add, by little and little, the pètunzè, and grind well, in the same way we directed when speaking about the clay

The greatest care should be taken in the preparation of the enamel, for the least negligence in the manipulation becomes very prejudicial; the little particles of the colouring substances, badly divided, get on the surface of the teeth, and produce spots, which prove that the operation of grinding has been incomplete.

If, on the contrary, all the ingredients have been perfectly mixed and divided, the enamel will be every where even, and the teeth will then have the greatest beauty.

The enamel, like the clay, is kept in a vessel of porcelain, constantly moistened.

Paste, No. 2.

Kaolin,	- - -	6 ounces.
Earth of Vanvres,	-	1 ounce, 4 drachms.
Oxide of titanium,	-	1-2 drachm, 14 grains.
Oxide of gold,	- -	1-8 grain, good weight.
Filings of platina,	-	2 grains.

Mix, and grind like it is directed above.

Enamel, No. 2.

Pètunzè, - - -	7 ounces.
Kaolin, - - -	3 drachms.
Oxide of titanium, -	1-2 drachm, 24 grains.
Oxide of gold, - -	1-8 grain, good weight.

Grind all these things, &c.

Paste, No. 3.

Kaolin, - - -	6 ounces.
Earth of Vanvres, -	1 ounce, 4 drachms.
Oxide of titanium, -	1-2 drachm, 24 grains.
Oxide of gold, - -	1-4 of a grain.
Filings of platina, -	2 grains.

Grind, &c.

Enamel, No. 3.

Pètunzè, - - -	7 ounces.
Kaolin, - - -	3 drachms.
Oxide of titanium, -	1-2 drachm, 24 grains.
Oxide of gold, - -	1-4 of a grain.

Grind, &c.

Paste, No. 4.

Kaolin, - - -	6 ounces.
Earth of Vanvres, -	1 ounce, 4 drachms.
Oxide of titanium, -	1-2 drachm, 34 grains.
Oxide of gold, - -	1-4 of a grain.
Filings of platina, -	2 grains.

Grind, &c.

Enamel, No. 4.

Pètunzè, - - -	7 ounces.
Kaolin, - - -	3 drachms.
Oxide of titanium, -	1-2 drachm, 34 grains.
Oxide of gold, - -	1-4 of a grain.

Grind, &c.

Paste, No. 5.

Kaolin, - - -	4 ounces.
Earth of Vanvres, -	4 drachms.
Oxide of titanium, -	1-2 drachm, 26 grains.
Oxide of zinc, - -	32 grains.
Oxide of gold, - -	1-4 of a grain.
Filings of platina, -	1 grain.

Grind, &c.

Enamel, No. 5.

Pètunzè, - - -	4 ounces, 2 drachms.
Kaolin, - - -	1 1-2 drachms.
Oxide of titanium, -	1-2 drachm, 26 grains.
Oxide of zinc, - -	32 grains.
Oxide of gold, - -	1-4 of a grain.

Grind, &c.

Paste, No. 6.

Kaolin, - - -	4 ounces.
Earth of Vanvres, -	4 drachms.
Oxide of titanium, -	1-2 drachm, 26 grains.

Oxide of zinc, - - 32 grains.
Filings of platina, - 1 grain.

Grind, &c.

Observation.—The Paste No. 6, inserted with the enamels No. 6 and 17.

Enamel, No. 6.

Pètunzè, - - - 4 ounces, 2 drachms.
Kaolin, - - - 1 1-2 drachms.
Oxide of titanium, - 1 drachm.
Oxide of gold, - - 1-4 of a grain.

Grind, &c.

Paste, No. 9.

Kaolin, - - - 1 ounce, 4 drachms.
Earth of Vanvres, - 2 drachms.
Oxide of titanium, - 1-2 drachm.
Filings of standard gold, 2 grains.
Filings of platina, - 2 grains.

Grind, &c.

Enamel, No. 9.

Pètunzè, - - - 2 ounces.
Kaolin, - - - 24 grains.
Oxide of titanium, - 16 grains.
Filings of standard gold, 2 grains.

Grind, &c.

Paste, No. 10.

Kaolin, - - - 6 ounces.
Earth of Vanvres, - 1 ounce, 4 drachms.

Oxide of titanium, - 2 drachms, 16 grains.
Oxide of gold, - - 1-4 of a grain.
Filings of platina, - 2 grains.
Grind, &c.

Observation.—The paste No. 10, inserted with the enamels Nos. 10, 11 and 12.

Enamel, No. 10.

Pètunzè, - - - 7 ounces.
Kaolin, - - - 3 drachms.
Oxide of titanium, - 2 drachms, 16 grains.
Oxide of gold, - - 1-4 of a grain.
Grind, &c.

Enamel No. 11.

Pètunzè, - - - 7 ounces.
Kaolin, - - - 3 drachms.
Oxide of titanium, - 2 drachms, 16 grains.
Oxide of gold, - - 1-4 grain, good weight.
Grind, &c.

Enamel, No. 12.

Pètunzè, - - - 7 ounces.
Kaolin, - - - 1 1-2 drachms.
Earth of Vanvres, - 1 1-2 drachms.
Oxide of titanium, - 2 drachms, 16 grains.
Oxide of gold, - - 1-4 grain, good weight.
Grind, &c.

Paste, No. 13.

Kaolin,	- - -	6 ounces.
Earth of Vanvres,	- -	1 ounce, 4 grains.
Oxide of titanium,	-	2 drachms, 26 grains.
Oxide of gold,	- -	1-4 grain, good weight.
Filings of platina,	- -	2 grains.

Grind, &c.

Enamel, No. 13.

Pètunzè,	- -	7 ounces.
Kaolin,	- - -	3 drachms.
Oxide of titanium,	-	3 drachms, 26 grains.
Oxide of gold,	- -	1-4 grain, good weight.

Grind, &c.

Paste, No. 14.

Kaolin,	- - -	6 ounces.
Earth of Vanvres,	-	1 ounce, 4 drachms.
Oxide of titanium,	-	2 1-2 drachms.
Oxide of gold,	- -	1-4 grain, good weight.
Filings of platina,	-	2 grains, grind, &c.

Observation.—The paste No. 14, is inserted with the enamels Nos. 14, 15 and 16.

Enamel, No. 14.

Pètunzè,	- - -	7 ounces.
Kaolin,	- - -	3 drachms.
Oxide of titanium	-	2 1-2 drachms.
Oxide of gold	- -	1-4 grain, good weight.

Grind, &c.

Enamel, No. 15.

Pètunzè, - - -	7 ounces.
Kaolin, - - -	1 1-2 drachms.
Oxide of titanium, -	2 1-2 drachms.
Earth of Vanvres, - -	1 1-2 drachms.
Oxide of gold, - -	1-4 grain, good weight.

Grind, &c.

Enamel, No. 16.

Pètunzè, - - -	7 ounces.
Kaolin, - - -	3 drachms.
Oxide of titanium, -	2 1-2 drachms.
Oxide of gold, - -	1-4 grain, good weight.

Grind, &c.

Paste, No. 17.

Kaolin, - - -	3 ounces.
Earth of Vanvres, -	5 drachms.
Oxide of manganese, -	25 grains.
Oxide of titanium, -	25 grains.
Oxide of gold, - -	1-4 grain, very exact.
Filings of platina, -	1 1-2 grains.

Grind, &c.

Observation.—The paste No. 17, is inserted with the enamels Nos. 17 and 18.

Enamel, No. 17.

Pètunzè - - -	4 ounces.
Kaolin, - - -	1 drachm.

Oxide of manganese,	-	25 grains.
Oxide of titanium,	-	25 grains.
Oxide of gold,	- -	1-4 grain, very exact.

Grind, &c.

Enamel No. 18.

Pètunzè,	- - -	4 ounces.
Kaolin,	- - -	1 drachm.
Oxide of manganese,	-	34 grains.
Oxide of titanium,	-	34 grains.
Oxide of gold,	- -	1-4 grain, very exact.

Grind, &c.

Paste No. 19.

Kaolin,	- - -	1 ounce. 4 drachms.
Earth of Vanvres,	-	2 drachms.
Oxide of titanium,	-	1-2 drachm, 9 grains.
Filings of standard gold,		2 1-2 grains.
Filings of platina,	-	3 grains.

Grind, &c.

Enamel, No. 19.

Pètunzè,	- - -	2 ounces.
Kaolin,	- - -	24 grains.
Oxide of titanium,	-	1-2 drachm, 9 grains.
Filings of standard gold,		2 1-2 grains.

Grind, &c.

Paste No. 20.

Kaolin, - - -	6 ounces.
Earth of Vanvres, -	1 ounce, 4 drachms.
Oxide of titanium, - -	2 1-2 drachms, 20 grs.
Oxide of gold, - -	1-2 grain, very exact.
Filings of platina, -	2 grains.

Observation.—The paste No. 20, is inserted with the enamels, Nos. 20 and 21.

Enamel, No. 20.

Pètunzè, - - -	7 ounces.
Kaolin, - - -	3 drachms.
Oxide of titanium, -	2 1-2 drachms, 20 grs.
Oxide of gold, - -	1-2 grain, very exact.

Grind, &c.

Enamel, No. 21.

Pètunzè, - - -	7 ounces.
Kaolin, - - -	1 1-2 drachms.
Earth of Vanvres, -	1 1-2 drachms.
Oxide of titanium, -	3 drachms.
Oxide of gold, - -	1-2 grain, good weight.

Grind, &c.

Paste, No. 22.

Kaolin, - - -	1 ounce, 4 drachms.
Earth of Vanvres, -	2 drachms.
Oxide of titanium, -	1-2 drachm, 19 grains.
Filings of standard gold,	3 grains.

Filings of platina, - 2 1-2 grains.

Grind, &c.

Enamel, No. 22.

Pètunzè, - - -	2 ounces.
Kaolin, - - -	24 grains.
Oxide of titanium, -	35 grains.
Filings of standard gold,	3 grains.

Grind, &c.

Paste, No 23.

Kaolin, - - .	6 ounces.
Earth of Vanvres - -	1 ounce, 4 drachms.
Oxide of titanium, -	3 drachms.
Oxide of gold, - -	1-4 grain, good weight.
Filings of platina, -	2 grains.

Grind, &c.

Enamel No. 23.

Pètunzè, - - -	7 ounces,
Kaolin, - - -	3 drachms,
Oxide of titanium, -	3 drachms,
Oxide of Gold, - -	1-4 of a grain, good weight,

Grind, &c.

Paste No. 24.

Kaolin, - - -	3 ounces,
Earth of Vanvres, -	6 drachms,
Oxide of titanium, -	1 1-2 drachms,
Oxide of Gold, - -	1-2 a grain, very exact,
Filings of Platina, -	1 grain.

Grind, &c.

Enamel No. 24.

Pètunzè, - - - 4 ounces 2 drachms,
Kaolin, - - - 1 1-2 drachms,
Oxide of Titanium, - - 1 1-2 drachms 10 grains,
Oxide of Gold, - - 3-4 of a grain, very exact,
Grind, &c.

Paste No. 25.

Kaolin, - - - 8 ounces,
Earth of Vanvres, - 1 ounce 4 drachms,
Oxide of Titanium, - 2 drachms 12 grains,
Ammoniated muriate of
platina, - - - 1-4 of a grain, very exact,
Oxide of Gold, - - 1-4 of a grain, good weight,
Grind, &c.

Observation.—The paste No. 25 is inserted with those of the enamels Nos. 25 and 26.

Enamel No. 25.

Pètunzè, - - - 8 ounces 4 drachms,
Kaolin, - - - 4 drachms,
Oxide of Titanium, - 2 drachms 12 grains,
Ammoniated muriate of
platina, - - - 1-4 of a grain, very exact,
Oxide of Gold, - - 1-4 of a grain,
Grind, &c.

Enamel No. 26.

Pètunzè, - - - 8 ounces 4 drachms,
Kaolin, - - - 4 drachms,

Oxide of Titanium, - 2 1-2 drachms,
Ammoniated muriate of
platina, - - - 1-4 of a grain,
Oxide of Gold, - - 1-2 a grain,
Grind, &c.

Paste No. 27.

To make sets of a single piece, after the first process:
Kaolin, - - - 1 ounce 4 drachms,
Kaolin having been once put into a porcelain furnace, } 4 drachms,
Earth of Vanvres, - 4 drachms,
Earth d'encollage,* 4 drachms,
Oxide of Gold, - - 2 1-2 grains,
Grind, &c.

I thought it convenient to make the paste of a rose colour, that the gums might have their proper colour.

The only precaution which one must take after the piece is moulded, is, to keep back a little of the paste, having the number of the enamel which we wish to employ, and to lightly mark the teeth by means of a pencil. This coat, once dried, is enamelled in the way we spoke of in paragraph 18 of this section.

Enamel No. 27.

Used for enamelling the parts of pieces with which the gums are figured.

Pètunzè, - - - 2 ounces,

---

* This earth, called d'encollage, is to be had from the manufacturers of porcelain; it incorporates itself into the pastes which they make use of to execute the most difficult flowers, without which would break their extreme delicacy. This earth is nothing more than Kaolin mixed with a little gum Arabic.

Kaolin, - - - - 3 drachms,
Oxide of Gold, - - 3 grains,

Grind, &c.

See the manner of using this enamel, Section V. paragraphs 1 *and* 2.

Paste No. 28.

Proper for making single pieces, but without gums.

Kaolin, - - - 2 ounces,
Kaolin once put into the potters' porcelain furnace, } 2 ounces,
Earth of Vanvres, - 2 ounces,
Earth d'encollage, - 1 ounce 4 drachms,
Oxide of Titanium, - 2 1-2 drachms,
Oxide of Gold, - - 3-8 of a grain,
Filings of Platina, - - 3 grains,

Grind, &c.

This paste can be enamelled with all the enamels indistinctly, that is, at the option of the artist; but he ought to be acquainted with all the tints, to be able to make a proper use of the enamel which he wants.

Without this particular knowledge, he will be liable to make wrong tints of pieces, which will not be like those of the natural teeth.

All the formulas of pastes and enamels which we use, are known by a number; in using, the number of the enamel which corresponds with that of the paste, and that which is used for enamelling the teeth made with the paste, having the same number. This plan has appeared necessary to us to establish order in our work. But we ought to observe, also, that, for increasing the number of the tints, the pastes may be enamelled with the enamels in which the numbers do not correspond. It is by this means we obtain a vast number of shades, which would be difficult to obtain by other means.

Having, at length, given various formulas for the, composition of the pastes and enamels which serve to establish the different shades of the teeth, and to actually suit every mouth, we shall now speak of the manner in which the moulds are made intended for modelling the teeth.

§ XII.—*Manner of Making the Moulds that are used for Incorruptible Teeth.*

We have observed in the second section of this work, that the teeth made of porcelain, are wanting, generally, in shape, which is never natural; for we cannot repeat it too much, the exact imitation depends upon three indispensable conditions: 1st. the shape; 2d. the position; 3d. the colour. And it is certain, if the artificial teeth want any of these conditions, they will not completely imitate the natural ones: but if, on the contrary, they come up to it, they approach the natural ones as much as possible.

To arrive at this point, it is necessary to have moulds that faithfully represent the natural teeth. For that purpose, punches of iron must be made, imitating in fineness of shape, the true teeth, and augmenting their diameter at least one third more than is natural, which admits of their retracting when submitted to the baking process.

These punches serve to stamp the little moulds of copper which are soldered to a band of white iron, after having been first prepared and stamped.

§ XIII.—*Manner of Making the Cramps of Incorruptible Teeth.**

The cramps which are introduced into incorruptible teeth, are of such importance for solidly mounting them on the backs, that the way to fix these cramps is not altogether a matter of indifference.

All the dentists are so well aware of the necessity of fixing them firmly, that each one prepares them in the manner which appears to him the most advantageous; but he has certain difficulties to overcome which are not always crowned with success. We have seen, on many occasions, teeth made by them, wherein the cramps were not solid, and where the teeth were easily separated. This remark is made by all those who use the incorruptible teeth, which has varied them into numberless shapes by the introduction of cramps; for our part, we think it useless to single out here those that are good for nothing, and we will limit ourselves to speaking of those which we use, and which we have adopted after having been convinced they are better than all the others.

To make cramps, take platina wire of a middling thickness, pass it through the screw hole of a vice, then plate it lightly: at length, being flattened sufficiently, without taking it out of the vice, which ought to rest upon its sides, cut the cramps of a sufficient length, and if you do not find the notch of the vice sharp enough, cut it more with the file; the cramps made in this manner can be well fixed in the tooth, and will never come out without breaking. *See at length the manner of modelling incorruptible teeth.*

---

* These are little pivots of metal, placed in the tooth before baking, which, after the baking, allow of being soldered to plates for insertion in the tooth.

We may, if we will, make cramps more simple than those we have spoken of. Draw out a platina wire to a middling thickness, after which it must be flattened; cut the cramps of a sufficient length, before cutting out each piece, with a cutting pincers.

There is another excellent way of making cramps, to which no objection can be made; it well fills up all the conditions; it is a misfortune it can only be employed for teeth furnished with talons or pivots. It consists in making screws of platina wire of a convenient size, then cut each vice about two lines in length; then prepare, with a file, the end which corresponds to the summit of the talon, and a hole is pierced in the middle. This hole is made for receiving a pin which is also soldered to the plate. *See the manner of mounting teeth with talons, Section V. paragraph* 8. This same hole which I have carefully bored through, serves again to pass through a screw, which permits me to mount, sometimes, incorruptible teeth on gold bases.

§ XIV.—*Manner of Modelling Incorruptible Teeth.*

The operation which has for its consideration the modelling of the teeth, appears to be, at first sight, of the least importance, and of no moment; it is, nevertheless, very essential, and requires to be well done. We shall give different precautions, and to which much attention should be given.

Before modelling the teeth, the paste should be made very unctuous, well kneaded with the fingers; and, that it may not become too liquid, it is necessary to put a certain quantity on a dry plate, that all the humidity may be absorbed; then they fill all the moulds or matrices with one of the pastes which we have prescribed. It is a practice, by means of a little square piece of platina, to give to the posterior part of the tooth, a verticle groove, on the sides of which are sunk (while the paste remains soft) two cramps, made with platina wire prepared for this purpose. It is also necessary, that the tooth may be more susceptible of being firmly soldered, to implant a third cramp a little lower than the two first, and in the middle of the groove upon the side of the triturating surface.

After this manner as many teeth may be moulded as are wished.

They are left to dry in their moulds: they may then be detached very easily; it is sufficient to unfold the band that the teeth may fall out.

§ xv.—*Of Incorruptible Teeth with Talons.*

Ever since the making of incorruptible teeth has been thought of, the necessity of making them with talons has always been felt; that is to say, equal, in all respects, to natural teeth.

If the dentists who have adopted them, had not made any to the teeth they fabricate, and contented themselves only with imitating the exterior surface, which is what they pretend to, than in making the incorruptible teeth thus, there would be more facility in mounting; and altogether less trouble in adjusting them to the mouth, because the teeth which are opposed to the artificial piece, finding less obstacle in the way, would not misplace, and consequently derange them. But the artist who, in his labours, would equal nature as much as possible, ought he to give up the work, because he meets with obstacles? No, certainly not; he ought, on the contrary, to redouble his efforts and his patience.

The subject with which we are occupied is well worth the trouble; and having also given it all our application, it is with some satisfaction that we communicate the means we have employed for making teeth with talons, susceptible of being mounted on plates like natural teeth, not on riveted pins, but on soldered pins; also by means of the screws, which we were one of the first to adopt, for mounting natural teeth, because this process is the best and most firm, although differing from the opinions of certain dentists.

To arrange teeth with talons, take a piece of paste, knead it between the fingers, and give it the shape of a crown of the tooth; put this tooth in a matrice,* in order that it may imitate nature. Introduce, in the mean time, in the middle of the talon and near the top, a screw of small dimensions, and about a line and a half long; this screw having been previously pierced in its centre, is intended to simulate the dental canal in the incorruptible tooth.

It is in the hole of this screw that the pin is soldered, after the tooth has been adjusted on the plate or on the screw, for it is on the screw the teeth ought to be mounted.

§ XVI.—*Manner of Making Incorruptible Grinding Teeth.*

If the perfect imitation of incisor and canine teeth was difficult, those of the grinders was yet more so. It is not to be wondered at that these last have not been imitated, and that the dentists have been limited to making the square plates with which they replace the grinding teeth; but this way of supplying them is inconvenient and arbitrary. Our first care has been to find out a way of imitation that approaches nearest to nature: to attain which, see here, what we have done.

In one of the preceding paragraphs, we recommended the

---

* I call matrice the moulds in which I model the teeth.

steel punches which exactly represent the shape of the natural teeth. We have made them that imitated grinding teeth of all sizes. We used the precaution to make them of an equal diameter at the top of their crowns, as well as at their collars, in order that the teeth moulded in the matrices made with these strong punches, when they became dried, might be easily taken out.

We have introduced into their interior, and by the part that ought to rest on the plate, a single cramp of the smallest screw, and two to the largest. We have again made to those we have implanted, a third cramp, on their exterior surface, to supply the vacancy, and adapt it to proper levers for fixing sets of teeth: in one word, we have made, and we are sure they can be made of all sorts of shapes, before they have undergone the baking process. In modelling they are straightened, and given the finest proportions, in order that they may have a most perfect imitation. In fine, nothing is impossible for an intelligent artist to do.

§ XVII.—*Manner of Hardening Incorruptible Teeth.*

What is called hardening, is performed by first exposing the teeth to a strong charcoal fire: after that, having put them in a crucible placed in a mass of live charcoal, which is left to entirely consume, and when the crucible is cold, the teeth are taken out, which must be carefully scraped.

By this preliminary baking, the cramps have already acquired by this means a certain solidity, which permits their being handled without fear of breaking them.

§ XVIII.—*Manner of Enamelling Incorruptible Teeth.*

The beauty of our teeth consists principally in the manner in which they are enamelled. The precise plastering of the enamel is no less necessary to their preservation, and is what protects them from exterior causes; for which reason one cannot bestow too much care in its preparation. If the paste has not been well ground, the enamel ought to be the more attended to. We have already made known the manner of preparing it; it now remains for us to speak of the manner of applying it to incorruptible teeth.

Presuming it to be in a state of extreme division, it may be applied to the exterior surface of the teeth, by means of a feather pencil.

Each tooth is fixed on the end of a match furnished with wax for modelling it; this wax is to hold the tooth by means of the cramps which penetrate; then there is laid on the surface of the tooth a sufficient quantity of enamel; care must be taken that the enamel is neither too thick nor too thin, for in either case the enamelling will be badly done.

The teeth are placed, one by one, on a platina grate, made expressly to facilitate their drying.

After being sufficiently dried, and the enamel adhered to the paste, they are put with care in a box, to be taken to the potter's porcelain furnace; they are shut up again in a casket sprinkled with sand, and in placing one along side of the other, they must not touch one another, for fear that during the baking, they will adhere together during the fusion of the enamel, which may happen in despite of all our pains.

It is here we repeat, it must be recommended to the potter to put the casket to the charge, for the reasons which we have assigned in the preceding paragraph.*

In the application of enamel, there exists another method, which we have equally employed. It is this: make enamel of the same consistence as that one the paste; put a certain portion in the bottom of the mould; put again upon the enamel a sufficient quantity of paste; fill up the mould as usual; make the grooves of which we have spoken, and put on the cramps.

The teeth moulded thus, need not undergo the operation of hardening; they are then put in a porcelain furnace, without having previously undergone a preparatory baking.

In the mean while, having spoken of the processes in the manipulation of divers pastes, and of enamels to suit them, as well as the manner of modelling the teeth, we believe it will be useful to give here the formulas proposed by M. Delabarre, in order to present, in the same compass, all that belongs to the confection of incorruptible teeth, and let every one judge to what extent we have simplified the processes.

Pastes proper for making the bases, according to M. Delabarre.

"The amalgams following," says this practician, "fill up all the desirable conditions."

White Paste.

Paste of the manufactories of porcelain,	20	parts,
Sand, grey or white silex, - -	1	part.

*At Paris they are baked with advantage at the manufactory of Mad. Crèmière, Menil-Montant street, No. 48.

Coloured Paste.

Paste of Porcelain, - - - -	20 parts,
Sand, - - - - - - -	1 part,
Alumine or infusible earth, - -	1-2 a part,

Whatever oxide you will, 150 décigrammes by 1-2 kilogrammes.

Sprinkle it with water and mix it well on glass with a muller, or on a porcelain plate, or, finally, in a mill.

Mass of white Enamel used for the Composition of Colouring Enamels.

Glazing of porcelain makers, - -	5 to 6 parts,
Porcelain earth, - - - -	3 parts.

This mixture is not more, in its present state, than half fused, but the oxides which are put in to colour it, give it that colour which it ought to have.

"Take any portion you will of this amalgam, join with it some centigrammes of metallic oxide with thirty grammes, and in order to vary the shades to advantage, make a reunion of the different oxides. Grind on glass for some time, in order that the colouring matter may well mix.

"Among the oxides that resist the heat of the porcelain fire, the best, says M. Delabarre, (and are, in consequence, less got at in the fabrication of calliodontes,*) the following may be mentioned, which are used on account of their colouring properties."

---

* This denomination was proposed by Ricci: M. Delabarre has adopted it; in mean while it appears to us wrong, because it does not designate clearly enough artificial incorruptible teeth; and why introduce a new denomination, while that which is most generally known is so precise.

Oxides arranged according to the degree of colouration they give to the enamels.		For 4 grammes.		Colours in.
	Cobalt to	0 grammes	0000535	blue.
	Platina	0 grammes	0000535	dark blue.
	Gold	0 grammes	00134	violet and red.
	Bismuth	0 grammes	00268	blue gray.
	Mercury	0 grammes	00268	gray.
	Silver	0 grammes	00268	yellow-white.
	Iron	0 grammes	00669	yellow-red.
	Manganese	0 grammes	01338	gray.
	Uranium	0 grammes	05350	pale yellow.
	Titanium	0 grammes	10700	pale yellow.
	Antimony	0 grammes	21400	yellow.

"As to the remainder, there is nothing absolute in the table which I have just presented," says M. Delabarre, "it is for the artist to make trials.

"In making the application, as above, I present some examples of the composition of coloured enamels."

Enamel composed after the manner which I have spoken of:

	4 grammes.	Millim.	
Oxide of titanium -	0 - -	32100	Mix them on glass, with water charged with gum Arabic.
Enamel composition	4 - -		
Red oxide of iron -	0 - -	03560	
Enamel composition -	4 - -		
Black oxide of iron -	0 - -	01338	
Oxide of manganese	0 - -	05350	
White oxide of lead -	0 - -	02675	

M. Delabarre, like other dentists, having felt the necessity of making pieces to embellish the gums, in order to remedy the depression of the edge of the alveolus, and thus make the artificial teeth of a natural length, has thought of making a paste which may serve for the base of incorruptible teeth, already baked in the furnace of the porcelain manufacturer. This paste is made very fusible by the addition of a solvent, in order to be able to vitrify it in a furnace with a current of air constructed in a chimney. *See a description of this furnace in his work*, vol. i. page 128.

This is the formula he uses for this purpose:

"Porcelain paste	- -	7 parts.
Calcined gypsum	- -	1 part.
White sand	- - -	1-20 of the mass.

Which oxide you please, 150 grammes by kilogrammes. Grind perfectly.

See how M. Delabarre expresses himself in making application of the following composition.

"I make use of the calliodontes very thin, and without cramps, but they are first baked by a porcelain fire. I proportion them in shape of the teeth on a grind-stone of stone: therefore this is a kind of inlaid work. When I wish to make a set of teeth with gums, I take of the above paste, I place it on the model, and let it dry; after that, I notch in the front little hollow places, in which I resemble it to joiner's work, which I size with a little gum-water; I insert a little collar of paste, which I carve in imitation of the festoons of the gums; afterwards I put a light coat of porcelain coverings, equally melted with gypsum, and sometimes with a little of the crystal of Mount Cenis.

"This joined work reunites with so much solidity in baking, that the percussion which would break the whole would not separate one part from the others.

"It is well to assure oneself of the solidity of the smallest sized pieces, in fixing upon them, before baking a base or bottom of platina, which is always understood, which will prevent them from falling into pieces, if they crack in the furnace, and which will facilitate the reunion, by means of enamel and a new application of the fire. In fine, if one or many of the teeth spoken of becomes deranged, it will be easy to carry them at once to the wheel of the lapidary, and to substitute others. For the rest, this accident may be foreseen and avoided by lifting up the pieces, which is done by the porcelain artists.

This paste is employed again by M. Delabarre, in the following manner, and he thus expresses himself:

"When I mount a set of teeth on a plate, I apply the paste here spoken of, behind the teeth, and afterwards in their interstices, in a manner to form them solely in front of the points of the gums, and on an inclined plane behind.

When there exists much sinking of the alveolus, pivots are then soldered to a stamped plate; after that, all the teeth being cut out after suitable dimensions, they are strung by the little pivots which are fixed behind, taking care that the edge of the masticator accords with the opposite row of teeth, after which the solder is melted; they are then tried in the mouth, their defects corrected, which then becomes quite easy, after that it is removed to adjust the pivots, in order to make them give the teeth the declivity we wish, or I might say, that it was very useful. Then a bottom or base is soldered, or circular bars, which, by keeping them in their respective separations, gives them much solidity. In fine, they are garnished with white earth, which is put around the edges of each tooth in the plate.

"These divers pieces are baked before they are enamelled, because they always make blemishes in several places: they are then covered over with new earth. In fine, the preparation may be extremely thin, and in consequence be much lighter in the pieces of large dimensions, and having less height before; at length, when there yet remains some good teeth, they should be fixed to the best advantage for patients. The paste which is put in the interstices agglutinates, and makes it quite solid, giving much beauty to the work."

In resuming the subject, it will be seen, that by the addition of a mineral solvent, the material of the porcelain is rendered much more fusible than that which we make. The dentists might make themselves sufficiently acquainted with these facts to bake it for imitating the gums.

"In this last case, the calliodontes, which might have been vitrified at the fire of the manufacturers, on trial, does not differ from that which has been placed in their furnaces."

To colour the base which shapes the gum, see in what manner it is handled by M. Delabarre; he expresses himself thus:

"I properly bake the bar—if any crevices are formed in it, I stop them up with earth, a little more delicate than the first; then I place a covering over it while the fusibility is going on, and raise the heat to the degree that is calculated for its semi-vitrification. I incorporate a small quantity of the muriate of gold, I put it in the furnace, and I stop the heat the moment I obtain the shade I wish; for it is essential to not forget that the more the pieces are submitted to its action, the less the colour is deepened."

In reproducing here the proceedings of M. Delabarre, we ought not to omit observing, that the last, having for its discussion the confection of artificial gums, was susceptible of rendering, in practice, the greatest services, if its execution did not require the most particular care, and a number of precautions of which few artists are capable.

In the following section we shall speak of the best means of mounting incorruptible teeth, to be then fixed and set in the mouth, without the least possible injury to the solidity of the natural teeth, to which they should be attached either with ligatures or elastic blades.

Porcelain teeth are mounted and fastened in the mouth, in nearly the same manner as those from animal material. They are soldered to plates, by means of a platina talon, or claw, which is put in the porcelain tooth previously to the baking. If inserted on fangs of teeth with pivots, these are in nearly all cases made of platina or gold. If ligatures are intended to be used, holes are made through the porcelain piece, into which the ligature is passed.

DENTAL SURGERY.

It is purposed in this part of our work to take a general notice of the different substances and preparations used by surgeon-dentists and physicians in the treatment of the teeth, gums &c. of which I will enumerate the following:

I.—Acids.

II.—Alkalies and Saponaceous substances.

III.—Astringents.

IV.—Stimulants, Anodynes, Narcotics, &c.

V.—Caustics.

VI.—Mechanical Substances.

CHAPTER I.

DENTAL PHARMACY.

It will readily occur to every reflecting mind, that in the exceedingly variegated treatment of the teeth, gums, &c. both for the cure of their diseases, and the preservation of their health and beauty, that a great variety of medicines and substances will be used. This is the case to a very considerable extent. It is not my intention to give the history of all the different substances used, or their therapeutic application, any farther than is indispensable to a correct understanding of their effects upon the teeth, gums, &c.; leaving the particular history of these substances to be studied in the different valuable works upon the materia medica. I wish to embody in this work all the formula of dental medicines that may be useful, which are to be found in the works of the different authors who have written upon this subject; besides many new formula of my own, with the mode of preparing them, with observations upon their modes of exhibition, and upon their indications and utility or pernicious qualities, &c. I am not aware that any work of this kind, is now extant upon this subject in the English language, and I flatter myself, that this part of our work, will be found useful to the dentist the physician, and the public at large. I have chosen to give many formula of medicines, which are pernicious, or may be so, if not properly used, in order to place physicians and surgeon-dentists upon their guard against using these pernicious substances. For I consider that truth and propriety, are both better illustrated by exhibiting their opposites.

SECTION I.

ACIDS.

The acids were formerly used to a considerable extent; but as in all sciences and arts, the progress of knowledge, the increase of experience and correct principles, dissipate early prejudices and pernicious customs, and pave the way to those judicious modes of practice which prove honorable to the profession, and useful to all mankind. This is the case with the acids: their use is now nearly exploded, and should be almost entirely, by every judicious practitioner of the dental art. We have previously noticed when speaking of the composition of enamel, that it was, as regards the circulation, extraneous, and acted upon only by chemical or mechanical agents. We also noticed that it was composed chiefly of the carbonate of lime, a little animal matter, with a large proportion of phosphoric acid. "Now," says Mr. Lord, "by examining the tables of elective attraction, we shall find that there are four, and only four acids, that precede the phosphoric in their affinity for lime; the oxalic, sulphuric, tartaric, and succinic."* Not only these, but all the acids, appear to exert a baneful influence upon the teeth, by weakening and dissolving the enamel, and by inflaming the substance of the tooth. The muriatic, nitric, tartaric, and even the concentrated acetic, are capable of injuring or destroying the teeth. All the quack remedies advertised in the form of lotions to clean the teeth and remove the tartar, have acids for their bases, and clean the teeth by removing a portion of their substance. Although they render the teeth white and of a chalky appearance at first, yet soon they become darker than before, and if the use of acids is persisted in for any length of time, destruction of the teeth will follow.

There can hardly be a doubt that even the milder acids, if used to any considerable extent, will exert a baneful influence upon the teeth.

---

* See Good's Study of Medicine, Vol. I. pages 34—35.

The strong acids have been used to destroy the nerves of the teeth; but as they are apt to injure the sound teeth, their use is almost entirely abandoned.

Acids are occasionally prescribed for medical purposes; in which case they ought to be passed through the mouth by means of a tube, as a quill, &c.; by which precaution they will be prevented from injuring the teeth.

Persons who erect the acid contents of their stomachs into their mouths, ought to rinse their teeth very frequently with some alkaline fluid; as, if they do not, their teeth are often injured by the acid of the stomach.

I will in this place, introduce the observations of Mr. Pepys, in his communication to Mr. Fox, containing the analysis of the human teeth, and the effects of some of the acids upon them, and close with the remarks of Dr. Blake and Mr. Wooffendale, upon the weaker acids, cream of tartar, and the acetic acid, from which may be inferred the injurious consequences of all.

* Bone, it has been observed, when exposed to the action of acid menstrua, becomes dissolved; that is to say, the solid or constituent substance of it is abstracted, and a gelatinous matter is left of the form of the original bone.

Nitric, muriatic, and acetic acids are capable of producing this change, which is accompanied with a liberation of an aeriform fluid, that precipitates lime in lime water, changes vegetable blues red, and, by its gravity, is known to be carbonate acid gas. These acid solutions yield a copious precipitate with pure ammonia, which is again soluble in either of the acids. After the precipitation by pure ammonia, the solution of the carbonate of ammonia, will still produce a new precipitate.

---

* Fox, Natural History of the Teeth, page 93.

* The great solubility of the phosphate of lime, in even the weakest of the acids, is very extraordinary: phosphate of lime mechanically suspended in water, is speedily and completely dissolved, by passing a copious stream of carbonic acid gas through it.

Sulphuric acid, of the specific gravity 1.83, appears at first to have no action: in the course of an hour small bubbles are perceived, the roots became blackened, and in twelve hours the enamelled part bursts, cracks, and separates, accompanied with an evident formation of selenite by the action of the acid on the lime which enters into the composition of the teeth.

Nitric and muriatic acid, of the specific gravity 1.12, act instantly on the tooth, accompanied with an evolution of a quantity of small air bubbles from the whole of the surface. About eight times their weight of these acids, are sufficient for the solution of the solidifying principles of the teeth. The mass left undissolved has nearly the original form of the tooth, is flexible, semi-transparent, and easily divided with the nail.

The dilute acetous acid (distilled vinegar) has a very trifling action, but when concentrated, acts both on the phosphate and carbonate of lime.

Boiling nitric acid, acts strongly on the teeth, with the evolution of carbonic acid, and a considerable quantity of azotic gas. The gelatine and solid substance are dissolved as the surfaces present themselves, but the operation being stopped at any part of the process, the residuum is firm and hard, but reduced in size, proportioned to the time the tooth has been acted upon.

---

* Fox, Natural History of the Teeth, pages 94 to 96.

Mr. Blake observes,* "The tooth-powders commonly sold, consist in a great measure of the cream of tartar, by the use of which, I have seen the teeth completely deprived of their cortex striatus, and the patients rendered quite miserable; for the bony part of the tooth in such cases, becomes sensible to the slightest touch, and also to the slightest changes of temperature in the atmosphere, or other fluids received into the mouth. Cream of tartar alone, has been recommended by Mr. Hunter as a tooth-powder, because, as he says, at the same time that it acts mechanically, it has likewise a chemical power, and dissolves this adventitious matter."†

To ascertain the bad effects of cream of tartar as a tooth-powder, I made the following simple experiment, which will at once explain how very detrimental the use of it must be, even in the smallest proportion. I placed a tooth in a solution of cream of tartar and water, and allowed it to remain in it for about twelve hours. When taken out, I observed that the surface of the cortex striatus was quite rough, and according as it became dry, it appeared sprinkled over with an immense number of small crystals, though very few were observable on the root. The formation of these crystals can be easily accounted for; the acid of tartar has a greater affinity to calcareous earth, than it has to the vegetable alkali, with which it is combined in cream of tartar; a double elective attraction of course takes place when a tooth is immersed in a solution of it; the acid of tartar combines with the lime, and forms a salt nearly insoluble in water, and which is deposited in the form of crystals on the body of the tooth; whilst the other portion, the vegetable alkali, and phosphoric

* Blake. History of the Teeth in Man, pages 156 to 159.

† Nat. Hist. Part II. page 69.

acid, &c. combine and remain dissolved in the mixture. Likewise in cream of tartar, the vegetable alkali is super-saturated with the acid of tartar, so that even in powder and without a complete decomposition of it, we see how readily it may act as a solvent for the cortex striatus, which is seemingly the chief part acted on by it, the bony part, as already mentioned, being covered with scarcely any of the crystals. When a tooth is placed in dilute acid of tartar, the body of it becomes covered in the same space of time with much larger crystals.

Mr. Wooffendale remarks,* "Cream of tartar, when used for cleaning the teeth, has the effect of destroying them in a two-fold degree; by friction, by which the teeth are cut or scratched by its roughness; and by its chemical power of dissolving them; as acids do, whether vegetable or mineral."

"I have several times taken a common wine-glassful of common household vinegar, into which I have introduced a sound, well enamelled human tooth: on taking it out, sixteen or eighteen hours after, I have found several hollows in the enamel, evidently corroded by the vinegar, in appearance something like is seen in iron when pitted with rust. All the teeth used in this experiment, were not corroded alike in the same time. When I have found the dissolution go fast forwards, I have, in sixteen or eighteen hours, taken the tooth out of the vinegar, and immersed it in Florence oil, where it has remained three or four days. On examining it then, I have found the dissolution stopped; and on returning it into the vinegar, the tooth has not appeared to be in the least affected by it for many hours."

---

* Practical Observations on the Human Teeth. By R. Wooffendale. London, 1783.

SECTION II.

ALKALIES AND SAPONACEOUS SUBSTANCES, &c.

The alkalies, alkaline and saponaceous substances are considerably used in cleaning the teeth, and in the composition of dentifrices. The carbonates of potash and soda are extremely useful in cleaning the teeth and mouth, and removing a filthy and disordered state of the gums; to dissolve the thick, clammy mucus, especially in sickness, and fevers, &c. Castile or Spanish soaps, in small quantities, are excellent substances which with a brush and soft water to clean the teeth. They give a peculiar sweetness to the breath. A brush drawn over a cake of pure Windsor or Spanish soap and then applied to the teeth will do much to preserve their health and beauty.

The ashes of burnt tobacco are often used with great advantage. The mild vegetable alkalies used in any form, if not used to excess, will be found very useful in preserving the health and beauty of the teeth, gums, and mouth. Dr. J. Green, professor of chemistry in Jefferson College, Philadelphia, in his lectures upon the super-carbonate of soda, mentions its useful qualities in removing the tooth-ache, which he considers to depend upon the formation of an acid within the carious portion of the tooth, and acting upon its nerve: the alkali neutralizes the acid, and thereby relieves the pain by removing the cause.

The kali purum is used as a caustic in destroying the nerve.

Quick lime has been used for the same purpose.

SECTION III.

ASTRINGENTS.

When speaking of diseases of the gums, in almost every case, in their curative treatment, we mentioned the utility of astringents in hardening them and promoting their healthy action, and inducing their union to the teeth when they have been divided or operated on after removing the tartar. We noticed that unless the tartar was completely removed, little permanent good could be expected from the use of astringents. In applying them to the teeth and gums, they are apt to blacken the former; consequently they should be washed clean with soft water after using the astringent. Astringents are used in the form of lotions, powders &c., and the class of them is very numerous. If properly used, they harden the gums, and cure a spongy, ulcerated state of them. They are used to cure scurvy of the gums, in cancrum oris; to arrest hæmorrhage after dental operations and extraction of the teeth, and after excision of tumours from the gums. They are used to relieve tooth-ache, and to reduce the sensibility of exposed nerves of teeth we wish to plug. The number of astringent substances are very great. Those generally used are the gallæ, (nut-gall,) of which the fresh Alleppo is the best, the oak bark, myrtle bark, the red peruvian bark, gum kino, the sulphates of copper, of alumine, (alum,) the mineral acids, and the acetic acid, &c. &c.

When judiciously used, they are exceedingly useful; promote a healthy state of the gums, and are almost indispensable in treating diseases of the soft parts about the mouth. They exert no pernicious influence upon the teeth, and are very useful in removing an irritable state of them.

SECTION IV.

OF STIMULANTS, ANODYNES, NARCOTICS, &c.

Stimulants are very often used in treating diseases of the teeth, gums, &c. In some instances we find a peculiarly debilitated state of the gums, when their vital powers appear to be very weak, indicated by a want of colour, being much lighter than usual, and a want of blood and active circulation in them. In this state, stimulant applications, and the use of a soft brush, so as to excite friction and gentle irritation of them, will often relieve this state of things. *Mr. Fox mentions a case of this kind, when the gums had so far lost their vitality as to appear white, without colour, and to allow of being pared off with a scalpel without exciting any pain. We also use stimulants to relieve tooth-ache, which they do by soothing the nerve, exciting counter irritation, or by promoting a flow of saliva, so as to induce a kind of evacuation from the adjacent parts.

The class of stimulants is very numerous and extensive: those chiefly used are nitrous and sulphuric ether, alcohol, rum, brandy. Mr Atkinson mentions his using rum in a case of tooth-ache, held in the mouth and changed every few minutes for twenty-four hours, so as to use more than a quart in that time, and with success.† Most of the essential oils have at times, been used and applied to pained teeth and nerves, as those of cloves, cinnamon, peppermint, horsemint, tanzy; also the cageput oil. Acrid aromatic substances are occasionally used, by chewing them, so as to promote a flow of

---

*See Fox, Part II, page 92. † See Duval, Note by Atkinson, page 125.

saliva, as the root of the peteveria alliacea, used in the West-Indies, called the Guinea-hen weed, from the fondness of that bird for it. Also the bulbs of most aliaceous plants; the seselis vulgare, common hartwort, or laserpitium silex Lin. which has long been celebrated as a sialagogue and remedy for the tooth-ache.* Camphor is also often of great use. Errhines are often used with success. All the essential oils are put on little pieces of cotton, and introduced into the cavity of the tooth. Anodynes and narcotics are occasionally used in treating diseased teeth, as opium, henbane, the leaves of the datura stramonium, (thorn apple plant,) tobacco in extract, tincture, or fumigation. Electricity and magnetism are at times used in diseases of the teeth, and recommended by some as being very useful. Mr. Charles Bew mentions a case, where a quack applied the fumigation of henbane seeds to draw worms from inflamed teeth, supposed to create the inflammation.†

SECTION V.

OF CAUSTICS.

Caustics are occasionally used in the course of our opertions upon the teeth, &c. as with a view of destroying the nerves of the teeth, and to cure or remove tumours of the gums, and to relieve their irritability in scorbutic affections, cancrum oris, &c. Those commonly used are the kali purum, (caustic potash,) the nitric and vitriolic acids, and the lunar caustic (argentum nitratum.) Of the use of the latter,

---

* See Good, vol. I, page 29. † Bew on the teeth, page 55.

and its qualities, we have already spoken. We noticed it as being the best of all caustics for purposes in dental surgery. When applied to irritable gums, it removes diseased irritability almost like a charm. We apply it to irritable denuded surfaces of the bony substance of the teeth with great advantage; and in some rare cases, to destroy the nerves of the teeth when inflamed.

Caution should be observed in applying the violent caustics to inflamed nerves or lining membrane of the teeth, as, in some constitutions, and under some states of the system, the irritation and dreadful anguish they occasion are apt to induce dangerous consequences.

I will present the reader with a case where fatal consequences resulted from the improper, and, no doubt, excessive use of a caustic preparation, which occurred in London some years ago, that came under the notice of Mr. William Fowler, and was published in the London Medical and Physical Journal, Vol. III. page 55.

Case.

A gentleman whom I attended was afflicted with the tooth-ache in the first dens molaris. Being much alarmed at the idea of extraction, he applied (unknown to me) to a Mrs. ——, who at that time was esteemed famous for the cure of the tooth-ache without drawing. She had applied her nostrum to the tooth twice within the space of three days, and on the fourth he came to me, complaining of a sore mouth, telling me where he got relief, and that the liquid which had been used was very caustic.

From the appearance of the violent inflammation which had taken place from the diseased tooth to the epiglottis, I advised him to consult some medical gentleman of eminence immediately, with which advice, I am sorry to say, he did not comply. Not hearing from him on the third day, I called, (en passant) but he was too ill to be seen; a derangement of intellects had taken place. I called again four days afterwards, and was informed that he died raving on the preceding day. I had every reason to believe that the fluid which had been inserted into the tooth with a view of destroying the nerve, had produced this tragical end.

SECTION VI.

MECHANICAL SUBSTANCES.

In some instances the teeth become stained by foreign matters lodged upon them, as we have before mentioned; and it is at present, and has been a practice from time immemorial, to use substances possessing mechanical properties with which to rub the teeth; which removes the foreign matter and restores them to their wonted whiteness. The substances used of this description are the bolar earths, prepared chalk, pummice-stone, pulverized sea-shells, pulverized fish-bone, cream of tartar, powdered barks, charcoal in fine powder, &c.

I wish in this place to make one general remark with respect to dentifrices possessing considerable mechanical properties, that if not used with the utmost prudence and caution they may be productive of the worst consequences. The substance of the tooth is liable to be rubbed away, the gums to be removed from the necks of the teeth, which always renders them more or less liable to caries. This remark also applies to hard brushes, used so indiscreetly as to rub away the gums from the necks of the teeth. I am at this time acquainted with a gentleman, who by a continued excessive and imprudent use of improper dentrifices and hard brushes, has removed the gums from the necks of nearly all his molar, bicuspid, and canine teeth, which has induced superficial caries in almost every one of these teeth.

I conclude these remarks with the observations of Dr. Blake on this subject, who says,* "From the foregoing observations it is perfecly evident, that the most simple and best prepared tooth-powder, frequently applied to the teeth, must be injurious, as they all tend to wear the cortex striatus. Even at present, many people are not content with tooth-powder alone, but form it into a paste, with syrup or honey, by which its action is much increased. Such preparations clean the teeth sooner than the others; they also much sooner wear off the cortex striatus, and destroy its beautiful polish, which never after can be regained.

We have already, in speaking of acids, remarked the bad effects of the cream of tartar, separately or alone, used as a dentifrice.

Charcoal pulverized, has, from its antisceptic properties, &c. been used as a dentifrice, and could we be always sure of suitable charcoal, and reduced to the tenuity of fine flour, it would no doubt be an excellent dentifrice. The Areca nut, when charred and ground, is said to afford a fine alkialescent and soft carbonaceous powder, possessing highly valuable properties, and as, without doubt, substances equally as good as this may be obtained for a carbonaceous dentifrice, I will give the reader an account of it from the observations of Dr. Reece and James Lynd, M. D.† Dr. Reece says, "It pre-

* Blake, History of the Teeth, &c. page 157.

† See Hertz, pages 47 to 50.

serves and renders the enamel of the teeth more clear, and destroys fetor arising from carious or decayed teeth, and on account of its being slightly alkalescent, also proves a powerful remedy for removing incrustations of the teeth."

From Dr. James Lind, late
*Head Hospital-Surgeon on the Bengal Establishment**

"The betel nut is called Areca by the Portuguese, Dutch, and other Low Europeans, who do not understand the Hindostan and Persian languages. In the latter it is called suparey, having no soporific quality, any more than the fragrant flower or betel leaf, nor have I seen it grow wild, or twine round trees in jungles, in the many campaigns and journies which I have made during twenty-five years, in the East India Company's extensive dominions, and of our allies, twelve hundred miles from Calcutta.

"The areca is most highly useful as the very best dentifrice that can be used; for since modern chemistry has discovered the wonderful medicinal powers of charcoal, the areca or betel nut charcoal must be superior to any other for a dentifrice, which I can recommend, having used it twenty-five years.

"When I arrived in England, after a long voyage of seven months, supposing my teeth wanted the aid of a dentist, I applied to a respectable one in London, who was astonished to find teeth so sound in a person of my age; and also observed, that all the East-Indians who employed him, had better teeth than the people of England of similar age, and which I attribute to the use of the areca nut tooth-powder,

---

* Hertz, pages, 47 to 49.

which must be infinitely more efficacious than charcoal prepared from any other vegetable substance whatever.

" The natives of India rub their teeth up and down with brushes made of chewed ends of fibrous soft wood, dragon's blood, canes, and mallow roots, which clean the interstices of the teeth ; whereas the common tooth-brushes, by rubbing in a horizontal direction, only wear off the enamel from the prominent parts of the teeth, which the famous dentist, Mr. Berdmore, has cautioned us not to do, and I have contrived a brush to prevent it.

"The dentifrice prepared by powdering charcoal, cannot be equal in virtue to the mungun prepared from the areca, betel nut, or suparey, however they may puff it off by quackish advertisements."

James Lind, M. D.

London, Jan. 11th, 1806.

Sir Mark Wood Baronet, M. P., Mr. Van Lynden*, and Mr. R. Winstanley, have given a most decided testimony in favour of the superiority of the prepared areca, for a dentifrice, over every other.†

Mr. Koecker objected to charcoal, from, as he observes, " its cutting quality ;" by which, I suppose, he means that when not reduced to a very fine powder, it is apt to injure the gums by insinuating itself between them and the teeth. I think this will seldom occur if the mouth be sufficiently rinsed with water after using the charcoal, and this reduced to a sufficiently fine powder.

* Late resident in a high official capacity at Ceylon, under the Dutch Government.

† See Hertz, pages, 50 to 51.

CHAPTER II.

FORMULÆ OF DENTAL MEDICINES.

In the application of the different medicines, medical and mechanical substances, &c. used by physicians and dentists, it will be readily acknowledged that a considerable variety must obtain both in the combinations of these medicines and their mode of exhibition. Of their several properties I have spoken before. I will, in this place, only remark that many of the old formulæ are given more as matters of curiosity than utility, and many forms of improper medicines are given, in order to guard the dentist against them.

SECTION I.

DENTIFRICES, &c.

℞.—Peruvian bark, - - ℥iii.
Armenian bole, - - ʒi.
Prepared chalk, - - ℥ss.
Ol. Bergamot, - - xx gts.

Mix and triturate.

℞.—Prepared chalk, - - ℥ii.
Sc'm alba, - - ʒi.
Orris Root, - - ℥ss.
Red saunders, - - do.
Ol. lavender, - - 10 gts.

Mix and triturate.

℞.—Pulverized fish bone, - ʒiii.
Cream tart. - ʒss.
Orris root, - - - ʒi.

Mix and triturate.

℞.—Pulverized charcoal, - ℥viii.
Carb. sodæ, - ʒii.
Cinchona bark, - - ℥ii.
Pulverized cloves, - ʒss.
Orris root, - - - ʒi.
Aqua rosa, - - - ʒi.
Essential oil, - - xxv gts.

Mix and triturate.

℞.—Armenian bole, - - 4 ozs.
Prepared chalk, - - 4 do.
Orris root, - - - 1 do.
Cortex peruvianus, - ¼ do.
Orris root, - - - ʒi.
Ol. cinnamon, - - xx gts.

Antiscorbutic Dentifrice.

℞.—Pulvis gallæ, - - ʒii.
Cort. Peru, - - ʒiv.
Red saunders, - - ℥i.
Ol. anise, - - - xx gts.

*" Take Dragon's blood,
Red saunders,

* B. Martin, pages, 128, 129.

Red coral,
Cochineal,
Rock alum,

Of each equal parts: after having reduced them to powder, one ounce must be mixed with three of clarified honey of roses, and bake it until it becomes of a thick consistence and middling solid; to be spread on a small piece of linen cloth coarse and fine, which ought to be applied to the gums, which is used as a powerful remedy for strengthening them."

*Another Powder for the Teeth.**

Take Hematite stone calcined,
Red coral ā ā ½lb,
Bones of the feet of sheep calcined,
Egg-shells, seeds or mother of Pearl,
Crab's eyes, ā ā ℥iv.

Prepare them on a pophyry stone. Take again of

Calcined Egg-shells,
Cuttle Fish-Bone,
Bole Armenic,
Red Earth, ā ā ss. lb.
Dragons' Blood in tears, ʒxii.
Alum Calcined,
Cinnamon, ā ā ℥ij.
Decripitated Salt, ℥i.

Rub them in a mortar, and pass them through a fine sieve, and that they may all be in an impalpable powder, and well mixed together, pass them a second time through the sieve."

The quantities that are given for making this composition, may suit those dentists who find themselves in a way of mak-

* Fauchard.

ing large sales. Those who are particular, may reduce the quantities to suit their wants, by keeping just proportions. When this powder is wanted to be made use of, a small quantity is put on a fine sponge a little moistened with water, with which the teeth are rubbed."

*Powder to Cleanse and Whiten the Teeth.**

"Take ℥vi of pumice stone, well calcined and reduced to powder. This powder is passed on the porphyry stone, moistened from time to time with rose-water, or that of myrtle; it is dried again to reduce it to an impalpable powder, and the following ingredients put in: Plate Lac, Dragon's Blood, Dried Bone, Bole Armenic, of each, ℥iij; Cinnamon, Cloves, Florentine orris, Rock Alum calcined, of each ʒi, all reduced to a subtile powder. It is used with a prepared root, in which the brush is dipped in this powder."

Another Powder for the same Use, and for strengthening the Gums.

Take Red Coral, and Tartar of wine, of each, ℥vi,
Dragon's Blood, Dried Bone, and
Bole Armenic, of each ʒi,
Cloves, Cinnamon, Florentine orris, and
White Salt, of each, ʒiij.

The whole ought to be well mixed, reduced to powder, and passed through a sieve of the finest cloth.

This powder is used at the end of a root, made as a little brush, or with a small piece of very fine sponge, a little moist-

* M. Bourdet, Tom. 2, page 301, 302, 303.

ened. People who are very careful of their teeth, and, in consequence, have them but little discoloured, use it once a month. Those whose teeth are easily tarnished, or who have soft or spongy gums, make use of it every time their teeth have lost their whiteness, without having the least fear of destroying the enamel, or altering the gums, as many people have supposed."

*M. Beaumé's Powder for the Teeth.**

Take Prepared Pumice-stone,	-	ʒi.
do. Red Earth,	- -	ʒi,
do. Red Coral,	- -	ʒi,
Dragon's Blood,	- -	ʒss.
Cream of Tartar,	- -	ʒiss.
Cinnamon,	- - -	ʒij.
Cloves,	- - - -	xxiv grains.

Make a powder, which mix intimately together.

"This powder is used to cleanse and whiten the teeth, to keep them clean, to prevent the inconveniences which sometimes happen by the accumulation of tartar. It is used with a brush, on which the bristles are wide apart and rather hard, in order that it may easily pass in the interstices of the teeth."

Lalande's Dentifrice Powder.†

Take Pumice Stone,	- -	ʒi.
Red Coral,	- - -	ʒi.
Sandal Citrin,	- -	ʒss.
Cream of Tartar,	- -	ʒiiss.

* Le Maire, page 208. † Le Maire, page 207.

Cinnamon,	- - -	ʒi.
Cloves,	- - -	ʒi.
Myrtle,	- - -	xviij grains.
Musk,	- - -	vi grains.
Benzoic Acid,	- -	iv grains.

Pulverize and porphyrize all the ingredients together, and put in Fine Lake, ʒiij. Mix all well for use.

Louseland's Dentifrice Powder.

Take Red Bark, selected and pulverized,		℥ij.
Red Saunders wood,	do. -	ʒi.
Volatile Oil of Cloves,	- -	xii drops.
do. do. Bergamotte,	-	viij drops.

Properly mix together.

It cleans the teeth well, constringes the gums, and gives a pleasant smell to the breath.

*Dentifrice Powder of M. Gariot, Surgeon-Dentist to the King of Spain.**

Take Red earth, prepared	- -	ʒvi
Cream of Tartar,	- -	ʒij.
Cloves,	- - - -	xxiv grains

This powder is used for lightly rubbing the teeth by means of a brush, which ought to be neither too hard nor too soft.

---

* Le Maire, page 207.

Another of the Same.

Take Red Coral,	- - - -	℥iv.
Dragon's Blood,	- - -	℥i.
Fine Carmine,	- - -	xxxvi grains.
Lemon peel,	- - -	ʒij.

This powder has the property of giving to the lips and gums a fine rose colour, which lasts for a considerable part of the day.

Powder.

* Though it is certain there are many formulas of powders used for cleaning the teeth, they may all be comprised in three classes. The first is the strongest, and comprehends substances which are neither improper nor inconvenient in their use ; I put in the second class, such as are hurtful to the teeth, either by their nature, by wrong proportions in combining them, or their bad preparation ; the third class embraces a small number of substances prepared and combined with discernment, and very proper to be used about the teeth and gums."

The formula which I am going to give, I have corrected by such as are most in vogue ; I have neutralized the excess of acid, which tends to make the teeth sensible, and to change their colour most ; I have augmented the quality, by the addition of bark, and of aromatics.

* Maury, pages 79—80—81—82.

Detersive Powder.

Take Red Bark,	- - -	℥ij.
English Magnesia,	- -	lbss.
Cochineal,	- - -	℥iss
Calcined Alum,	- -	℥i.
Cream of Tartar,	- -	lbss.
Essential Oil of English Mint,		ʒv.
Do. do. of Cinnamon,		ʒiij.
Spirit of Amber, musk rose,		ʒi.

Reduce separately to an impalpable powder the first five ingredients; porphyrise then the alum with the cochineal, in order to brighten the colour; put in the cream of tartar and the bark; place then the essences in another vessel with the magnesia; and when they have been absorbed, mix them with the first powder, and pass them through a very fine seive.

Use.

This powder perfectly cleans the teeth, without hurting the enamel; it strengthens the gums, and colours them a fine rose, and agreeably refreshes the mouth. The teeth and gums are rubbed with it by means of a brush two or three times a week, and if necessary every day, without any inconvenience. For young people of from 12 to 18 years, it is sufficient to use it once a week.

As it is soluble, take care to wet only what is to be made use of, and to be careful about keeping it in a dry place.

Another Powder.

Take Charcoal of white wood,	-	℥viij.
Bark,	- - - - -	℥iv.

White Sugar, - - - ℥viij.
Essential Oil of Mint, - ʒiij.
Do. do. of Cinnamon, ʒij.
Spirit of Amber, musk rose, . ʒss.

Reduce to an impalpable powder and mix them.

SECTION II.

ODONTALGIC PILLS.

In applying medicines to the exposed nerves of the teeth, either to relieve tooth-ache, or prepare the nerves of teeth for receiving the presence of metallic stoppings, it is often convenient and indispensable to form our medicines into pills, so as to fill the cavity of a tooth in this way, from which fluid medicines would immediately pass off. I give a few forms of these. In their exhibition, the pills are to be adapted to the size of the cavity in the decayed tooth, and after it is introduced it should be covered with a piece of wax, so as to prevent the pill from being dissolved in the liquor of the mouth.

℞. Pulvis Gallæ, - - ʒii.
Opium, - - - ʒss.
Pulvis Camphoræ, - ʒjs.
Tinct. Daturæ Stramonii q. s. to reduce the substances to pills.

℞. Hydrargyrus Cum Sulphure, xx grs.
Opium, - - - [illegible]
Spiritus Camphoræ, q. s. to pill.

℞. Ol. Cassiæ, - - - v gts.
Do. Cloves, - - v gts.
Pulvis Gallæ, q. s. to pill.

This is a valuable extemporaneous preparation, as is the following.

℞. Ol. Cagaput, - - iii gts.
Opium, - - - iii grs.
Pulvis Camphoræ, - ii grs.
Triturate and pill.

℞. Pulvis Gallæ, - - ʒi.
Carb. Sodæ, - - xx grs.
Triturate and pill.

℞. Opium, - - -
Camphor, ā ā - - xx grs.
Tincture Belladonna, q. s. to pill.

℞. Pulvis Gallæ, pro re natar,
Aqua to pill, -

SECTION III.

PASTES, OPIATES, ELECTUARIES, ODONTALGIC MIXTURES, ANTI-SCORBUTIC TINCTURES, WASHES, &c. &c.

In this country these kinds of preparations have not been much used, whilst with the French and continental physicians and dentists, they are much in repute. I give a few formulæ of them, many of which are very useful.

℞. Olei Hyosciam,	- -	℥i.
Opii Thebaici,	- -	℥ss.
Extract Belladonna,	-	
" Camphoræ, ā ā	-	viii gts.

This is given by Dr. Handel of Metz, and has obtained great repute on the continent.*

℞. Nitrous Ether,	- -	5 parts,
Pulvis Aluminæ,	- -	2 do.
Misce.		

This remedy is given from memory, and I think it was announced to a society of medicine in London by a Dr. Blake, and represented as almost infallible in the cure of odontalgia. I have used it with indifferent success.

℞. Camphor,	- -	
Opium, ā ā	- -	℥i.

Pure Alchohol, q. s. to dissolve the ingredients.

This is a valuable remedy, especially if the tooth-ache is excited by cold.

℞. Antiscorbutic Tincture,	-	
Pulvis Gallæ	- -	℥iii.
Camphor,	- - -	℥i.
Best Port Wine,	- -	ii. lbs.

Misce.—Let it stand in a warm situation three days, and it will be fit for use.

Another.

℞. Saturated Decoction,	-	
Of the Cortex Querci,	-	ii. lbs.

---

* See Murphy, page 116.

Tinctura Thebaici, ℥i
Mix.

*Plaster for the Aching of the Teeth.**

"Take the gums or resins of Jacamoque and of Caregne, of each ℥i; dissolve them with a gentle heat in a sufficient quantity of mastic oil; put in a drachm of the extract of laudanum; all being well incorporated together, take it off the fire; let it become cool, and make plasters on taffeta or black velvet of the size of a French farthing; they are applied on each side of the temporal arteries, and remain there until they fall off themselves; then others are applied, and worn as long as may be necessary."

Paste to dissipate Defluxions and appease Pains in the Teeth.

Take Root of Pyrethrum, Black Pepper,
Ginger, Staphisaigre, Mace, Cloves,
Cinnamon, of each, ʒss. Marine Salt, ℥i.

Reduce them all to a fine powder, put them in a glazed earthen vessel, pour over them twelve ounces of good red vinegar, boil them with a gentle fire, stirring them all the time with a wooden spatula, until reduced to the consistence of thick honey; then it is taken off the fire, and kept in a fine earthen water-pot. For using this paste, the size of a small bean is put in small fine cloth, which is placed between the gum and the cheek of the side where the pain and defluxion is.

"The effect of this remedy is, to make the spittle flow more freely than the smoking or mastication of tobacco, which

---

* Fauchard, pages 165 and 166.

is very disagreeable. The paste is taken off when the pain in the tooth is appeased, or when the fluxion begins to diminish, and renewed again, if necessary. If it is held in the mouth a little too long, it heats the insides of the cheek, and sometimes excites little blisters, which easily disappear by washing the mouth with lukewarm water."

*Opiate for the Teeth.**

Take Red Coral, - - - - -	ʒiij
Dragon's Blood in tears, -	ʒi
Seeds of Mother of Pearl and Cuttle fish-bone, ā ā -	ʒss.
Crab's eyes, Bole Armenia, Red Earth, Calcined Hematite, or Precious Stone, ā ā -	ʒiij.
Calcined Alum, - - -	ʒi.

Reduce them all to an impalpable powder, and incorporate with them a sufficient quantity of clarified honey of roses, and make an opiate of a soft consistence; taking care that this mixture is made in a vessel twice as large as it ought to be to contain the whole, on account of the fermentation of the ingredients, which takes place much more in summer than in winter; and during the fermentation, care should be taken to stir this composition once or twice a day with a wooden spatula."

Four or five drops of the oil of cinnamon, and as much of cloves may be put in it, which give it a good odour and increases its virtues also."

"This opiate is admirable for cleansing and whitening the teeth, strengthening and constringing the gums, too often re-

---

* Fauchard, pages 75 to 82.

laxed by scorbutic affections or by other acrid humours, into which they are often infiltrated; besides which, this opiate can never cause any bad effects to the enamel of the teeth.

To keep and preserve the teeth and gums, about the size of a pea of this opiate is put on a piece of fine sponge, and the teeth rubbed up and down, and down and up, outside and inside, once or twice a week. If the gums require to be the more strengthened, the same opiate is used on the end of the fingers, with which they are rubbed two or three times a day, and so for eight or ten days in succession. The two following opiates may also be used for whitening the teeth; they are very good for this purpose."

Another Opiate for the Teeth.

Take Prepared Coral, - - - -	℥ij.
Gum Shell Lac, Dragon's Blood, Catechu or Japan earth, ā ā -	℥i.
Cinnamon, Cloves, Root of Pyrethrum, ā ā - - - -	ʒvi.
Red Saunders, Cuttle Fish-bone, Calcined Egg-shells, ā ā - -	℥ss.
Decripitated Salt, - - -	ʒi.

Reduce them all to powder, and sift them through a linen sieve, as fine as silk, then mix them in a marble mortar, with a sufficient quantity of the honey of roses.

Another Opiate for the Teeth.

To make the other opiate, take Hartshorn, Ivory, the bones of the feet of sheep, the wood of rosemary, of crusts of bread, ā ā ℥ij; burn them separately, and reduce them to charcoal; of red earth, the dry rind of pomegranate, tartar of Montpellier, ā ā ℥ss. cinnamon, ʒij. Reduce all to a fine powder, sift and incorporate it with a sufficient quantity of the honey of roses. These opiates are enclosed in fine earthen-ware glazed pots, to be used as occasion may require."

"The powders, may be more convenient for some persons. I will give here two of excellent composition.

Powder for Cleansing and Whitening the Teeth.

"Calcine, or reden by the fire twelve ounces of pumice-stone; reduce it to powder in a mortar, and prepare it on the porphyry stone.

Take again, Fine or common lake, ℥vi; Cuttle-fish-bone, ℥iv; Bole Armenic, Red earth, and Calcined Alum, of each, ℥ij; Cinnamon, ʒij; Cloves, ʒi.

Reduce these drugs to powder in a covered mortar, and pass them through a very fine and covered sieve. When this powder is sifted, you join that of the pumice-stone, porphyrized; and in order that all may be well mixed together, and that this powder be extremely fine, pass again once through the sieve; then you put it up.

"It is used by means of a small sponge a little moistened.

"It may also be made into an opiate by mixing it with a sufficient quantity of the clarified honey of roses."

*Antiscorbutic Gargle.**

Take sarsaparilla, esquine, and shavings of guaiacum, of each, ℥ij. Infuse them as described before, for the space of twenty-four hours, in a half septier of myrtle-water, with

* M. Bourdet, Tom II, pages 319, 320.

as much distilled plantain-water. Strain then the liquor; put in ℥viij. cinnamon-water, ℥iv. of the strong spirit of scurvy-grass, wherein is dissolved, ʒi. sal ammoniac, ʒij. tincture of myrrh, ʒij. tincture of aloes, and ʒi tincture of cloves. Incorporate them well together, and make the patient rinse his mouth with it.

When the scorbutic ulcers are deep, and the sphacelus and gangrene have affected the gums, and the jaw carious, at the same time the operations are performed which I have described, the ulcers are opened at the same time, after having let out the pus, and the contiguous parts are bathed with the following composition."

Spirituous Water for Scorbutic and Gangrenous Ulcers.

Take strong spirit of scurvy-grass and tincture of guaiacum, ā ā ℥iv; wherein is dissolved ʒi. sal. ammoniac, ʒi. camphor, and ʒij. of good theriac diluted in ʒij. tincture of myrrh, ʒij. tincture of aloes, and ʒij. tincture of cloves, all well mixed together.

It is not sufficient to touch the ulcers very often with a linen rag or sponge: a tent must be dipped in it, and kept there, if the ulcer is deep, or little compresses or pledgets, which are kept in continually.

*Another Opiate for soft Gums: spongy, relaxed, swelled, &c.**

"Take red coral, tartar of wine,
dried bone, ā ā ℥ij.

* M. Bourdet, Tome II, page 305.

Thyme, rosemary, and marjoram,
very dry, and in powder, ā ℥i.
Cloves and cinnamon, ā ā ℥ij.
Sal. ammoniac, rock alum, ā ℥i. Dissolved in a little of the tincture of guaiacum made with spirits of wine.

The whole being well incorporated together, with a sufficient quantity of clarified honey of roses, and put in a proper vessel for the space of twelve or fifteen days, and preserved in fine earthen-ware pots. It is used in the same way as the preceding, every morning, until the gums are restored; then every third or fourth day, in order to keep them in a good state."

*Paste for Easing Pains of the Teeth**

Persons to whom all the ordinary remedies cannot give ease to spoiled teeth should have them extracted; or, if they are not willing to support the operation for curing them, may use with confidence the following paste, which will almost always succeed in easing severe pains caused by exposure of the nerve.

"Take Opium,	- - -	iij grains,
Cloves in powder,	-	x grains,
Gall nuts, do. do.	-	x grains,
Red earth,	- -	xv grains,
Camphor,	- -	x grains, and of

Anodyne drops as much as may be necessary to make these powders of the consistence of a thick paste. The hole in the tooth is well filled up with it on going to bed, the night is generally passed without pain, and it is banished for a greater or less time by this palliative."

---

* M. Bourdet, Tome II, page 312.

*Lalande's Odontalgic Elixir.**

Take Essential oil of cloves,	- -	ʒi.
Do. do. of thyme,	- -	ʒss.
Thebaic extract,	- - -	℥ii.
Alcohol of roses,	- - -	℥ij.
Frontignan wine,	- - -	℥iij.

Digest for the space of eight days, and filter for use. A few drops are put into the mouth, which is held on the painful side, which is rejected immediately when the pain has ceased."

Ether Dentifrice of the same.†

"Take Sulphuric ether,	- - -	℥ij.
Laudanum,	- - - -	℥ss.
Camphor,	- - - -	ʒi.
Oil of thyme,	- - - -	ʒss.
Oil of rosemary,	- - -	ʒss. Mix.

A small piece of cotton is dipped in this mixture, and is placed directly in or on the side of the painful tooth."

Dentifrice Electuary of the same.‡

"Take Pumice stone,	- - - -	ʒij.
Dried bone,	- - - -	ʒii.
Red coral,	- - - -	ʒij.
Florentine orris,	- - -	℈ij.
Calcined alum,	- - -	℈ij.
Pulverised cinnamon,	- -	℈ij.

* Le Maire, page 195, † Le Maire, page 195. ‡ Le Maire, page 196.

Rock alum, - - - - ℥i.
Cochineal, - - - - ʒi.

Pulverise and porphyrise all these substances, each separately: then make according to art an electuary, with a sufficient quantity of Narbonne honey, with which you have previously made a syrup. Let it ferment for the space of forty-eight hours, taking care to stir it from time to time, and put in

Alcohol of cloves, - - XXIV drops,
Alcohol of musk, - - X drops.

Triturate the mixture again, and put it in tin boxes, or pots of fine earthen-ware convenient for use."

*Cologne Water.**

" Take Rect. spirits of wine, - - lbs. vi.
Spirit of rosemary, - - lb.i ℥. x.
Compound water of balm, - lbs. i.
Essential oil of bergamotte, - ℥i. LIV grains,
Essential oil of cedrat, - ʒi.
Essential oil of lemons, - ʒij.

These ingredients are all put into a large bottle; the mixture is shaken, and the water is made. If it is wanted in a more delicate state, it must be rectified in a water bath, with a gentle heat to draw it nearly all off, within about half a pint. This water is used for the toilette, and not as a medicament.

Madame de la Veillière's Water for the Teeth.†

" Take cinnamon, - - - ℥ij.
Cloves, - - - ʒvi.

* Le Maire, Dentiste des dames, page 192. † Ibid.

Recent rinds of lemons, -	℥xii.
Red roses, dried, - -	ʒi.
Scurvy grass, - - -	℥viij.
Alcohol, - - - -	lbs. iij.

Pound the cinnamon and cloves, divide the roses and rinds of lemons, bruise the scurvy grass; they are then macerated in the alcohol for the space of twenty-four hours; and distilled in a water bath."

*Vulnerary and Spirituous Water, or Water of D'arquebusade.**

"Take fresh leaves of sage, - -	ā ā ʒiv.
Do. do. of angelica, -	
Do. do. of absinthium,-	
Do. do. of sariette, -	
Do. do. of fennel, -	
Do. do. of mentastrum,	
Do. do. of hysop, -	
Do. do. of balm, -	
Do. do. of basilic, -	
Do. do. of rue, - -	
Do. do. of thyme, -	
Do. do. of marjoram, -	
Do. do. of rosemary, -	
Do. do. of origanum, -	
Do. do. of calamus, -	
Do. do. of serpolet, -	
Do. do. of lavender, -	
Rectified spirit of wine, -	lbs. viij.

These plants are all first grossly cut in pieces: they are then infused for ten or twelve hours in the spirit of wine,

* Le Maire, page 193.

followed by distillation in a water bath, to draw of all the spirituous liquor. It is preserved in a well stopped bottle. It is called by this name, Vulnerary Spirituous and D'arquebusade Water. It is very agreeable: It is used internally to prevent the bad consequences which sometimes follow from bruises and falls."

*Cadet's Odontalgic Mixture.**

Take sulphuric ether,	- - -	ʒi.
Liquid laudanum,	- -	ʒi.
Turlington's balsam,	- -	ʒi.
Essential oil of cloves,	-	ij drops,

Mix together.

"Some cotton is dipped in this mixture, and applied to the painful tooth."

Opiate of M. Gariot,

Surgeon to the king of Spain.

Take rock alum,	- - -	℥ss.
Dragon's Blood,	- -	ʒiij.
Cinnamon,	- - -	ʒi.
Mastic,	- - - -	ʒi.

"Reduce all to a fine powder, and take a sufficient quantity of the honey of roses, to make an opiate, which is used with success, after the mouth has been washed in water; of which a few drops of Le Maire's Elixir has been put in."

---

* Le Maire, pages, 204, 205.

Opiate for the Teeth.

Take of the above powder, (Baumè)		℥i.
	Painters' red lake, - -	ʒij.
	Narbonne honey, - -	℥iv.
	Mulberry syrup, - -	℥ij.
	Essential oil of cloves, -	ij drops.

Make an opiate, and make use of it like the powder with the brush I have described above.

*Vogler's Odontalgic Remedy.**

Take	mastic, - - -	ʒij. vij grains.
	Sandarac, - - -	ʒij. vij grains.
	Choice dragon's blood, -	xxxvi grains.
	Dried opium, - -	℥i.
	Volatile oil of rosemary,	viij. drops.
	Spirit of scurvy grass,-	a sufficient quantity.

After having separately pulverised the mastic, the sandarac, the dragon's blood, and the opium, they are mixed, and moistened with the volatile oil of rosemary, and are ground in a marble mortar; then the spirit of scurvy grass is put in by little and little, and in sufficient quantity to form a uniform mass of a soft consistence, both plastic and semi-ductile.

It is used against pains of the teeth, by applying and spreading on the gum a portion of this emplastic mass of the size of a pea.

Lalande's Dentifrice Elixir.†

Take	root of pyrethrum, -	℥i ʒij.
	Cloves, - - -	ʒss.

---

* Le Maire, page 210. † Le Maire, page 197.

Flowers of lavender, - ℥ij.
Cochineal, - - - ʒij.
Rock alum,- - - ʒij.
Brandy of 22 degrees,- lbs. iv. ℥iv.

Make an elixir according to art, of which put in a few drops in water when made use of.

Elixir for the Teeth.

By Abbè Argelat.

Take spirit of rosemary, - ℥viij.
Root of pyrethrum, - ʒi.

"Put these two ingredients into a matras, and let them infuse for the space of some days, and filter the liquor. The mouth is rinsed with a spoonful of this elixir mixed with twice as much water. It is proper to excite the saliva a little, and to remove from the gums little humours which collect about them, which might occasion some slight pains of the teeth."

*Parmentier's Astringent Gargle.**

Take oak bark, - - - ℥i.
River water, - - lb. i.
Sulphate of alumine, - ʒi.
Honey of roses, - - ℥i.

This gargle is particularly used when the gums are swelled and spongy. The gums shou'd be made to bleed well by means of a quill tooth pick before using it.

---

* Le Maire, pages 198, 202.

Plench Odontalgic Lotion.

Take root of pyrethrum, - ʒij.
Muriate of ammonia, - ʒi.
Extract of opium,- - grains ij.
Distilled water of lavender, ℥ij.
Distilled vinegar, - - ℥ij.

Digest this mixture for the space of some days, and filter. In pains of the teeth, a spoonful of this lotion is held in the mouth from time to time, and care taken not to swallow it.

* "If the gums are found ulcerated, without being excrescenced, there is no other operation to practice but the application of the following remedies: Take two drachms of rock alum in powder, one ounce of tincture of myrrh and aloes, with one drachm of camphor; put all into a half pint of brandy, and let the affected person frequently rinse his mouth with it, or by injecting it upon the ulcers only, by means of a syringe: these ulcers are again rubbed by means of a piece of linen rag rolled around a small stick, which is dipped in the lotion, and with which the gums are rubbed: this is the practice in the Hotel Dieu at Paris, in which most of the diseases of the mouth are treated; it should be remembered also, that when the disease is prolonged by any excrescences of the gums, they are extirpated. It should be remarked that these rubbings should be repeated very frequently, to derive any utility from them."

Detersive Opiate.†

"I here give the formulary of an opiate, because there are persons who prefer this kind of preparation.

---

* Le Dentiste Observateur, pages 98, 99. †Maury, pages 82, 83.

Take fine honey, - - - lbs. ij.
Calcined alum, - - ʒij.
Extract of bark, - - ℥i.
Essential oil of peppermint, ℥iss.
Do. do. of cinnamon, ʒss.
Spirit of amber, musk rose, ʒij.

"Reduce the honey by boiling down to one third; colour it with a little orcanet: mix into it the bark, and strain it through a fine cloth; when it is almost cold, incorporate the alum with it, but do not put in the essences until it is entirely cold.

Use.

It has the same properties as the detersive powder, and it may be used in the same manner.

*Liquors.**

"Since a long time, waters, liquors, spirits and elixirs of all those which have been discovered, the principal merit consist in those that keep the mouth fresh, and give it an agreeable smell. The following formula has enjoyed, until the present time, in the hands of its inventors, a merited reputation. Some changes may be observed, which I thought ought to be made, and I hope they will be of advantage."

Philodontic and Antispasmodic Liquor.

Take alcohol of 38 degrees, - - 2 litres.
Essential oil of English mint, ʒi.

* Maury, pages, 83, 84.

Neroli, - - -	ʒiij.
Essence of cinnamon, -	ʒij.
Spirit of amber, musk rose,	ʒij.
Sulphuric ether, - -	ʒss.

This liquor is coloured at pleasure, either with the tinctures of orcanet, of orcel, or of saffron: it is filtered then, and the ether is not put in until about the time it is put in flasks."

Use.

"People who take a particular care of their teeth, go in quest of this liquor, because it gives a very agreeable smell to the mouth. From eight to ten drops is put into a glass of water one third full, and a brush dipped in, with which the teeth and gums are rubbed. It removes the bad smell of the mouth, restores and hardens the gums, prevents caries of the teeth, and stops its beginning, if used with care."

*Elixir.**

Take Root of ratania, - -	℥viii.
Vulnerary alcohol, -	4 litres.
Essential oil of English mint,	ʒiv.
Do. do. of orange rind,	ʒi.

Put the bruised root in a matras; pour over it the vulnerary alcohol, and let it digest for the space of eigheeen days; filter it, and then put in the essences, which you will have previously dissolved in alcohol, ℥iv.

* Maury, pages 85, 86.

Use.

This elixir cures many diseases of the mouth; among others, the beginning of scurvy, apthos, spongy gums, which it prevents from bleeding.

From 15 to 20 drops of this elixir may be put in a glass of water one third full, held for some time in the mouth, and the teeth and gums rubbed with a brush. If this wash is repeated two or three times a day, the ulcers soon deterge, and cicatrize, the swelling and the dropping ceases; the bad smell of the mouth, and the teeth that are not very firm, are tightened, or if they not sheltered, as well as those which require a certain treatment, that give much disorder to the mouth,

*Calming Drops.**

Take Alcohol of 40 degrees,	-		℥iij.
Sulphuric Ether,	-		
Liquid Laudanum,	-	ā	℥i.
Turlington's Balsam,	-		
Essence of Cloves,	-		ʒiij.

This liquor must be kept in flasks hermetically sealed.

Use.

I believe I can give the calming drops as one of the most efficacious remedies against the mischief produced by caries, or any other affections of the mouth. When the carious part has been cleaned as much as possible with cotton, another piece of cotton is introduced into it, wetted with one

* Maury, pages 86, 87, 88.

or two of these drops, taking care to touch only the carious part. If the pains proceed from the caries, or from another cause, and have already produced a defluxion, a cataplasm is applied to the affected cheek, prepared with linseed and a decoction of poppy heads, to which is added fifteen or twenty of these drops; this application is renewed every three hours. If the gums are only affected, a gargle composed of six or eight of these drops, and of two spoonfuls of barley-water, will produce a sensible effect; but it must be repeated many times during the day, and kept for three or four minutes in the mouth.

Calming Grains.

Take Resinous extract of opium, -	ʒvi.
Frankincense, - - -	ʒiv.
Camphor, - - - -	ʒiij.
Essence of cloves, - -	ʒiss.
Virgin wax, - - -	ʒvi.

"Prepare according to art, small grains, the size of the head of a pin, which are introduced into the carious part.

Tooth-Brushes, Tooth-Picks, &c.

Tooth-brushes are perhaps indispensable in keeping the mouth and teeth in a healthy and clean state. By a judicious use of them, the gums are preserved in a healthy condition, and the teeth are rendered free from foreign matters, and preserved in a cleanly and neat condition. They are made of different shapes and different degrees of harshness. Hard and stiff brushes if the teeth are firm and sound, and applied to the teeth alone, may be used with advantage. But soft and limber brushes are applied to the gums, and teeth in an irritable, loose, and diseased state. The gums may be rubbed with a sponge to advantage, either dipped in pure water, or in some medicated liqour. Soft brushes are alone admissible for the teeth and gums of children.

Tooth-brushes may be made of different sizes and cut into different shapes, so as to clean the teeth inside and out, and adapted not only to regular teeth, but those which are irregular.

Tooth-Picks.

These are made of gold, silver, &c., and of tortoise-shell, ivory, quill, &c. The metallic tooth-picks are generally rejected. Those from the quill, &c. are prefered and recommended by nearly all dentists. The oldest dentists and writers on the teeth, affirm the utility of tooth-picks. They should have a place in every gentleman's pocket, and every lady's toilet; and should be always used after every meal, to remove every particle of food from between the teeth. They may at first make the gums bleed, but they will finally do for the gums between the teeth, what the brush does for them on the outside, that is, make them firm and healthy.

I cannot dismiss the subject, without urging the use of tooth-picks, as well as tooth-brushes; as without them, bits of food, mucus, tartar, &c., collect between the teeth, irritate the gums, and cause them to assume a spongy, inflamed, and swollen state, whilst their use obviates these unpleasant effects, and becomes an efficient adjuvant in producing a pleasant, sweet, and healthy state of the mouth.

FINIS.

A

LIST OF BOOKS,

With the Names of Authors who have written upon the Science of Odontotechny, from the Latin, German, Danish, Swedish, French, and English Languages.

Arenius. Dissertation on catarrh and its descents, such as odóntalgia, epiphora, and otalgia. Rostock, 1663.

Andrèe. Dissertation on diseases of the teeth rendering extraction necessary, and on their mechanical force and use. Leipsic, 1784.
do. on the first teething of children. Leipsic, 1790.

Allzey, do. on teething, and diseases attending it. Edinburgh, 1788.

Aurivillius. do. on difficulty of teething. Upsal, 1757.

Alberti. do. on the lateness of wisdom teeth. Halle, 1737.

Auzebi. Treatise on odontalgia. Lyons, 1771.

Audibran, Chambly. Essay on the art of the dentist. Paris, 1808.
Letters to dentists on porcelain teeth. Paris, 1808.
Joseph. A treatise, historical and practical, on the artificial incorruptible teeth. Paris, 8 vo. 1821.

Arnemann. System of surgery, 2d part, 3d division, on the diseases of the teeth. Gottingen, 1802.

Assur. Undervatelse om de mait vanliger tansguk domar. Stockholm, 1799.

Buchner. Dissertation on the care of the teeth, and keeping them sound, Halle, 1752.

Bauhinus. do. on odontalgia. Bas. 1660.

Brendel. do. on tooth-ach. Erf. 1697.

Branver. do. on do. Leid. 1692.

Beurliz. do. on difficulty of teething. Altd. 1720.

Blake. Treatise on the formation and structure of the teeth in man and in various animals. Edinb. 1798.

Bring. Observations on the modern doctrine of the teeth, especially those of man. Lond. 1793.

Beaupreau. Dissertation on the properties and preservation of the teeth. Paris, 1764.
Letter to Mr. Cachais on the diseases of the maxillary sinus. Paris, 1769.

Baurdet. Letter to Mr. D——. Paris, 1754.
Researches and observations on every branch of the art of the dentist. Paris, 1757.
Easy means for the care of the mouth and the preservation of the teeth. Paris, 1759.
Dissertation on the depositions of the maxillary sinus. Paris, 1764.
Easy methods to keep the mouth clean and the teeth healthy. Leips. 1766.

Bunon. Dissertation on the prejudices concerning the diseases of the teeth of pregnant women. Paris, 1759.
Essay on the diseases of the teeth. do. 1743.
Experience and demonstrations. do. 1746.

Botot. Advice to the people. Paris, 1789.

Baumes. Treatise on the first dentition. do. 1800.

Bucking. Complete directions for the extraction of teeth. Hendal, 1782.

Bodenstein. Medicine for the teeth. Franckf. 1576.

Brunner. Introduction to the necessary science of a dentist. Vienna and Leipzig, 1766.
On the cutting of the milk teeth. do. 1771.

Blumenthal. Short views on the natural history of the teeth. Stendal, 1800.
Becker. On the teeth and the surest remedies, &c. &c. Leipsig, 1807 & 1810.
Bennet. A dissertation on the teeth and gums. Lond. 1779.
Berdmore. do. on the disorders and deformities of the teeth and gums. Lond. 1770.
Bew. A popular treatise on the teeth, with an account of the cause of caries, 8 vo. Lond. 1819.
On tic douloureux. 8 vo. London.

Couring. Dissertation on the nature and pain of the teeth. Thelmst. 1672.
Crausius. do. on the tooth-ache. Jena. 1681.
Crause. do. on the sensibility of the teeth. do. 1704.
Cumme. Dissertation on the history of the teeth, treated pathologically and therapeutically. Thelmst 1716.
Courtois. The observing dentist. Paris 1775.
Caigné. Dissertation on the teething of infants of the first year. Paris, 1802.
Collinbush. Advice for all classes. 1789.
Courtois. Examination on the nature and diseases of the teeth. Gothca, 1778.
Campani. Odontalgia, ossia trattato sopra i denti de denti ecloro cura e la maniera di estragli. Florenza, 1789.
Chamont. Dissertation on artificial teeth. London, 1797.
Curtis. Treatise on the structure and formation of the teeth. London, 1769.
Curious observations on that part of chirurgery relating to the teeth. London, 1687.

Decastrillo. Colloquy on teething. Valladolid, 1557, and Madrid, 1570.
Defritsch. Dissertation on the teeth. Vienna, 1772.
Depré. do. on difficulty of teething. Erf. 1720.
Dubois-Dechemant. do. on the advantages of the new incorruptible teeth. Paris, 1788.
Drouin. On the diseases of the teeth. Strasburgh, 1761.
Dupont. Remedy for the tooth-ache. Paris, 1633.
Duval. Of accidents in the extraction of teeth. Paris, 1802.
Reflections on the tooth-ache. do. 1803.
The youth's dentist. do. 1805.
Historical researches on the art of the dentist among the ancients. Paris, 1808.
On fistulas of the teeth. Paris, 1812.
Dubois-Foucou. Exposition of new methods for the manufacture of composition teeth. Paris, 1808.
Letter addressed to the gentlemen dentists. Paris, 1808.
Duchemant. Dissertation on artificial teeth in general. London, 1797.
Deschamps. The younger, treatise on the diseases of the nasal fauces and of their sinus. Paris, An XI.
Delabarre, C. F. Odontology, or observations on the human teeth. Paris, 1815, in 8vo. 4 plates.
A treatise on the second dentition and a natural method of directing it, &c. Paris, 1819. 22 plates.
do. on the mechanical part of the art of the surgeon-dentist. 2 vols. 8vo. Paris, 1816. 42 plates.
Natural method of directing the second dentition with proofs of the growth of the jaw in all parts. 8vo. 5 plates. Paris 1826.
The sincere dentist. Bayreuth.
The careful do. Vienna, 1798.
Tooth-ache or certain remedies to cure it. Pirna, 1805.

Erastus. Tract on the teeth. Figuri, 1595.
Eustachius. Smallbook on the teeth. Venice, 1574.
Ehinger. Dissertation on the tooth-ache. Altd. 1718.
Eloy. do. on anti-tooth-ache remedies. Vienna, 1772.
Ethmuller. Medical, and surgical treatise on the diseases of the teeth. Leipsig, 1798.
Esswein. Observations on the teeth, &c. Charleston, S. C. 1820.
do. at the Havanna, in Spanish. 1827.

Frank. On restoring teeth to soundness. Heidelb, 1672.
Dissertation on the tooth-ache. Jena, 1692.
Fauchon. Tracts on vicious positions of the teeth. Paris, 1775.
Fleurimon. Methods for preserving the teeth sound and good. Paris, 1682.
Fauchard. The Surgeon-Dentist. Paris, 1728.-46.-86.
Treatise on the teeth. A. D. French translated by Buddeus. Berlin, 1733.
Fischer. On the different forms of the interior maxillary bone in different animals. Leipsic, 1800.
Fox. Account of the diseases, which affect children during the first dentition. Append. Natural history of the human teeth. Lond. 1803.
History of the diseases of the teeth and gums. London, 1806.
Fuller. A popular essay on the structure, formation and management of the teeth, illustrated by engravings. Lond. 1810.
Flagg. Observations on the teeth. Boston.
Fitch, Samuel S. Observations upon the importance of the teeth. 8vo. Philad. 1828.

Glaubrecht. Analectic dissertation on the tooth-ache, and its various remedies, especially the magnetic. Argent. 1766.
Goeckel. Epitome of the theory and practice of odontalgia. Nordl. 1688.
Grün. Dissertation on the tooth-ache. Jena, 1795.
Günz. do. on fetor of the gums, and observations on ulcerated teeth. Leips. 1753.
Gehler. Observations on the third teeth. Leips. 1786.
Gerauldy. The art of preserving the teeth. Paris, 1737.
Gilles, the flower of; remedies against the tooth-ache. Paris, 1622.
Grousset. Dissertation on dentition or the developement of the teeth in man. Paris, 1803.
Gariot. Treatise on the diseases of the mouth. Paris, 1805.
Gallette. On the art of the dentist. Mayence, 1803.
Present for persons of both sexes, to keep the teeth healthy and clean. Franckf. 1796.
Gardette, James. Transplanting of the teeth. Philad. 1821.
Guilleman and Schmiz. Eye and tooth doctor. Dresden, 1710.
Gerbi. Storia naturale de un puoro insitto. Florent. 1794.
Giraud. The good mother, or a treatise on the means of procuring for children a strong and lasting constitution, particularly by a happy teething. Brunswick 1790.
Gariot. System of the Physiology, Pathology, and Therapeutics of the mouth, with remarks by Angermann. Leips. 1806.
Gallette. Glances into the provinces of the science of a dentist. Maing, 1810.

Horstius. On the golden tooth. Leips. 1595.
Heister. Dissertation on the pain of the teeth. Altd. 1711.
Epistle on bones and teeth, found in different parts of the human body. Thelmst. 1743.
Heye. Dissertation on pain of the teeth. do. 1672.

Hauffmann. Dissertation on the teeth, their diseases and cure. Halle, 1698 and 1714.
Hilscher. do. on the tooth-ache. Jena, 1748.
Hauffmann. do. on anti-tooth-ache remedies. Halle, 1700.
Hubner. do. on supper taking. (Coenaesthesi.) do. 1794.
Hurhius. Tract on diseases of the eye, ear, and teeth. Leid. 1602.
Heeslop. Dissertation on the difficult and laborious teething of infants. Leid. 1702.
Hebensheit. do. on the second teething of youth. Leip. 1738.
Hunter. Natural history of the human teeth. Amst. 1778.
do. do. of the teeth and a description of their diseases. Leips. 1780.
do. do. of the teeth and their diseases. Lond. 1771.
Hersh. Practical remarks on the teeth. Jena, 1796 and 1801.
On the means of preserving the health of the teeth. Ronneburg and Leips. 1799.
Hurlock. Practical treatise upon dentition. Lond. 1742.
Hertz. A familiar dissertation on the causes and treatment of the diseases of the teeth. 8vo. London.
Hemard, Urbain. Dissertation on the true anatomy of the teeth, their nature and properties. Lyon, 1582.
Hebert. Citizen dentist. Lyon, 1778.
Hernandez. Semiology of the tongue, lips, and teeth. Toulon, 1708.

Ingolsetter. On the golden tooth of the Silesia boy. Leips. 1695.
Hersh. Practical remarks on the teeth. Jena. 1796 & 1801.
On the means to preserve the health of the teeth. Leyden, 1799.
Juncker. Dissertation on affections of the teeth. 2d. Difficulty of teething. 3d. On tooth-ache. 4th. On the four chief diseases of infants. Halle, 1740, 45, 46, and 58.
Janckeè. do. on extraction of the teeth. Leips. 1751.
On the bones of the mandible of children of seven years of age. Leips. 1751.
Jackson. Dissertation on the physiology and pathology of eruptions of the teeth. Edinb. 1772 and 78.
Gebaux. Dissertation on the teeth. 12 mo. London.
Josse. Analysis of the enamel of the teeth. Paris, year X. (Journal of medicine.)
Jourdain. Treatise on depositions in the maxillary sinus. Paris, 1761.
Essay on the formation of the teeth. Paris, 1766.
Treatise on the diseases and surgical operations of the mouth. Paris, 1778.
Jourdan and Maggiolo. Manual of the dentist's art. Nancy, 1807.
Junker. On head and tooth-ache, and the remedies against them. Brunswic, 1802.
Jourdain. On the surgical diseases of the mouth, and the parts connected therewith. 1784, (translated from the French,) Nurnberg.

Kemme. Dissertation treating the history of the teeth, physiologically, therapeutically, and pathologically. Helmst.
Kuchler. Dissertation on fistulous ulcers of the teeth. Leips. 1733.
Konen. Dissertation on the principal diseases of the teeth. Franck. 1793.
Kulencamp. Dissertation on the difficulty in teething of infants. Harderow, 1788.
Kraitterman. Sore eye and tooth doctor. Arnst. 1732.
Kuntzman. Short and theoretical treatise to preserve healthy, and remedy diseased teeth. Stutgard, 1772.
Koecker, Leonard. Principles of dental surgery. 8 vo. London, 1826.
Diseases of the jaws. do. 1828.
Laubmeyer. Dissertation on the teeth. Regiom. 1745.

Ludwig. On the enamel of the teeth. Leips. 1753.
Liddelius. On the golden tooth of the Silesian boy. Hamb. 1626.
Leichner. Dissertation on the sore pain of the teeth. Erf. 1688.
Laeselius. do. on pain of the teeth. Regiom. 1639.
Lehmann. do. tracing a catalogue of coleopteral medicines. Gotting. 1796.
Loescher. do. on the wisdom teeth and their diseases. Viteb. 1728.
Ludolff. do. on diseases of the gums. Erf. 1722.
Ludwig. do. on difficult teething. Leips. 1800.
Lècluse. Useful treatise to the public for taking care of the teeth. Nancy, 1750.
Essential directions for preventing and preserving the teeth from decay. Paris, 1755.
New elements of odontology, containing the anatomy of the mouth, and the abridged practice of the dentist, with many observations. Paris, 1754 and 1782.
Lemonnier. Dissertation on the diseases of the teeth. Paris, 1753 and 83.
Letter to Mr. Mauton. Paris, 1764.
Leroy de la Faudignère. Method for preventing and curing the diseases of the teeth and gums. Paris, 1766.
Lemaitre. Report made to the society of inventions and discoveries, on perfect sets of teeth. Paris, 1784.
Laforgue. Seventy articles relating to diseases of the teeth. Paris, year VIII.
Theory and practice of the dentist's art. Paris, 1802.
On semeology of the mouth. Paris, 1806.
Dissertation on the first dentition. Paris, 1809.
Theory and practice of the dentist's art, 2d edition. Paris, 1810.
Legros. The preserver of the teeth. Paris, 1812.
Lemaire. The ladies' dentist. do. 1812.
do. do. do. 1818.
Laforgue. Triumph of the first dentition, new and curious almanac. Paris, 1816.
Lentin. On the effect of the electric shock in tooth-ache. 1756.
Leroy, (Alphonse.) Means to keep children healthy, and particularly during the dangerous time of dentition to save their lives. Vienna, 1786.
Laforgue. Theory and practice of the dentist, from the French, with remarks by Angermann. Leipsic and Berlin. 1803.
Lavini. Tratto soma la quatita di denti col modo di codengli mantan erglic fortificaroti Fivenzi, 1740.
Lewis. Essay on the formation of the teeth, with a supplement containing the means of preserving them. Lond. 1772.

Meckel. Diss. an prosbi qui dentium translocationem sequunter, benerci sint, nec ne ? Halx. 1792.
Martin. Dissertation on the tooth-ache. Erf. 1680.
Moebius. do. on do. Jena, 1661.
Myrshen. do. do. do. Giess. 1693.
Mongin. Eyo pregnanti mulieri acutissimo dentis dolore laboranti ejusdem evubrïo? Paris, 1740.
Monarius. On affections of the teeth. Bas. 1578.
Muller. On the scorbutic bleeding of the gums. Altd. 1675.
Martin. Dissertation on the teeth. Paris, 1679.
Mouton. Essay on odontology. do. 1746.
Mahon. The observing dentist. do. year VI.
Mortet. Dissertation on the extraction of teeth with the aid of a new instrument. Paris, 1802.
Meyer. Treatise on the usual diseases of the teeth. Hanan, 1778.
Murphy, Joseph. Natural history of the human teeth, with a treatise on their diseases from infancy to old age. 8 vo. Lond. 1811.

Nicolai. Dissertations on the various affections of the teeth, and their nourishment in health. Jena. 1799.

Oettinger. Dissertation on the developement of the teeth. Erlang. 1770.
Ortlob. do. on the difficult teething of children. Leip. 1694.
Pacheus. Dissertation on pain of the teeth. Bas. 1707.
Pauli. do. do. do. Haffnia, 1579.
Planer. do. on the tooth-ache. Tub. 1685.
Palhe. do. whether tobacco helps the tooth-ache. Turonile.
Ploucquet. do. does the pain proceed from the inflammation of the nerves or of the tooth itself? Tub. 1794.
Paldamus. Dissertation on diseases of the teeth. Halle. 1799.
Pestorff. do. on difficult dentition. Ulti, 1699.
Pahl. do. on do. do. of infants. Leips. 1776.
Plenk. Doctrine of the diseases of the teeth and gums. Nap. 1781.
Poservits. Semiology of idiopathic and symptomatic apthx. Viteb. 1790.
Plisson. Observations on a new method of curing certain pains of the teeth. Lyon, 1788.
do. on an extraordinary disease of the gums. Lyons, 1791.
Pasch. Treatise from surgery on the teeth. Vienna, 1767.
Paff. do. on the human teeth and their diseases. Berlin, 1756.
Plenk. Doctrine of the diseases of the teeth, and of the gums, from the Latin, with remarks by Wasserberg. Vienna, 1779.
Palfyr. Naavrdenge Berchseyring van het benderen van's menschen Lychham. Gendt. 1702.
Parmly, L. S. Lectures on the natural history and management of the teeth. 8 vo. New York, 1821.
Eleazar. An essay on the disorders and treatment of the teeth. 8 vo. London and New York, 1822.

Rolfinck. Dissertation on tooth-ache. Jena, 1669.
Raer. do. on generating and rising of the teeth. Lyons, 1694.
Rabicki. do. on difficult teething. Regiom, 1803.
Ringelmann. On diseases of the bones and of caries, especially that of the teeth. Arnst. 1805.
Ricci. Principles of odontology. Paris.
Reymondon. Dissertation on dentition. do.
Rosset. do. do. do.
Riviere. Instructions for preserving the teeth. Paris, 1811.
Ryff. Useful advice, how to sharpen the eye, and how to preserve the teeth fresh and tight. Wurtsburg, 1548.
Ringelmann. Treatise on rheumatic tooth-ache. Wurtsburg, 1800.
Ritchter. Rudiments of surgery, 4th vol. of the diseases of the mouth. 1797 and 98.
Ruspini. A treatise on the teeth, their structure and various diseases. Lond. 1768 and 79.
Rousseau, L. F. E. M. A comparative anatomy of the dental system in man and various animals. Paris, 1828. 8 vo. 30 plates.
Dissertation on the first and second dentition. Paris, 1820.
Maury. Observations on the porcelain teeth. Paris, 1816.
Ramsbotham. Treatise on dentistry. Jamaica, W. I.

Scardovi. Dissertation on the teeth. Argent, 1645.
Shiers. do. do. Trageot, 1772.
Sebiz. On the teeth, contagion, &c. Argent, 1664.
do. do. (disp. IV.) do. 1645.
Schelhammer. Dissertation on stroking away tooth-ache. Kelio, 1701.
Sennertus. do. on the tooth-ache. Viteb. 1629.
Seisser. do. do. Lndg. Bat. 1675.
Strobebberger. do. on podagra and tooth-ache. Leip. 1630.
Siebold. History of tumours, hemmorrages, &c. cured. Herhip. 1788.
Schneidler. On the use of acids in scurvy. Ulm, 1791.
Schmeidel. Dissertation on difficult teething. Erl. 1751.

Streithein: do. on teething. Altd. 1638.
New and secret experiments for preserving the beauty of the teeth. Haye, 1706

Schmidt. A few words to those who wish to keep their teeth in good order. Dessau and Leyd. 1801.
Art to have good teeth from infancy up. Gotha. 1801.
Useful instructions how to preserve the teeth good. Dessau, 1805.
Theory and experience on the teeth. Leips. 1807.

Serre. History of the tooth-aches of the fair sex during pregnancy. Vienna, 1778.
Treatise on rheumatism and inflammation from which swellings and gum-boils proceed. 1791.
Practical representations of the teeth. Berlin. 1803.

Schäffer. The imaginary worms in teeth. Regensberg, 1751.

Sasse. On the difficult dentition of children. Lubben, 1802.

Stinberg. Admonitions and doubts against the doctrine of dentists on the difficult dentition in children. Hanov. 1802.

Starck. Treatise on excresences, with a translation of Ketelain and Shoozt, of the same. Jena, 1784.

Skinner. A treatise on the human teeth, concisely explaining their structure and cause of disease and decay. New York, 1801.

Tylhosby. Disquisition on two boys, one with a gold tooth and another with a big head, in Lithuania. Clivia.

Trecurth. Dissertation on the tooth-ache. Halle, 1688.

Thunberg. do. on the use of cajeput oil. Upsal, 1797.

Teske. New experiment in curing the tooth-ache by means of magnetic steel. Konigsburg, 1765.

Tolver. Treatise on the teeth. Lond. 1752.

Timaens. do. on the tooth-ache. do. 1769.

Vandermasson. On the necessity of care of the gums and teeth. Gotha, 1802.
The dentist for all classes. L. 1803.
N. B. How can parents ease the dentition of children?

Vater. Dissertation on the tooth-ache. Viteb. 1683.

Vanderbelen. do. do. do. Lovan, 1782.

Vesti. do. do. do. Erf. 1697.

Vacher. do. on accidental teeth. Paris, 1767.

Vigier. Tract on catarrh, rheumatism, and defects of the teeth. Geneva, 1620 and 24.

Valentini. Dissertation on looseness, loss and repairing of the teeth. Jena, 1798.

Vandermonde. Whether in the dentition of infants attended with convulsions or drowsiness, there should be a repeated use of cathartics? Paris, 1767.

Vase. Is hemmorrhage by the extraction, a fatal carelessness of the operator? Paris, 1735.

Warenius. Dissertation on catarrh, and tooth-ache proceeding from it. Genev. 1727.

Wagner. do. on difficult dentition. Jena, 1798.

Wedel. do. on dentition of infants. do. 1678.

Woost. On ulcers in the mouth of infants. Viteb. 1790.

Weyland. Dissertation on maxillary fetor, complicated with fistulous ulcer, near the inner angle of the eye. Argent. 1771.

Woffendale. Practical observations on the human teeth. Lond. 1783.

Walkey. On the diseases of the teeth their origin explained. Lond. 1793.
The Dentist for all classes. Leipsic, 1803.
Dentists' Manual. Vivna, 1807.
Weinhold. Remarkable changes in the jaws. Leipsic, 1810.

Zeidler. Dissertation on pain of the teeth. Leips. 1631.
Zirgler. On the chief diseases in the cavities of the bones of the forehead, also those of the upper and lower mandible. Rinteln, 1750.
Trenor. Tic douloureux. New York, 1824.
Structure, organization, and nourishment of the teeth. New York, 1826.

Zabarnagen. Councils how to preserve the teeth. Ewf. 1614.
Zakbockjen. Bevattende de middelen om de Gozondeit der tamden to bewaven. Arnheim, 1804.

DIRECTIONS FOR PLACING THE PLATES.

PLATE I. to be placed between pages 24 and 25.
II. " " " 350 and 351.
III. " " " 426 and 427.
IV. " " " 432 and 433.
Synoptical Tables " " " 48 and 49.

EXPLANATION OF THE PLATES.

PLATE I. FIG. 1. A part of each maxilla showing a perfect set of teeth in their appropriate situation.
1. a. b. c. e. e. superior row of infant teeth.
2. a. b. c. e. e. inferior row of infant teeth.
3. a. b. c. e. e. e. superior row of adult teeth.
4. a. b. c. e. e. e. inferior row of adult teeth.

PLATE II. Different specimens of cleansing, plugging, and extracting instruments.

PLATE IV. Different forms of artificial teeth, prepared for insertion in the mouth.

ERRATA.

Page 70, seventh line from top, after "membranous," read "sacs"
129, seventh do. for "sawing," read "sowing"
149, twenty-second line from top, for "eroded," read "corroded"
185, fifth do. after "face," add "continued"
213, ninth do. for "cancroris," read "cancrum oris"
241, twenty-seventh do. for "ii or iii," read "ij or iij."
248, fifth from the bottom, for "their," read "them."
260, fifth from top, for "have," read "prove."
301, eleventh from top, for "an." read "art."
312, ninth do. for "Philadelphia," read "Pennsylvania"
324, fourteenth do. for "him," read "Mr. Koecker"
347, fifteenth do. for "by," read "in."
thirtieth do. for "probably," read "palpably"
twenty-first do omit the word "all"
348, twelfth do for "Medor," read "preda," and omit the period before it.
365, Note Mr. Fox is referred to by mistake
374, fifth line from bottom, for "Zufa," read "Tufa."
383, fifth line from top, for "abandoned," read "abraded."
390, sixteenth do. after "bicuspid," add "or"
408, sixteenth do. for "natures," read "matters."
436, fourth line from bottom, for "manina," read "marina."
455, eighth line from top, for "he," read "she."
463, sixteenth do. for "pestiors," read "portions."
487, first from bottom, for "like it is," read "as"

Some other mistakes; as the occasional use of the word "when," that should have been "where." They are left to the indulgence of the reader.

Lightning Source UK Ltd.
Milton Keynes UK
UKHW022010150119
335599UK00010B/617/P